Management of Diabetic Retinopathy

Developments in Ophthalmology

Vol. 60

Series Editor

F. Bandello Milan

Management of Diabetic Retinopathy

Volume Editors

Francesco Bandello Milan
Marco A. Zarbin Newark, NJ
Rosangela Lattanzio Milan
Ilaria Zucchiatti Milan

77 figures, 64 in color, and 30 tables, 2017

KARGER

Basel · Freiburg · Paris · London · New York · Chennai · New Delhi · Bangkok · Beijing · Shanghai · Tokyo · Kuala Lumpur · Singapore · Sydney

Francesco Bandello
Department of Ophthalmology
University Vita-Salute
San Raffaele Scientific Institute
Via Olgettina, 60
IT–20132 Milan (Italy)

Marco A. Zarbin
Institute of Ophthalmology and Visual Science
New Jersey Medical School
Rutgers University
6th Floor Doctors Office Center
90 Bergen Street
Newark, NJ 07103 (USA)

Rosangela Lattanzio
Department of Ophthalmology
University Vita-Salute
San Raffaele Scientific Institute
Via Olgettina, 60
IT–20132 Milan (Italy)

Ilaria Zucchiatti
Department of Ophthalmology
University Vita-Salute
San Raffaele Scientific Institute
Via Olgettina, 60
IT–20132 Milan (Italy)

Library of Congress Cataloging-in-Publication Data

Names: Bandello, F. (Francesco), editor. | Zarbin, Marco A., editor. | Lattanzio, R. (Rosangela), editor. | Zucchiatti, Ilaria, editor.
Title: Management of diabetic retinopathy / volume editors, Francesco Bandello, Marco A. Zarbin, Rosangela Lattanzio, Ilaria Zucchiatti.
Other titles: Management of diabetic retinopathy (Bandello) | Developments in ophthalmology ; v. 60. 0250-3751
Description: Basel ; New York : Karger, 2017. | Series: Developments in ophthalmology, ISSN 0250-3751 ; vol. 60 | Includes bibliographical references and index.
Identifiers: LCCN 2017009946| ISBN 9783318060416 (hard cover : alk. paper) | ISBN 9783318060423 (e-ISBN)
Subjects: | MESH: Diabetic Retinopathy--therapy | Macular Edema | Diabetic Retinopathy--diagnostic imaging
Classification: LCC RE661.D5 | NLM WK 835 | DDC 617.7/3--dc23
LC record available at https://lccn.loc.gov/2017009946

Bibliographic Indices. This publication is listed in bibliographic services, including Current Contents® and Index Medicus.

www.karger.com
Printed on acid-free and non-aging paper (ISO 9706)
ISSN 0250–3751
e-ISSN 1662–2790
ISBN 978–3–318–06041–6
e-ISBN 978–3–318–06042–3

Contents

List of Contributors

Daniela Bacherini
Department of Surgery and Translational Medicine
Careggi University Hospital, Eye Clinic
University of Florence
Largo Piero Palagi, 1
IT–50139 Florence (Italy)
E-Mail daniela.bacherini@gmail.com

Francesco Bandello
Department of Ophthalmology
University Vita-Salute
San Raffaele Scientific Institute
Via Olgettina, 60
IT–20132 Milan (Italy)
E-Mail bandello.francesco@hsr.it

Maurizio Battaglia Parodi
Department of Ophthalmology
University Vita-Salute
San Raffaele Scientific Institute
Via Olgettina, 60
IT–20132 Milan (Italy)
E-Mail battagliaparodi.maurizio@hsr.it

Neelakshi Bhagat
Institute of Ophthalmology and Visual Science
New Jersey Medical School
Rutgers University
6th Floor Doctors Office Center
90 Bergen Street
Newark, NJ 07103 (USA)
E-Mail bhagatne@njms.rutgers.edu

Adriano Carnevali
Department of Ophthalmology
University of 'Magna Graecia'
Viale Europa, Germaneto,
IT–88100 Catanzaro (Italy)
E-Mail adrianocarnevali@live.it

Giuseppe Casalino
Department of Ophthalmology
University Vita-Salute
San Raffaele Scientific Institute
Via Olgettina, 60
IT–20132 Milan (Italy)
E-Mail peppecasalino@gmail.com

Maria Vittoria Cicinelli
Department of Ophthalmology
University Vita-Salute
San Raffaele Scientific Institute
Via Olgettina, 60
IT–20132 Milan (Italy)
E-Mail cicinelli.mariavittoria@hsr.it

Marco Codenotti
Department of Ophthalmology
University Vita-Salute
San Raffaele Scientific Institute
Via Olgettina, 60
IT–20132 Milan (Italy)
E-Mail codenotti.marco@hsr.it

Florence Coscas
Hôpital de Créteil
Département d'Ophtalmologie de Créteil
Université Paris XII, Val de Marne-France
Centre d'Exploration Ophtalmologique de l'Odéon
FR–75006 Paris (France)
E-Mail coscas.f@gmail.com

Gabriel Coscas
Hôpital de Créteil
Département d'Ophtalmologie de Créteil
Université Paris XII, Val de Marne-France
Centre d'Exploration Ophtalmologique de l'Odéon
F–75006 Paris (France)
E-Mail gabriel.coscas@gmail.com

Luigi Antonio De Vitis
Department of Ophthalmology
University Vita-Salute
IRCCS Ospedale San Raffaele
Via Olgettina, 60
IT–20132 Milan (Italy)
E-Mail l.devitis@studenti.unisr.it

Ugo Introini
Department of Ophthalmology
University Vita-Salute
San Raffaele Scientific Institute
Via Olgettina, 60
IT–20132 Milan (Italy)
E-Mail introini.ugo@hsr.it

Lorenzo Iuliano
Department of Ophthalmology
University Vita-Salute
San Raffaele Scientific Institute
Via Olgettina, 60
IT–20132 Milan (Italy)
E-Mail iuliano.lorenzo@hsr.it

Rosangela Lattanzio
Department of Ophthalmology
University Vita-Salute
San Raffaele Scientific Institute
Via Olgettina, 60
IT–20132 Milan (Italy)
E-Mail lattanzio.rosangela@hsr.it

Xintong Li
Institute of Ophthalmology and Visual Science
New Jersey Medical School
Rutgers University
6th Floor Doctors Office Center
90 Bergen Street
Newark, NJ 07103 (USA)
E-Mail xintli@gmail.com

Anat Loewenstein
Department of Ophthalmology
Tel Aviv Medical Center
Weitzman 6 St.
Tel Aviv, 64239 (Israel)
E-Mail anatl@tlvmc.gov.il

Marco Lupidi
Department of Biomedical and Surgical Sciences
Section of Ophthalmology
'S. Maria della Misericordia' Hospital
University of Perugia
IT–06156 Perugia (Italy)
E-Mail dr.marco.lupidi@gmail.com

Gisella Maestranzi
Department of Ophthalmology
University Vita-Salute
San Raffaele Scientific Institute
Via Olgettina, 60
IT–20132 Milan (Italy)
E-Mail maestranzi.gisella@hsr.it

Silvia Maestroni
Complications of Diabetes Unit
Diabetes Research Institute
IRCCS San Raffaele Scientific Institute
Via Olgettina, 60
IT–20132 Milan (Italy)
E-Mail maestroni.silvia@hsr.it

Paola Maffi
Internal Medicine and Transplant Unit
IRCCS San Raffaele Scientific Institute
Via Olgettina, 60
IT–20132 Milan (Italy)
E-Mail paola.maffi@hsr.it

Edouardo Midena
Department of Ophthalmology
University of Padova
Via Giustiniani, 2
IT–35128 Padova (Italy)
E-Mail edoardo.midena@unipd.it

Elad Moisseiev
Department of Ophthalmology
Tel Aviv Medical Center
Weitzman 6 St.
Tel Aviv, 64239 (Israel)
E-Mail elad_moi@netvision.net.il

Lekha Mukkamala
Institute of Ophthalmology and Visual Science
New Jersey Medical School
Rutgers University
6th Floor Doctors Office Center
90 Bergen Street
Newark, NJ 07103 (USA)
E-Mail lravindraraj99@gmail.com

Luisa Pierro
Department of Ophthalmology
University Vita-Salute
San Raffaele Scientific Institute
Via Olgettina, 60
IT–20132 Milan (Italy)
E-Mail pierro.luisa@hsr.it

Elisabetta Pilotto
Department of Ophthalmology
University of Padova
Via Giustiniani, 2
IT–35128 Padova (Italy)
E-Mail elisabetta.pilotto@unipd.it

Giuseppe Querques
Department of Ophthalmology
University Vita-Salute
IRCCS Ospedale San Raffaele
Via Olgettina, 60
IT–20132 Milan (Italy)
E-Mail querques.giuseppe@hsr.it

Alessandro Rabiolo
Department of Opthalmology
University Vita-Salute
IRCCS Ospedale San Raffaele
Via Olgettina, 60
IT–20132 Milan (Italy)
E-Mail rabiolo.alessandro@hsr.it

Stanislao Rizzo
Department of Surgery and Translational Medicine
Careggi University Hospital, Eye Clinic
University of Florence
Largo Piero Palagi, 1
IT–50139 Florence (Italy)
E-Mail stanislao.rizzo@gmail.com

Riccardo Sacconi
Department of Ophthalmology
University Vita-Salute
San Raffaele Scientific Institute
Via Olgettina, 60
IT–20132 Milan (Italy)
E-Mail ric.sacconi@gmail.com

Antonio Secchi
Internal Medicine, Vita-Salute San Raffaele University
IRCCS San Raffaele Scientific Institute
Via Olgettina, 60
IT–20132 Milan (Italy)
E-Mail secchi.antonio@hsr.it

Ashish Sharma
Lotus Eye Hospital and Institute
Coimbatore, TN, 641014 (India)
E-Mail drashish79@hotmail.com

Valentina Turco
Complications of Diabetes Unit
Diabetes Research Institute
IRCCS San Raffaele Scientific Institute
Via Olgettina, 60
IT–20132 Milan (Italy)
E-Mail turco.vnt@gmail.com

Marco A. Zarbin
Institute of Ophthalmology and Visual Science
New Jersey Medical School
Rutgers University
6th Floor Doctors Office Center
90 Bergen Street
Newark, NJ 07103 (USA)
E-Mail zarbin@earthlink.net

Gianpaolo Zerbini
Complications of Diabetes Unit
Diabetes Research Institute
IRCCS San Raffaele Scientific Institute
Via Olgettina, 60
IT–20132 Milan (Italy)
E-Mail zerbini.gianpaolo@hsr.it

Ilaria Zucchiatti
Department of Ophthalmology
University Vita-Salute
San Raffaele Scientific Institute
Via Olgettina, 60
IT–20132 Milan (Italy)
E-Mail ilaria.zucchiatti@gmail.com

Preface

Diabetic retinopathy is the leading cause of blindness among working-age individuals in the industrialized world. Our understanding of the pathogenesis of this condition continues to evolve as does the treatment of its sight-threatening complications: diabetic macular edema and proliferative diabetic retinopathy. This book provides the latest information on the pathogenesis and diagnosis of diabetic retinopathy. In addition, the results of all relevant randomized clinical trials that serve as the basis for modern treatment of diabetic retinopathy are reviewed. The impact of modern diagnostic (e.g., optical coherence tomography-angiography) and therapeutic (e.g., small-gauge vitrectomy) technology is reviewed. Most importantly, this book does not simply provide a convenient summary of this critical information. Because data from randomized trials usually cannot be directly translated into clinical practice (e.g., due to limitations of patient enrollment or other aspects of study design), the data are analyzed and interpreted by highly experienced clinicians with the goal of facilitating application of these results to routine clinical practice. Ophthalmology residents, fellows, and practicing clinicians will find this book to be a useful reference when seeking evidence-based treatment strategies for various complications of diabetic retinopathy. Members of the pharmaceutical industry will find this overview useful when attempting to identify new avenues for drug development and unmet therapeutic needs in the management of diabetic retinopathy at all stages of the disease. Members of the insurance industry and overseers of national health policy will find this book to be a useful reference when trying to establish evidence-based guidelines for therapeutic intervention in managing the complications of diabetic retinopathy.

Francesco Bandello, Milan
Marco A. Zarbin, Newark, NJ
Rosangela Lattanzio, Milan
Ilaria Zucchiatti, Milan

Bandello F, Zarbin MA, Lattanzio R, Zucchiatti I (eds): Management of Diabetic Retinopathy.
Dev Ophthalmol. Basel, Karger, 2017, vol 60, pp 1–5 (DOI: 10.1159/000459641)

The Burden of Diabetes: Emerging Data

Paola Maffi[a] • Antonio Secchi[b]

[a]Internal Medicine and Transplant Unit, and [b]Internal Medicine, Vita-Salute San Raffaele University, IRCCS San Raffaele Scientific Institute, Milan, Italy

Abstract

In recent times, the global prevalence of diabetes has increased substantially, reaching 8.3% in 2014, which corresponds to 387 million patients. Studies in Europe and USA have shown increased incidence of type 1 Diabetes (T1D) over time at a rate of 3–5% per year. Another most worrying feature of the rapid increase of diabetes is the emergence of type 2 Diabetes (T2D) in children, adolescents, and young adults. The well-known behavioral risks factors and epigenetic mechanisms recently observed require an integrated approach to prevent T2D. Diabetes significantly influences the patient' survival, quality of life, and development of organ system degeneration. Epidemiological studies have shown increased mortality in diabetic patients, especially women, which increased approximately fivefold, whereas cardiovascular mortality increased 20- to 30-fold when compared to the normal population. Diabetes is the leading cause of end-stage renal disease and vision loss in developed countries. Around 40% of T1D and T2D start on renal replacement therapy. While after 40 years of diabetes, the cumulative proportion of patients with any retinopathy and advanced retinopathy was 84.1 and 50.2%, respectively. However, the most prevalent chronic complication of diabetes is neuropathy. Distal Symmetric Polyneuropathy occurs in at least 20% of people with T1D after 20 years and in 10–15% of newly diagnosed T2D, increasing to 50% after 10 years. Cardiovascular Autonomic Neuropathy may be present in up to 60% of patients after 15 years and is an independent risk factor for cardiovascular mortality.

Diabetes mellitus has become a large worldwide public health concern. In recent years, the global prevalence of diabetes mellitus has increased substantially, reaching 8.3% in 2014, which corresponds to 387 million patients [1].

The number of people with diabetes worldwide has more than doubled during the past 20 years. Epidemiological data predict an inexorable and unsustainable increase in global health expenditure attributable to diabetes, so disease prevention should be given high priority.

In 2004, a report from the University of Edinburgh provided estimates of global prevalence of diabetes in the year 2000 and projections for 2030 [2]. Data on diabetes prevalence by age and sex from a limited number of countries were extrapolated from all 191 countries of World Health

Organization member states and applied to United Nations' population estimates for the period. The prevalence of diabetes for all age groups worldwide was estimated to be 2.8% in 2000 and 4.4% in 2030. The authors of the study suggested that there were 171 million people with diabetes in 2000, which was projected to rise to 366 million in 2030. It appears that these reports have consistently underestimated the global burden given that the 2011 IDF report [3] estimated a total of 366 million people with diabetes already, a number previously forecasted for 2030. The meteoric rise of the global estimate, a greater than twofold increase, to the current estimate of 415 million [4], provides a firm basis for this claim.

These studies did not discriminate between type 1 diabetes (T1D) and type 2 diabetes (T2D).

Recent studies in Europe and USA showed increased rates of T1D incidence over time with great geographical heterogeneity. They showed that the incidence of T1D is increasing at a rate of 3–5% per year. This gives a doubling time for the incidence of T1D of 14–23 years [5].

Another most worrying feature of the rapid increase of diabetes is the emergence of T2D, particularly in children, adolescents, and young adults. Although the role of traditional risk factors for T2D, such as genetic, lifestyle, and behavioral risk factors, has been given attention, recent research has focused on identifying the contributions of epigenetic mechanisms and the effect of intrauterine environment. An integrated approach is needed to prevent T2D that must recognize its heterogeneity [6].

The burden of diabetes is not only related to the matter of therapy aimed at glycemic control, but also significantly influences the patient's survival, quality of life, and development of organ system degeneration (cardiovascular disease [CVD], nephropathy, retinopathy, neuropathy).

T1D is consistently associated with increased mortality, though the excess risk may have recently decreased [7]. Large differences in T1D mortality are observed internationally, with a slightly higher mortality in Europe than in the US. Excess mortality also differs by sex, with women having greater mortality than men [8]. A systematic review of all causes of mortality has shown that a significant and clinically meaningful sex difference exists in the excess risk of mortality (in particular, vascular mortality conferred by T1D to the detriment of women). In individuals with T1D, the excess risk of all-cause mortality was 37% higher in women than in men. For macrovascular outcomes (including cardiovascular and renal diseases), the excess risk of mortality in women compared to men was even more extreme. Mortality rates from other causes, neoplastic diseases or accident and suicide, were similar in both women and men. However, the excess vascular mortality recorded in women compared with men with T1D might be due to women having an overall greater cumulative lifetime exposure to hyperglycemia because of poorer glycemic control compared with men [9].

A steady increase was observed when mortality across all age groups was considered.

The Pittsburgh Epidemiology of Diabetes Complications (EDC) Study [10], demonstrated that the total and CVD mortality and hospitalized CVD are significantly increased in this contemporary US cohort of young adults with long-standing T1D. It is considered a prospective cohort study of childhood-onset (<17 years old) T1D diagnosed or seen within 1 year of diagnosis followed since 1986–1988, initially with biennial examinations for 10 years and thereafter with biennial questionnaires and further examinations at 18 and 25 years post baseline. The analyses were restricted to EDC participants who were <45 years old during the January 1, 1996 to December 31, 2012 follow-up period (n = 502); the results were compared to data for the 1996–2012 age-matched background Allegheny County, Pennsylvania, population obtained through the Allegheny County Health Department. The results demonstrated that in T1D cohort compared with the age-matched background population, the total mortality increased approximately fivefold, whereas CVD mortality increased 20- to 30-fold. Hospitalized CVD events increased eightfold, with revascularization procedures accounting for much of the increased risk. For all outcomes, the relative risk in women was larger than that for men. Another recent report, from the Swedish National Diabetes Register, showed that even for patients with T1D who had on-target glycemic control for the past 8 years, both total and cardiovascular mortality were increased compared with the general population [11]. When examined by age and sex, regardless of glycemic control, the study reported that men 18–49 years old had 3- to 4-fold greater total mortality than the general population, whereas women in the same age group had more than fourfold greater total mortality.

The burden of diabetes chronic complications is well documented in longitudinal long-term follow-up studies. The Diabetes Control and Complications Trial and the Epidemiology of Diabetes Interventions and Complications study (DCCT/EDIC) represent the largest epidemiological and intervention studies on T1D treatment and on the related development of retinopathy, nephropathy, neuropathy, and CVD [12]. Early interventions designed to optimize glycemic control have been shown to reduce the development and progression of these complications. Besides, participants in the DCCT with further follow-up in the EDIC study demonstrated that intensive diabetes therapy compared with conventional therapy during the DCCT, had beneficial effects from a period of intensive glycemic control and persisted beyond the completion of the intervention trial, despite similar levels of glycemic control in the two treatment groups during EDIC. This phenomenon was referred as "metabolic memory" [13, 14]. The UK Prospective Diabetes Study (UKPDS), a large long-term intervention trial in T2D, showed the effects of intensive treatment, as opposed to the conventional approach, on the reduction of diabetes-related events, micro and macrovascular [15, 16].

Diabetic kidney disease (DKD) represents a relevant burden on people's health and significantly contributes to the increase in cardiovascular risk among diabetic patients.

Moreover, DKD is the leading cause of end-stage renal disease in the Western world in patients starting renal replacement therapy. It affects 40% of T1D and T2D patients [17]. When incipient nephropathy is considered, in terms of microalbuminuria, the cumulative incidence in patients with T1D is 12.6% over 7.3 years EURODIAB [18]. The incidence of microalbuminuria in T2D is 2.0% per year, and the prevalence 10 years after diagnosis is 25% in the UKPDS [19].

The increase in albuminuria has been found to be a strong predictor of a more rapid decline in renal function and an increase in cardiovascular and all-cause mortality [20].

Diabetic retinopathy is a leading cause of vision loss in developed countries and it also represents a relevant burden on health and quality of life. Apart from its effects on vision, the presence of diabetic retinopathy also signifies a heightened risk of life-threatening systemic vascular complications [21].

In the past, one of the first largest epidemiological study on this problem, the Wisconsin Epidemiological Study of Diabetic Retinopathy, had demonstrated an almost 100% risk of developing at least mild retinopathy over a course of 30 years of diabetes, with 50% of patients having sight-threatening retinopathy [22].

Subsequently, an European study with the aim of analyzing the risk profile under real-life conditions, defines the risk profile for diabetic retinopathy in a large cohort of patients with T1D as: any retinopathy was present in 27.4% and advanced retinopathy (severe non-proliferative or proliferative diabetic retinopathy) in 8.0% of the cohort. After 40 years of diabetes, the cumulative proportion of patients with any retinopathy and advanced retinopathy was 84.1 and 50.2%, respectively [23].

Diabetic neuropathies, a heterogeneous group of conditions that affect different parts of the nervous system, are the most prevalent chronic complications of diabetes.

Estimates of the incidence and prevalence of Distal Symmetric Polyneuropathy (DSPN), accounting for about 75% of diabetic neuropathies, vary greatly, but evidence from several large observational cohorts and the DCCT/EDIC suggests that DSPN occurs in at least 20% of people with T1D after 20 years of disease duration. DSPN may be present in at least 10–15% of newly diagnosed patients with T2D, with rates increasing to 50% after 10 years of disease duration [24]. DSPN is the most important cause of foot ulceration, and it is also a prerequisite in the development of Charcot neuroarthropathy (CN). Foot ulceration and CN are both recognized as late complications of DSPN [25]. These late complications drive amputation risk and economic costs of diabetic neuropathy and are also predictors of mortality.

Cardiovascular Autonomic Neuropathy (CAN) prevalence increases substantially with diabetes duration, and prevalence rates of at least 30% were observed in the DCCT/EDIC cohort after 20 years of T1D duration. In T2D, the prevalence of CAN also increases with diabetes duration and may be present in up to 60% of patients after 15 years. A timely diagnosis of CAN may have important clinical implications, as CAN is an independent risk factor for cardiovascular mortality, arrhythmia, silent ischemia, any major cardiovascular event, and myocardial dysfunction. In addition, CAN independently predicts the progression of diabetic nephropathy and chronic kidney disease in diabetes [26].

In conclusion, considering the increasing incidence of diabetes, type 1 and 2, and its devastating consequences, any effort aimed at identifying the treatable causes, early treatment and even prevention, would be a top priority of biomedical research and Health Authorities.

References

1 IDF Diabetes Atlas – ed 6 (Database on the Internet) 2013. http://www.idf.org/diabetesatlas (accessed July 13, 2015).
2 Wild S, Roglic G, Green A, Sicree R, King H: Global prevalence of diabetes: estimates for the year 2000 and projections for 2030. Diabetes Care 2004;27:1047–1053.
3 Whiting DR, Guariguata L, Weil C, Shaw J: IDF diabetes atlas: global estimates of the prevalence of diabetes for 2011 and 2030. Diabetes Res Clin Pract 2011;94:311–321.
4 IDF Diabetes Atlas – ed 7. Brussels, Belgium, International Diabetes Federation, 2015.
5 Forlenza GP, Rewers M: The epidemic of type 1 diabetes: what is it telling us? Curr Opin Endocrinol Diabetes Obes 2011;18:248–251.
6 Zimmet PZ, Alberti KG: Epidemiology of diabetes-status of a pandemic and issues around metabolic surgery. Diabetes Care 2016;39:878–883.
7 Morgan E, Cardwell CR, Black CJ, McCance DR, Patterson CC: Excess mortality in Type 1 diabetes diagnosed in childhood and adolescence: a systematic review of population-based cohorts. Acta Diabetol 2015;52:801–807.
8 Huxley RR, Peters SA, Mishra GD, Woodward M: Risk of all-cause mortality and vascular events in women versus men with type 1 diabetes: a systematic review and meta-analysis. Lancet Diabetes Endocrinol 2015;3:198–206.
9 Huxley R, Barzi F, Woodward M: Excess risk of fatal coronary heart disease associated with diabetes in men and women: meta-analysis of 37 prospective cohort studies. BMJ 2006;332:73–78.
10 Miller RG, Mahajan HD, Costacou T, Sekikawa A, Anderson SJ, Orchard TJ: A contemporary estimate of total mortality and cardiovascular disease risk in young adults with type 1 diabetes: the pittsburgh epidemiology of diabetes complications study. Diabetes Care 2016;39:2296–2303.
11 Lind M, Svensson AM, Kosiborod M, Gudbjörnsdottir S, Pivodic A, Wedel H, Dahlqvist S, Clements M, Rosengren A: Glycemic control and excess mortality in type 1 diabetes. N Engl J Med 2014;371:1972–1982.
12 Diabetes Control and Complications Trial (DCCT)/Epidemiology of Diabetes Interventions and Complications (EDIC) Study Research Group: Intensive diabetes treatment and cardiovascular outcomes in type 1 diabetes: the DCCT/EDIC study 30-year follow-up. Diabetes Care 2016;39:686–693.
13 The Diabetes Control and Complications Trial/Epidemiology of Diabetes Interventions and Complications Research Group: Retinopathy and nephropathy in patients with type 1 diabetes four years after a trial of intensive therapy. N Engl J Med 2000;342:381–389.

14 Writing Team for the Diabetes Control and Complications Trial/Epidemiology of Diabetes Interventions and Complications Research Group: Sustained effect of intensive treatment of type 1 diabetes mellitus on development and progression of diabetic nephropathy: the epidemiology of diabetes interventions and complications (EDIC) study. JAMA 2003;290:2159–2167.
15 Intensive blood-glucose control with sulphonylureas or insulin compared with conventional treatment and risk of complications in patients with type 2 diabetes (UKPDS 33). UK Prospective Diabetes Study (UKPDS) Group. Lancet 1998;352:837–853.
16 Effect of intensive blood-glucose control with metformin on complications in overweight patients with type 2 diabetes (UKPDS 34). UK Prospective Diabetes Study (UKPDS) Group. Lancet 1998; 352:854–865.
17 National Kidney Foundation: KDOQI clinical practice guideline for diabetes and CKD: 2012 update. Am J Kidney Dis 2012;60:850–886.
18 Chaturvedi N, Bandinelli S, Mangili R, Penno G, Rottiers RE, Fuller JH: Microalbuminuria in type 1 diabetes: rates, risk factors and glycemic threshold. Kidney Int 2001;60:219–227.
19 Adler AI, Stevens RJ, Manley SE, Bilous RW, Cull CA, Holman RR: Development and progression of nephropathy in type 2 diabetes: the United Kingdom prospective diabetes study (UKPDS 64). Kidney Int 2003;63:225–232.
20 Fox CS, Matsushita K, Woodward M, Bilo HJ, Chalmers J, Heerspink HJ, Lee BJ, Perkins RM, Rossing P, Sairenchi T, Tonelli M, Vassalotti JA, Yamagishi K, Coresh J, de Jong PE, Wen CP, Nelson RG; Chronic Kidney Disease Prognosis Consortium: Associations of kidney disease measures with mortality and end-stage renal disease in individuals with and without diabetes: a meta-analysis. Lancet 2012;380:1662–1673.
21 Cheung N, Mitchell P, Wong TY: Diabetic retinopathy. Lancet 2010;376:124–136.
22 Klein R, Klein BE, Moss SE, Davis MD, DeMets DL: The Wisconsin epidemiologic study of diabetic retinopathy. II. Prevalence and risk of diabetic retinopathy when age at diagnosis is less than 30 years. Arch Ophthalmol 1984;102:520–526.
23 Hammes HP, Kerner W, Hofer S, Kordonouri O, Raile K, Holl RW; DPV-Wiss Study Group: Diabetic retinopathy in type 1 diabetes – a contemporary analysis of 8,784 patients. Diabetologia 2011; 54:1977–1984.
24 Pop-Busui R, Boulton AJ, Feldman EL, Bril V, Freeman R, Malik RA, Sosenko JM, Ziegler D: Diabetic neuropathy: a position statement by the American diabetes association. Diabetes Care 2017; 40:136–154.
25 Boulton AJ: The pathway to foot ulceration in diabetes. Med Clin North Am 2013;97:775–790.
26 Astrup AS, Tarnow L, Rossing P, Hansen BV, Hilsted J, Parving HH: Cardiac autonomic neuropathy predicts cardiovascular morbidity and mortality in type 1 diabetic patients with diabetic nephropathy. Diabetes Care 2006;29:334–339.

Paola Maffi, MD
Internal Medicine and Transplant Unit
IRCCS San Raffaele Scientific Institute
Via Olgettina, 60
IT–20132 Milan (Italy)
E-Mail paola.maffi@hsr.it

Bandello F, Zarbin MA, Lattanzio R, Zucchiatti I (eds): Management of Diabetic Retinopathy.
Dev Ophthalmol. Basel, Karger, 2017, vol 60, pp 6–15 (DOI: 10.1159/000459642)

The Eye as a Window to the Microvascular Complications of Diabetes

Gianpaolo Zerbini[a] · Silvia Maestroni[a] · Valentina Turco[a] · Antonio Secchi[b]

[a]Complications of Diabetes Unit, Diabetes Research Institute, and [b]Internal Medicine, Vita-Salute San Raffaele University, IRCCS San Raffaele Scientific Institute, Milan, Italy

Abstract

Although microvascular complications of diabetes (retinopathy, neuropathy, and nephropathy) affect different organs, they are strongly correlated to each other. Based on recent data, their onset and progression could be directly monitored, focusing our attention only on the eye. When confirmed and standardized, this approach could allow one to simplify the way in which we follow the progression of different diabetic complications, and thus establish new strategies aimed at preventing, treating and, hopefully, inducing the remission of microvascular complications of diabetes.

Diabetic Retinopathy

Diabetic retinopathy (DR) is a microangiopathic disease, mainly affecting the retinal arterioles, capillaries, and venules, although larger vessels may also be involved [1, 2].

It usually takes several years (sometimes decades) to move from the diagnosis of diabetes to the detection of retinal microaneurysms, the established first clinical sign of DR [3, 4]. This "silent" period, if coupled with the presence of a valid biomarker of predisposition to DR, might represent the best moment to start a therapeutic strategy aimed at preventing the development of DR.

The ideal biomarker should be non-invasive, able to predict the development of the disease before the appearance of the first clinical signs, and, if possible, serve as an indicator of a causal mechanism. In this case, the biomarker could also, at least potentially, become a surrogate end point in both drug development and preventative treatment [5].

Unfortunately, we are still far from identifying a specific marker able to predict the development of DR, but some recent clinical findings could be of help to achieve this objective.

A number of clinical studies in the last few years have demonstrated that some preclinical dysfunctions such as neuronal loss [6] and pericyte dropout do actually occur early in the diabetic retina [7].

Neuronal cells are the major component of the retina, and several reports have demonstrated that the neuroretinal function (measurable by electroretinogram [ERG], dark adaptation test, contrast sensitivity, and color vision test) is compromised long before the onset of vascular lesions in diabetic patients [8, 9]. Moreover, histology performed in post-mortem diabetic retinas demonstrated increased apoptosis in ganglion cells in humans, and animal models have demonstrated accelerated apoptosis of retinal neurons, glial activation, impaired glial cell metabolism, and microglial cell activation [10, 11].

The link between diabetes-driven neuronal dysfunction and vascular disease is not easy to explain, but we have to take into account the existence, in the central nervous system, of a physical and biochemical interaction between neurons, glia, and specialized vasculature tissues known as neurovascular unit, a structure that maintains homeostasis [11].

Pericytes are contractile smooth muscle cells that regulate blood flow; they are also involved in the control of proliferation and repair of endothelial cells inside the retinal vascular system. The loss of pericytes is followed by the loss of capillary endothelial cells, and is associated with the formation of retinal microaneurysms [4, 7].

Pericytes and/or neuron loss could potentially represent a good biomarker of the subsequent development of DR, but unfortunately histological samples are needed to count their number.

A possible alternative to evaluate and quantify neuronal and vascular dysfunctions in the retina in the preclinical phase of DR comes from the recent development of novel in vivo imaging and functional tests capable of evaluating the thickness of the neuroretinal layers (Optical Coherence Tomography [OCT]) and the myogenic response of retinal vessels (Digital Vessel Analyzer [DVA]).

Optical Coherence Tomography

Retinal neurodegeneration in diabetic patients is caused by different mechanisms. Hyperglycemia disrupts the delicate metabolic environment inside the retina and alters the function of the insulin receptor (essential for neuronal development, growth, and survival), leading to neural apoptosis. In addition, molecular factors such as increased oxidative stress, inflammatory cytokines, and glutamate excitotoxicity contribute to the process of neuronal damage and death [11].

Atrophy of ganglion cells and degeneration of retinal nerve fibers in histologic retinal sections of patients with 40 years of diabetes was described for the first time in the 1960s [12, 13].

At first, neurodegeneration could be observed only in autopsy samples and hence could not be used as a marker of DR, but this dysfunction is now commonly diagnosed due to the clinical implementation of OCT.

OCT imaging allows the cross-sectional visualization of retinal layers and the quantitative mapping of total retinal thickness at 3 micron level of resolution. OCT technology is used routinely for the detection of anatomical abnormalities within the retinal layers. Of interest, this methodology is still increasing its potential as several software programs for image segmentation have been developed recently allowing the high-definition measurement of the thickness of individual retinal layers [14].

Based on this technology, several studies have demonstrated a thinning of the retinal ganglion cell layer [15, 16], the retinal nerve fiber layer (RNFL) [16], and the inner retinal layers (ganglion cell layer + inner plexiform and inner nuclear layers) [17] in the macula of type 1 diabetic patients (T1DM) with minimal signs of DR.

The most interesting finding, however, was the reduction of the total retinal thickness described in the macula of T1DM with no clinical signs of DR [17–20].

The total retinal thinning is associated with a reduction in the signal amplitude of the multifocal ERG in young individuals with T1 and T2DM without DR [20], while another study has shown a reduction of RNFL and ganglion cell layer [21] in adolescent T1DM patients with no DR.

The thinning of retinal layers, detected in diabetic patients without DR, correlates with retinal dysfunctions that were shown to precede the appearance of clinical signs of DR [9], thus suggesting that the thinning of retinal layers could also precede the vascular alterations of this complication.

Unfortunately, there was no follow-up on patients affected by the thinning of retinal layers, and the lack of longitudinal data represents the major limiting factor of these studies.

The only longitudinal study (4 years follow-up) performed so far on 45 T1DM with no or minimal DR demonstrated a progressive thinning of the RNFL in the macula and a thinning of the parafoveal ganglion cell layer + inner plexiform layer. These dysfunctions are independent of HbA1C, DR grade, or progression of DR, suggesting that progressive neuroretinal degeneration was primarily related to diabetes duration [22].

Dynamic Vessel Analyzer

Retinal hemodynamic measurements are an attractive approach to identify abnormalities that may precede the development of clinical DR because they relate directly to the vessels, and can be performed non-invasively in humans. For this reason, several studies have been performed to investigate the relationship between retinal arteriolar and venular caliber, and the incidence of DR in resting conditions [5]. The results of these studies have only been partially successful [22], suggesting that to detect vascular abnormalities in case of DR a functional challenge must be applied [23].

Postural change exploits the response of retinal hemodynamics to a change in posture from sitting to reclining. First, baseline measurements (retinal arterial diameter and blood speed) are obtained in the sitting position; the subjects are then asked to recline on their right side, and new measurements are taken after 30 min of reclining. The last set of retinal hemodynamic measurements was obtained 20 min after the subjects resumed the sitting position. In response to reclining, the retinal arterial diameter normally decreases due to the increased perfusion pressure induced by the postural change. This response is termed as "myogenic response" because it represents the intrinsic response of arterial smooth muscle cells [24, 25].

A few studies have demonstrated that T1DM patients without DR fail to show vasoconstriction after postural change, while blood speed and flow responses are highly variable, compared to control subjects [24]. Moreover, a follow-up study on T1DM demonstrated that patients with a defective myogenic response develop clinical DR in 4 years [25]. This study also shows that when the onset of DR occurs after short diabetes duration, the myogenic response is prominently defective. Conversely, when DR develops after long diabetes duration, the myogenic response is comparable with those of control subjects, suggesting that other factors may be involved in DR development [25].

Based on these premises, defective myogenic response should probably be considered as an accelerator of the development of DR, and for this reason may be a good risk marker of the complication.

The most important disadvantage of the postural change examination is that it is extremely difficult to standardize, especially when performed in older people with mobility problems. For these reasons, the "flickering light stimulation test" is used frequently to evaluate the myogenic response of retinal vessels.

This examination utilizes the dynamic retinal vessel analyzer (DVA, IMEDOS, Germany) to investigate the functional abnormalities that consist of reduced or absent dilation of retinal vessels in response to light stimulation.

The DVA allows the continuous non-invasive measurement of retinal vessel diameter, 25 times/s using stimulation tests of vessel function. By interrupting the green measuring light, the DVA generates a flicker light with a frequency of 12.5 Hz and with a bright-to-dark ratio of 25:1.

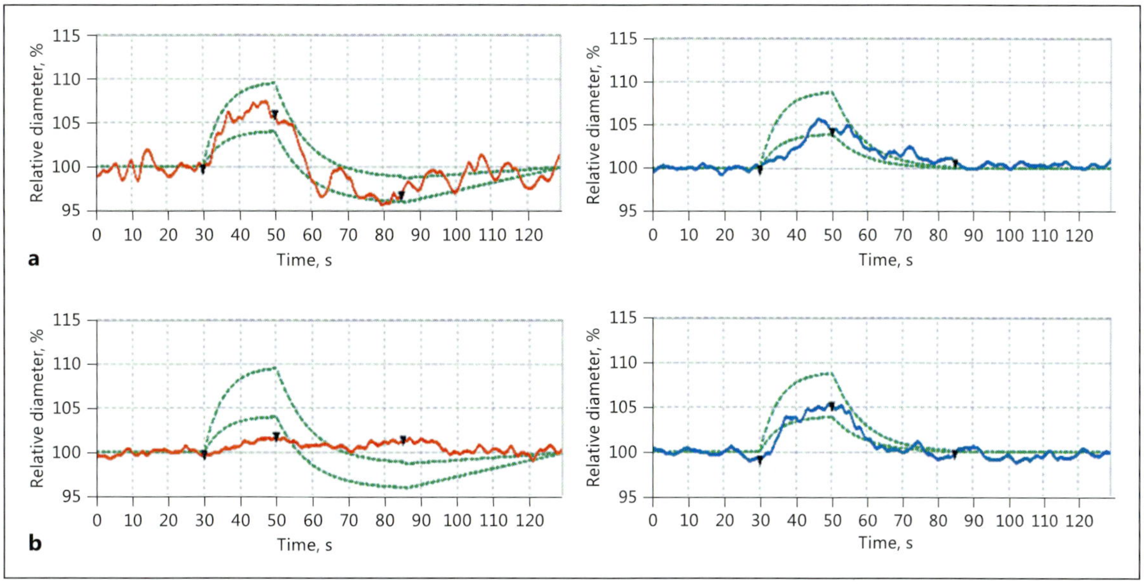

Fig. 1. DVA trace from (**a**) control subject showing dilatatory effect in both arterioles (left panel) and venules (right panel) during flicker stimulation; (**b**) patient with DR showing a reduced dilatatory effect.

The changes of vessel's diameters are measured during the entire duration of the flickering light stimulation test [26].

The examination consists of a 50 s baseline vessel diameter measurement, followed by provocation with flicker light performed for 20 s, and by a final observation for 80 s after the end of the flicker exposure, repeated 3 times [5, 26].

Flickering light stimulates the activity of the neural retina, and the increased metabolic demand activates auto regulatory mechanisms that dilate retinal blood vessels through the release of nitric oxide by neuron and endothelial cells [27], and consequently enhance blood flow. This process enables the retina to regulate blood flow in response to neural activity and is called neurovascular coupling [28].

Whereas in healthy individuals retinal arterioles and venules increase their diameter by 4 and 5%, respectively, in response to diffuse luminance flicker, T1DM patients with no sign of DR show response to this stimulus of 2.7 and 3.1%, respectively [29], and this parameter worsens with the progression of the disease [26]. Same results were obtained in a study on T2DM patients [30].

An example of flickering analysis is shown in Figure 1.

Response to flicker correlates with pattern ERG and oscillatory potential in healthy subjects and patients with diabetes and no DR [28], suggesting that the impairment of flicker-induced responses may be partly attributed to the inner retinal dysfunction that occurs early in diabetes.

Conversely, another study showed that reduced flicker response occurs before pattern ERG abnormalities in T1DM patients with no DR [31], demonstrating that flickering is not influenced by abnormal neural activity in early stage of the disease. All these results are independent of glycated hemoglobin and blood pressure.

Conclusions

Currently, we have 2 possible candidate markers for predicting the development of DR, but unfortunately both show some limitations.

It has been demonstrated that retinal neurodegeneration, as evaluated by OCT, precedes the clinical evolution of DR, but all the studies performed so far fail to answer the question whether a marked thinning of the RNFL or of the ganglion cell layer may predict the development of DR or if they are just independent phenomena. A recently published study performed on T2DM patients demonstrates that the thinning of the ganglion cell complex is a predictive marker of the development of diabetic neuropathy (DN) rather than a marker of DR [32].

Conversely, myogenic response evaluated with postural change was shown to predict the progression toward clinical DR, but the study was performed only in 13 patients [25].

To resolve the issue and to clarify whether retinal abnormalities detected by OCT and/or DVA may actually predict the subsequent development of clinical DR, a longitudinal study in which retinal thinning, flicker response, and functional analysis by ERG are evaluated in parallel in the same patients appears to be mandatory.

Diabetic Neuropathy

DN, which may be asymptomatic in up to 50% of cases, is one of the most common complications of diabetes. The clinical manifestations of DN cannot be restricted to a single disease, but are rather the result of several entities with different natural histories, findings, and outcomes, reasonably explained by a pool of different disorders having independent causes and pathogenic mechanisms.

The variety of syndromes affecting the peripheral nervous system in case of diabetes have been organized in a number of different classifications during the last few years, with those based on clinical manifestations of DN being the most commonly used [33]. From a clinical point of view, DN has been clearly defined as a chronic symmetric sensorimotor polyneuropathy, usually beginning after years of chronic hyperglycemia.

Typically, the first diabetes-driven neural dysfunctions are represented by a slight alteration of nerve conduction, reduced heart beat response to deep breathing, higher vibration threshold at toes, and decreased ankle reflexes [34].

Longitudinal data from the Rochester cohort have shown that both duration and magnitude of exposure to hyperglycemia are strictly related to the severity of the clinical manifestations of DN, to the point that severe hyperglycemia can actually result in acute reduction of nerve conduction velocity and axonal shrinkage [35].

Chronic hyperglycemia could lead to the injury of Schwann cell (myelin), neurons, or axons on one hand or to the damage of micro-vessels (that would secondarily end up by causing nerve fiber injury) through several putative mechanisms on the other.

It has been shown that chronic hyperglycemia directly affects the phospholipid and/or fatty acid metabolism with a consequent inhibition of the polyol pathway, resulting in an insufficient utilization of glucose, sorbitol, and fructose that tend to accumulate in peripheral tissues [34].

Chronic hyperglycemia also reduces the availability of myo inositol and Na^+ K^+ ATPase in a number of organs, thus causing an alteration of conduction velocity and probably axo-glial dysjunction [36].

Another effect of chronic hyperglycemia is the accelerated glycosylation of proteins, with the consequent increased formation of advanced glycation end-products and their pathologic accumulation in various tissues. Hyperglycemia also affects both fast and slow axonal transport, with the latter conceivably resulting in a reduction of caliber and integrity of nerve fibers [36]. Hence, sensory testings and electrophysiology are often unable to demonstrate and quantify precisely the benefits of therapeutic interventions. Electrophysiology carefully assesses the damage of large nerve fibers, but is not so accurate with small nerve fibers, which are usually affected quite early in the case of diabetes [37] but in contrast to large fibers, are also able to undergo self-repair even in case of advanced neuropathy [38].

A precise and reproducible quantification of the damage to small nerve fibers should therefore be the main target to correctly assess neural degeneration and regeneration in diabetic patients. The direct morphologic examination of nerve fibers in sural nerve biopsies and the evaluation of the density of intra-epidermal nerve fibers in skin-punch biopsies may allow one to quantify accurately the damage and repair of nerve fibers, but both procedures are invasive and unsuitable for patients.

Ideally, a test aimed at early detection of DN should be at the same time non-invasive and quantitative and capable of detecting changes (also small changes) along time as in the case of preventive or therapeutic interventions. A recently identified technology, for example, corneal confocal microscopy (CCM), seems to fulfill these attributes, being at the same time non-invasive, quantitative in case of small fiber pathology, and particularly sensitive as it allows one to stratify neuropathic severity [39]. This novel approach is able to accurately define the extent of corneal nerve damage and repair, 2 parameters that tightly correlate with peripheral nerve function [40]. In this regard, Tavakoli et al. [41] have recently shown that CCM identifies small nerve fiber damage and accurately quantifies the severity of DN in its very early stages. They have also shown that dysfunctions seen with CCM correlates with intraepidermal nerve fiber loss [42], and that this technique is able to detect early nerve fiber regeneration after pancreas transplantation [43, 44].

The cornea is the only human organ allowing one to study directly and in vivo the unmyelinated nerve fibers. Studies in diabetic patients have shown that the progressive increase of the clinical severity of neuropathy is associated with a progressive reduction of corneal nerve fiber length [45], paralleled by a decreased corneal sensitivity [46]. Furthermore, deficits in corneal nerve fiber length have been shown to correlate with a reduced intra-epidermal nerve fiber density as seen in skin biopsies [45]. Before the discovery of in vivo CCM, detailed histological analysis of the human cornea was possible only by postmortem examination using light and electron microscopies. CCM has been developed further in the last few years, and allows one to analyze in situ details of the corneal architecture such as the corneal epithelium, Bowman's membrane, stroma, and endothelium at a resolution of 1–2 μm [47].

The specific damage to unmyelinated C-class nerve fibers that densely innervate the cornea is responsible for most of the symptoms and signs experienced by diabetic patients affected by peripheral neuropathy [47]. In the context of using corneal nerve morphology as a surrogate for peripheral neuropathy, the study and quantification of 4 key parameters: (1) nerve fiber density (NFD), (2) nerve branch density (NBD), (3) nerve fiber length (NFL), and (4) tortuosity coefficient (TC), have not only allowed one to detect and stratify peripheral neuropathy in its early stages [45], but also to demonstrate the repair of affected nerves after simultaneous pancreas and kidney transplantation [48]. NFD is defined as the total number of main nerve fibers per frame divided by the area of the frame in square millimeters. NBD is defined as the total number of main nerve branches divided by the area of the frame. NFL is the total length of nerve fibers. TC is a mathematical computation of the nerve fiber tortuosity [43].

After careful analysis of the corneal nerve density and morphology, a strong correlation has been found between reduction in fiber density/branching and severity of somatic neuropathy [49]. Changes in corneal nerve tortuosity can also be detected in DN, and increased nerve tortuosity might by itself represent a morphological marker of nerve regeneration because sciatic-nerve-crush experiments have demonstrated that regenerating nerves are characterized by increased tortuosity, particularly in older animals [40].

The early diagnosis of DN is essential for both stratifying patients for risk and to set up a preventive strategy for the complication itself. The capability of CCM to carefully identify and define the extent of nerve damage (even when still at a preclinical level) could represent a new non-invasive way to accurately diagnose DN in its very early stages and to quantify its progression or regression in the presence of an innovative preventive approach [45].

In conclusion, CCM is an ideal surrogate marker for early diagnosis, stratification of severity, and assessment of therapeutic efficacy of new treatments in human DN [44]. CCM may represent a novel tool, allowing one to expedite drug development programs for therapies deemed to be beneficial in the treatment of diabetic DN.

Diabetic Nephropathy

The renal complication of diabetes, known as diabetic nephropathy (DNeph), affects approximately 30% of T1DM and, if untreated, leads invariably to end-stage renal disease. From a functional point of view, the evolution of DNeph is characterized by the progressive increase of urinary albumin excretion rate (or microalbuminuria) paralleled by the reduction of glomerular filtration rate [50, 51].

Recent clinical evidences suggest that, despite the continuous improvement of clinical protocols aimed at controlling the glucose metabolism and blood pressure, the risk of developing end-stage renal disease as a consequence of DNeph has not changed significantly during the last 20 years [52, 53]. In general, these findings suggest that the cellular/molecular mechanisms leading to the development of DNeph are probably not yet fully understood and that further studies are needed to identify in advance patients predisposed to develop this complication (at stages that precede the appearance of microalbuminuria) and, in parallel, to develop new drugs able to prevent the onset of DNeph rather than to modulate its progression. A major problem with the correct diagnosis of DNeph (particularly, in type 2 diabetes) arises from the fact that diabetes-driven morphologic changes at glomerular level can be appreciated only invasively by performing renal biopsies [54]. The possibility to indirectly monitor the evolution of DNeph through the study of vascular and neural components of the retina would significantly simplify the way this complication could be treated.

DR almost invariably precedes the development of DNeph [51, 55], in line with a strong connection between the 2 complications. Search for DR in a diabetic patient with a pre-existing diagnosis of microalbuminuria is often a way to confirm the presence of DNeph. Diabetes by itself may in fact increase the incidence of a number of non-diabetic renal diseases, and the coexistence of DR and microalbuminuria could be of help in clarifying the clinical scenario [56].

DR is considered synonymous with endothelial dysfunction, and the concurrence between DR and DNeph suggested that the same abnormality could also underlie the development of the renal complication of diabetes. The hypothesis that the 2 complications might share a similar pathogenesis based on endothelial dysfunction [57, 58], ischemia, and consequent proliferation of incompetent new vessels in the retina [3] and in the glomerulus [59, 60] was raised a few years ago and confirmed by the clinical evidence that both complications are positively influenced by anti-angiogenic treatment [59–61].

Further confirmation of the strong link between the 2 complications comes from the recent demonstration that retinal vessel caliber predicts the development of DNeph [62] (along with other microvascular complications of diabetes) raising once again the possibility that retinal and glomerular microvessels might share the same dysfunctions (and in the same temporal order) in case of diabetes.

Another possible link between the retina and the glomerulus (and, consequently, between DR and DNeph) is represented by the recent demonstration that the podocyte, despite its mesodermic origin, shares with neurons a number of common characteristics, including the presence of neuron-like functional synaptic vesicles [63, 64]. In particular, neuronal proteins involved in synaptic vesicle recycling, for example, dynamin, synaptojanin, and endophilin, seem to play a major role in the formation and maintenance of podocyte foot processes [65, 66]. As described earlier in the chapter dedicated to DR [17–20], early retinal degeneration has been suggested as the possible first diabetes-driven dysfunction that will lead, years later, to the development of clinical manifestations of DR, and the possibility that a similar "neurodegeneration" of the podocyte might subsequently lead to the development of DNeph cannot be presently ruled out [67].

Also, in the near future the possibility of monitoring the progression of DNeph through a careful evaluation of retinal morphology and function appears to be quite realistic as a result of increased clinical capability to diagnose both complications and of the significantly improved technologic devices used in the field of ophthalmology.

Conclusion

Although the different microvascular complications of diabetes differ for target organ and natural history, they nonetheless tend to cluster in the same individuals, suggesting a possible common background. By offering the unique possibility to monitor at the same time the progression of different complications of diabetes, the eye may rapidly become a useful tool for setting up a strategy focused on the simultaneous prevention of retinopathy, neuropathy, and nephropathy.

References

1 Scott I, Flynn H, Smiddy W: Diabetes and Ocular Disease: Past, Present, and Future Therapies, ed 2. American Academy of Ophthalmology Monograph. New York, NY, Oxford University Press, 2010.
2 Mazzeo A, Beltramo E, Iavello A, Carpanetto A, Porta M: Molecular mechanisms of extracellular vesicle-induced vessel destabilization in diabetic retinopathy. Acta Diabetol 2015;52:1113–1119.
3 Martín-Merino E, Fortuny J, Rivero-Ferrer E, García-Rodríguez LA: Incidence of retinal complications in a cohort of newly diagnosed diabetic patients. PLoS One 2014;9:e100283.
4 Frank RN: Diabetic retinopathy. N Engl J Med 2004;350:48–58.
5 Ikram MK, Cheung CY, Lorenzi M, Klein R, Jones TL, Wong TY; NIH/JDRF Workshop on Retinal Biomarker for Diabetes Group: Retinal vascular caliber as a biomarker for diabetes microvascular complications. Diabetes Care 2013;36:750–759.
6 Kern TS, Barber AJ: Retinal ganglion cells in diabetes. J Physiol 2008;586:4401–4408.
7 Beltramo E, Porta M: Pericyte loss in diabetic retinopathy: mechanisms and consequences. Curr Med Chem 2013;20:3218–3225.
8 Pescosolido N, Barbato A, Stefanucci A, Buomprisco G: Role of electrophysiology in the early diagnosis and follow-up of diabetic retinopathy. J Diabetes Res 2015;2015:319692.
9 Reis A, Mateus C, Melo P, Figueira J, Cunha-Vaz J, Castelo-Branco M: Neuroretinal dysfunction with intact blood-retinal barrier and absent vasculopathy in type 1 diabetes. Diabetes 2014;63:3926–3937.
10 Antonetti DA, Barber AJ, Bronson SK, Freeman WM, Gardner TW, Jefferson LS, Kester M, Kimball SR, Krady JK, LaNoue KF, Norbury CC, Quinn PG, Sandirasegarane L, Simpson IA; JDRF Diabetic Retinopathy Center Group: Diabetic retinopathy: seeing beyond glucose-induced microvascular disease. Diabetes 2006;55:2401–2411.
11 Antonetti DA, Klein R, Gardner TW: Diabetic retinopathy. N Engl J Med 2012;366:1227–1239.
12 Wolter JR: Diabetic retinopathy. Am J Ophthalmol 1961;51:1123–1141.
13 Bloodworth JM Jr: Diabetic retinopathy. Diabetes 1962;11:1–22.
14 Terry L, Cassels N, Lu K, Acton JH, Margrain TH, North RV, Fergusson J, White N, Wood A: Automated retinal layer segmentation using spectral domain optical coherence tomography: evaluation of inter-session repeatability and agreement between devices. PLoS One 2016;11:e0162001.
15 van Dijk HW, Verbraak FD, Stehouwer M, Kok PH, Garvin MK, Sonka M, DeVries JH, Schlingemann RO, Abràmoff MD: Association of visual function and ganglion cell layer thickness in patients with diabetes mellitus type 1 and no or minimal diabetic retinopathy. Vision Res 2011;51:224–228.
16 van Dijk HW, Verbraak FD, Kok PH, Garvin MK, Sonka M, Lee K, Devries JH, Michels RP, van Velthoven ME, Schlingemann RO, Abràmoff MD: Decreased retinal ganglion cell layer thickness in patients with type 1 diabetes. Invest Ophthalmol Vis Sci 2010;51:3660–3665.

17 van Dijk HW, Kok PH, Garvin M, Sonka M, Devries JH, Michels RP, van Velthoven ME, Schlingemann RO, Verbraak FD, Abràmoff MD: Selective loss of inner retinal layer thickness in type 1 diabetic patients with minimal diabetic retinopathy. Invest Ophthalmol Vis Sci 2009;50:3404–3409.
18 Chen Y, Li J, Yan Y, Shen X: Diabetic macular morphology changes may occur in the early stage of diabetes. BMC Ophthalmol 2016;16:12.
19 Park HY, Kim IT, Park CK: Early diabetic changes in the nerve fibre layer at the macula detected by spectral domain optical coherence tomography. Br J Ophthalmol 2011;95:1223–1228.
20 Bronson-Castain KW, Bearse MA Jr, Neuville J, Jonasdottir S, King-Hooper B, Barez S, Schneck ME, Adams AJ: Adolescents with type 2 diabetes: early indications of focal retinal neuropathy, retinal thinning, and venular dilation. Retina 2009;29:618–626.
21 El-Fayoumi D, Badr Eldine NM, Esmael AF, Ghalwash D, Soliman HM: Retinal nerve fiber layer and ganglion cell complex thicknesses are reduced in children with type 1 diabetes with no evidence of vascular retinopathy. Invest Ophthalmol Vis Sci 2016;57:5355–5360.
22 Sohn EH, van Dijk HW, Jiao C, Kok PH, Jeong W, Demirkaya N, Garmager A, Wit F, Kucukevcilioglu M, van Velthoven ME, DeVries JH, Mullins RF, Kuehn MH, Schlingemann RO, Sonka M, Verbraak FD, Abràmoff MD: Retinal neurodegeneration may precede microvascular changes characteristic of diabetic retinopathy in diabetes mellitus. Proc Natl Acad Sci U S A 2016; 113:E2655–E2664.
23 Lorenzi M, Feke GT, Cagliero E, Pitler L, Schaumberg DA, Berisha F, Nathan DM, McMeel JW: Retinal haemodynamics in individuals with well-controlled type 1 diabetes. Diabetologia 2008;51:361–364.
24 Lorenzi M, Feke GT, Pitler L, Berisha F, Kolodjaschna J, McMeel JW: Defective myogenic response to posture change in retinal vessels of well-controlled type 1 diabetic patients with no retinopathy. Invest Ophthalmol Vis Sci 2010;51:6770–6775.
25 Tecilazich F, Feke GT, Mazzantini S, Sobrin L, Lorenzi M: Defective myogenic response of retinal vessels is associated with accelerated onset of retinopathy in type 1 diabetic individuals. Invest Ophthalmol Vis Sci 2016;57:1523–1529.
26 Mandecka A, Dawczynski J, Blum M, Müller N, Kloos C, Wolf G, Vilser W, Hoyer H, Müller UA: Influence of flickering light on the retinal vessels in diabetic patients. Diabetes Care 2007;30: 3048–3052.
27 Dorner GT, Garhofer G, Kiss B, Polska E, Polak K, Riva CE, Schmetterer L: Nitric oxide regulates retinal vascular tone in humans. Am J Physiol Heart Circ Physiol 2003;285:H631–H636.
28 Lecleire-Collet A, Audo I, Aout M, Girmens JF, Sofroni R, Erginay A, Le Gargasson JF, Mohand-Saïd S, Meas T, Guillausseau PJ, Vicaut E, Paques M, Massin P: Evaluation of retinal function and flicker light-induced retinal vascular response in normotensive patients with diabetes without retinopathy. Invest Ophthalmol Vis Sci 2011;52:2861–2867.
29 Mandecka A, Dawczynski J, Vilser W, Blum M, Müller N, Kloos C, Wolf G, Müller UA: Abnormal retinal autoregulation is detected by provoked stimulation with flicker light in well-controlled patients with type 1 diabetes without retinopathy. Diabetes Res Clin Pract 2009;86:51–55.
30 Lott ME, Slocomb JE, Shivkumar V, Smith B, Quillen D, Gabbay RA, Gardner TW, Bettermann K: Impaired retinal vasodilator responses in prediabetes and type 2 diabetes. Acta Ophthalmol 2013; 91:e462–e469.
31 Lasta M, Pemp B, Schmidl D, Boltz A, Kaya S, Palkovits S, Werkmeister R, Howorka K, Popa-Cherecheanu A, Garhöfer G, Schmetterer L: Neurovascular dysfunction precedes neural dysfunction in the retina of patients with type 1 diabetes. Invest Ophthalmol Vis Sci 2013;54:842–847.
32 Salvi L, Plateroti P, Balducci S, Bollanti L, Conti FG, Vitale M, Recupero SM, Enrici MM, Fenicia V, Pugliese G: Abnormalities of retinal ganglion cell complex at optical coherence tomography in patients with type 2 diabetes: a sign of diabetic polyneuropathy, not retinopathy. J Diabetes Complications 2016;30: 469–467.
33 Thomas PK: Classification, differential diagnosis, and staging of diabetic peripheral neuropathy. Diabetes 1997; 46(suppl 2):S54–S57.
34 Dyck PJ, Giannini C: Pathologic alterations in the diabetic neuropathies of humans: a review. J Neuropathol Exp Neurol 1996;55:1181–1193.
35 Dyck PJ, Kratz KM, Karnes JL, Litchy WJ, Klein R, Pach JM, Wilson DM, O'Brien PC, Melton LJ 3rd, Service FJ: The prevalence by staged severity of various types of diabetic neuropathy, retinopathy, and nephropathy in a population-based cohort: the Rochester Diabetic Neuropathy Study. Neurology 1993;43:817–824.
36 Boulton AJ, Malik RA, Arezzo JC, Sosenko JM: Diabetic somatic neuropathies. Diabetes Care 2004;27:1458–1486.
37 Malik RA, Veves A, Walker D, Siddique I, Lye RH, Schady W, Boulton AJ: Sural nerve fibre pathology in diabetic patients with mild neuropathy: relationship to pain, quantitative sensory testing and peripheral nerve electrophysiology. Acta Neuropathol 2001;101:367–374.
38 Malik RA, Veves A, Tesfaye S, Smith G, Cameron N, Zochodne D, Lauria G: Toronto Consensus Panel on Diabetic Neuropathy. Small fibre neuropathy: role in the diagnosis of diabetic sensorimotor polyneuropathy. Diabetes Metab Res Rev 2011;27:678–684.
39 Eaton SE, Harris ND, Rajbhandari SM, Greenwood P, Wilkinson ID, Ward JD, Griffiths PD, Tesfaye S: Spinal-cord involvement in diabetic peripheral neuropathy. Lancet 2001;358:35–36.
40 Malik RA, Kallinikos P, Abbott CA, van Schie CH, Morgan P, Efron N, Boulton AJ: Corneal confocal microscopy: a noninvasive surrogate of nerve fibre damage and repair in diabetic patients. Diabetologia 2003;46:683–688.
41 Tavakoli M, Quattrini C, Abbott C, Kallinikos P, Marshall A, Finnigan J, Morgan P, Efron N, Boulton AJ, Malik RA: Corneal confocal microscopy: a novel noninvasive test to diagnose and stratify the severity of human diabetic neuropathy. Diabetes Care 2010;33:1792–1797.
42 Quattrini C, Tavakoli M, Jeziorska M, Kallinikos P, Tesfaye S, Finnigan J, Marshall A, Boulton AJ, Efron N, Malik RA: Surrogate markers of small fiber damage in human diabetic neuropathy. Diabetes 2007;56:2148–2154.
43 Mehra S, Tavakoli M, Kallinikos PA, Efron N, Boulton AJ, Augustine T, Malik RA: Corneal confocal microscopy detects early nerve regeneration after pancreas transplantation in patients with type 1 diabetes. Diabetes Care 2007;30: 2608–2612.

44 Tavakoli M, Kallinikos P, Iqbal A, Herbert A, Fadavi H, Efron N, Boulton AJ, A Malik R: Corneal confocal microscopy detects improvement in corneal nerve morphology with an improvement in risk factors for diabetic neuropathy. Diabet Med 2011;28:1261–1267.

45 Hossain P, Sachdev A, Malik RA: Early detection of diabetic peripheral neuropathy with corneal confocal microscopy. Lancet 2005;366:1340–1343.

46 Tavakoli M, Kallinikos PA, Efron N, Boulton AJ, Malik RA: Corneal sensitivity is reduced and relates to the severity of neuropathy in patients with diabetes. Diabetes Care 2007;30:1895–1897.

47 Marshall AG, Lee-Kubli C, Azmi S, Zhang M, Ferdousi M, Mixcoatl-Zecuatl T, Petropoulos IN, Ponirakis G, Fineman MS, Fadavi H, Frizzi K, Tavakoli M, Jeziorska M, Jolivalt CG, Boulton AJ, Efron N, Calcutt NA, Malik RA: Spinal disinhibition in experimental and clinical painful diabetic neuropathy. Diabetes 2017, DOI: 10.2337/db16-1181. Epub ahead of print.

48 Malik RA, Kallinikos P, Abbott CA, van Schie CH, Morgan P, Efron N, Boulton AJ: Corneal confocal microscopy: a noninvasive surrogate of nerve fibre damage and repair in diabetic patients. Diabetologia 2003;46:683–688.

49 Kallinikos P, Berhanu M, O'Donnell C, Boulton AJ, Efron N, Malik RA: Corneal nerve tortuosity in diabetic patients with neuropathy. Invest Ophthalmol Vis Sci 2004;45:418–422.

50 Borch-Johnsen K, Andersen PK, Deckert T: The effect of proteinuria on relative mortality in type 1 (insulin-dependent) diabetes mellitus. Diabetologia 1985;28: 290–596.

51 Andersen AR, Christiansen JS, Andersen JK, Kreiner S, Deckert T: Diabetic nephropathy in type 1 (insulin-dependent) diabetes: an epidemiological study. Diabetologia 1983;25:496–501.

52 Gregg EW, Li Y, Wang J, Burrows NR, Ali MK, Rolka D, Williams DE, Geiss L: Changes in diabetes-related complications in the United States, 1990–2010. N Engl J Med 2014;370:1514–1523.

53 Tasci I, Basgoz BB, Saglam K: Glycemic control and the risk of microvascular complications in people with diabetes mellitus. Acta Diabetol 2016;53:129–130.

54 Najafian B, Mauer M: Morphologic features of declining renal function in type 1 diabetes. Semin Nephrol 2012;32:415–422.

55 He F, Xia X, Wu XF, Yu XQ, Huang FX: Diabetic retinopathy in predicting diabetic nephropathy in patients with type 2 diabetes and renal disease: a meta-analysis. Diabetologia 2013;56:457–466.

56 Dong Z, Wang Y, Qiu Q, Zhang X, Zhang L, Wu J, Wei R, Zhu H, Cai G, Sun X, Chen X: Clinical predictors differentiating non-diabetic renal diseases from diabetic nephropathy in a large population of type 2 diabetes patients. Diabetes Res Clin Pract 2016;121:112–118.

57 Karlberg C, Falk C, Green A, Sjølie AK, Grauslund J: Proliferative retinopathy predicts nephropathy: a 25-year follow-up study of type 1 diabetic patients. Acta Diabetol 2012;49:263–268.

58 Boelter MC, Gross JL, Canani LH, Costa LA, Lisboa HR, Três GS, Lavinsky J, Azevedo MJ: Proliferative diabetic retinopathy is associated with microalbuminuria in patients with type 2 diabetes. Braz J Med Biol Res 2006;39:1033–1039.

59 Yamamoto Y, Maeshima Y, Kitayama H, Kitamura S, Takazawa Y, Sugiyama H, Yamasaki Y, Makino H: Tumstatin peptide, an inhibitor of angiogenesis, prevents glomerular hypertrophy in the early stage of diabetic nephropathy. Diabetes 2004;53:1831–1840.

60 Ichinose K, Maeshima Y, Yamamoto Y, Kitayama H, Takazawa Y, Hirokoshi K, Sugiyama H, Yamasaki Y, Eguchi K, Makino H: Antiangiogenic endostatin peptide ameliorates renal alterations in the early stage of a type 1 diabetic nephropathy model. Diabetes 2005:54: 2891–2903.

61 Bandello F, Cicinelli MV, Parodi MB: Anti-VEGF molecules for the management of diabetic macular edema. Curr Pharm Des 2015;21:4731–4737.

62 Broe R, Rasmussen ML, Frydkjaer-Olsen U, Olsen BS, Mortensen HB, Hodgson L, Wong TY, Peto T, Grauslund J: Retinal vessel calibers predict long-term microvascular complications in type 1 diabetes: the Danish Cohort of Pediatric Diabetes 1987 (DCPD1987). Diabetes 2014; 63:3906–3914.

63 Rastaldi MP, Armelloni S, Berra S, Li M, Pesaresi M, Poczewski H, Langer B, Kerjaschki D, Henger A, Blattner SM, Kretzler M, Wanke R, D'Amico G: Glomerular podocytes possess the synaptic vesicle molecule Rab3A and its specific effector rabphilin-3a. Am J Pathol 2003; 163:889–899.

64 Rastaldi MP, Armelloni S, Berra S, Calvaresi N, Corbelli A, Giardino LA, Li M, Wang GQ, Fornasieri A, Villa A, Heikkila E, Soliymani R, Boucherot A, Cohen CD, Kretzler M, Nitsche A, Ripamonti M, Malgaroli A, Pesaresi M, Forloni GL, Schlöndorff D, Holthofer H, D'Amico G: Glomerular podocytes contain neuron-like functional synaptic vesicles. FASEB J 2006:20:976–978.

65 Soda K, Balkin DM, Ferguson SM, Paradise S, Milosevic I, Giovedi S, Volpicelli-Daley L, Tian X, Wu Y, Ma H, Son SH, Zheng R, Moeckel G, Cremona O, Holzman LB, De Camilli P, Ishibe S: Role of dynamin, synaptojanin, and endophilin in podocyte foot processes. J Clin Invest 2012;122:4401–4411.

66 Gu C, Lee HW, Garborcauskas G, Reiser J, Gupta V, Sever S: Dynamin autonomously regulates podocyte focal adhesion maturation. J Am Soc Nephrol 2017;28:446–451.

67 Srivastav K, Saxena S, Mahdi AA, Kruzliak P, Khanna VK: Increased serum urea and creatinine levels correlate with decreased retinal nerve fibre layer thickness in diabetic retinopathy. Biomarkers 2015;20:470–473.

Prof. Antonio Secchi
Internal Medicine and Transplant Unit, Vita-Salute University
IRCCS San Raffaele Scientific Institute
Via Olgettina, 60
IT–20132 Milan (Italy)
E-Mail secchi.antonio@hsr.it

Bandello F, Zarbin MA, Lattanzio R, Zucchiatti I (eds): Management of Diabetic Retinopathy.
Dev Ophthalmol. Basel, Karger, 2017, vol 60, pp 16–27 (DOI: 10.1159/000459687)

Emerging Insights into Pathogenesis

Edoardo Midena[a, b] · Elisabetta Pilotto[a]

[a]Department of Ophthalmology, University of Padova, Padova, and [b]GB Bietti Foundation, IRCCS, Rome, Italy

Abstract

Diabetic retinopathy (DR) is a frequent complication of diabetes mellitus (DM). Persistent hyperglycemia leads to the activation of multiple cellular pathways involved in the pathogenesis of DR, resulting in increased inflammation, oxidative stress, and vascular dysfunction. DR has been considered a "chronic, low-grade inflammatory disease of the retina". However, an increasing body of evidence suggests that inflammation and neurodegeneration both occur in human diabetes even before the development of clinical signs of DR. One of the first signs of inflammation in DM is the activation of retinal glia cells (RGC). RGC include microglia and macroglial cells (Müller cells and astrocytes). Activated RGC release cytotoxic substances responsible for the recruitment of leukocytes, blood-retinal barrier breakdown, direct glial dysfunction, and neuronal cell death. Recently, many inflammatory mediators, growth factors, and other molecules have been investigated in human vitreous and aqueous humor samples to better understand, in vivo, the multiple pathways and mechanisms leading to the pathogenesis of DR and its complications, such as diabetic macular edema, with potential for more tailored treatment. Moreover, non-invasive techniques, like optical coherence tomography, have allowed to detect new findings in the retinal layers, such as the hyperreflective intraretinal spots, which have been hypothesized to represent an in vivo marker of microglial activation, and early neural cell loss, confirming the hypothesis that neurodegeneration occurs early both in type 1 and 2 diabetes. These new emerging insights foster a better understanding of the pathogenesis of DR, which can no longer be considered as a pure retinal vascular complication of DM.

Introduction

The pathophysiology of diabetic retinopathy (DR) and diabetic macular edema (DME), which represents the leading cause of legal blindness among diabetic patients, is multifactorial and partly still unknown [1]. For many decades, DR and DME have been considered a pure microvascular complication of diabetes mellitus (DM): endothelial cell damage, pericyte loss, and secondary breakdown of the inner blood-retinal barrier were considered the only drivers in the pathogenesis of DR and DME. It is now known that other relevant factors may contribute to the pathogenesis of DR and DME, for example, hypoxia, leukostasis, and inflammation [2–4]. Moreover, an increasing body of evidence suggests that neurodegeneration and retinal glial cell activation occur even before the earliest clinical manifestation of diabetic retinal vasculopathy [5, 6].

This chapter summarizes the emerging insights, mainly obtained using in vivo investigation and retinal imaging techniques, which permit a better understanding of the pathogenesis of DR and DME.

Neuronal Cell Degeneration

An increasing body of evidence suggests that neurodegeneration of the retina (the result of a negative balance between neurotoxic and neuroprotective factors) is a critical component of DR and precedes the earliest clinical manifestation of diabetic retinal vasculopathy [7–10]. There are 2 basic hypotheses that account for loss of cells in the neural retina. First, the loss of blood-retinal barrier integrity, which initially manifests as an increase in vascular permeability, causes a failure to control the composition of the extracellular fluid in the retina, which in turn leads to edema and neuronal cell loss. Alternatively, diabetes has a direct effect on metabolism within the neural retina, leading to an increase in apoptosis, which in turn causes breakdown of the blood-retinal barrier [5]. It is not clear which hypothesis is more important, and, in fact, it is likely that vascular permeability and neuronal apoptosis are closely linked components of DR. However, the gradual loss of neurons suggests that the progress of the disease is ultimately irreversible, since these cells cannot usually be replaced.

In histologic sections of retinas of animal models and in postmortem human retinas, apoptotic cells have been observed in all retinal layers, suggesting the involvement of different types of neurons. However, increased apoptosis has been mainly observed in the inner retina, where retinal ganglion cells are located [11–14]. Numerous studies have demonstrated that diabetes, through the alteration of different metabolic pathways, induces functional deficits and even the loss of different types of retinal cells which extend from the inner to the outer retinal cells: ganglion cells, bipolar cells, amacrine cells, horizontal cells, and eventually photoreceptors [15]. This cell loss could explain the decrease in retinal thickness detected in diabetic eyes with or without clinical signs of DR compared to normal subjects, as reported by different authors [16–19]. Biallosterski et al. [16] found a significant reduction in the pericentral macular thickness in 53 diabetic patients with mild non-proliferative DR. Van Dijk et al. [20, 21] demonstrated, by spectral domain optical coherence tomography (SD-OCT), a decrease in the inner retinal thickness in the macula in diabetics with mild DR, suggesting that this phenomenon might be first due to ganglion cells loss in the pericentral areas and second to retinal nerve fiber layer (RNFL) thinning in the peripheral macula. Similarly, other authors have reported the thinning of RNFL and, in some cases, of the retinal ganglion cell-inner plexiform layer complex too, suggesting that retinal neurodegeneration is an early event in DM, representing a preclinical stage of DR [20, 22–24]. In fact, a decrease of RNFL thickness in the superior macular region in diabetics without DR or with minimal signs of DR has been documented in vivo, particularly among those with poor metabolic control [25–29].

Reduced RNFL thickness may be explained by progressive ganglion cell and astrocyte loss induced by diabetes. It may depend on a direct toxicity of hyperglycemia or on Müller cell dysfunction, in which the latter are unable to maintain adequate osmotic equilibrium between the intra- and extracellular matrices with consequent apoptosis of neuronal cells and progressive axonal degeneration [15, 30–34].

The hypothesis according to which neurodegeneration precedes vascular damage is confirmed by certain electrophysiological and psychophysical studies, which show that the alterations are present even before the microvascular damage becomes ophthalmoscopically or angiographically visible. Such retinal changes in function mainly consist of sensitivity loss, altered color perception, and failure of retinal recovery time [35, 36]. Moreover, it has been observed that in diabetic mice the oscillatory potentials of the electroretinogram have increased peak latencies and/or reduced amplitudes, suggesting a compromised inner retinal function secondary to altered neuronal transmission or to the combined loss of amacrine and ganglion cells [37].

Retinal Glial Cell Activation

The main retinal glial cells are Müller cells. Müller cells extend through the entire retina, from the photoreceptor inner segments to the internal limiting membrane. Müller cells are neuronal structural support cells and represent connection elements between the neurons and vascular cells, hence regulating neuronal nutrition, development, and metabolism. Moreover, they contribute to the local inflammatory response [38]. Müller cells are important in the metabolic support and nutrition of neurons, potassium and water homeostasis, protection against oxidative stress, contribution to neuronal signaling, re-cycling of photopigments, and release of neuroactive and vasoactive substances (increased vascular endothelial growth factor (VEGF)/decreased pigment epithelium-derived factor; matrix metalloproteinase (MMP) secretion and retinal development) [31, 32, 39]. They are particularly susceptible to diabetes-induced damage and are considered as key elements in the onset and the progression of DR [40]. Müller cells react to hyperglycemia by undergoing a reactive gliosis, a process characterized by 3 non-specific responses: hypertrophy, cellular proliferation, and an increase in intermediate filament proteins nestin, vimentin, and glial fibrillary acidic protein (GFAP).

The aquaporins (AQPs) are a family of integral membrane proteins with low molecular weight (about 30 kDa/monomer) arranged in tetramers, which mediate the transcellular flow of free water and, in some cases, of gas and solutes. The AQPs have a crucial task in preserving the ion- and osmotic equilibrium inside the central nervous system, neuroretina included, in response to different osmotic gradients and hydrostatic pressures [41]. Among the various AQPs, AQP1 and AQP4 have received the greatest attention, because it has been demonstrated that in the retina they facilitate the bidirectional flow of free water and also modulate the neuronal excitability [41].

GFAP and AQPs are biomarkers of early Müller cell activation. Recently, Vujosevic et al. [42] measured these specific biomarkers in the aqueous humor (AH) of diabetic patients compared to controls.

Mean GFAP concentration is significantly increased in diabetic patients with DR compared both to controls and diabetics without DR. In normal subjects, GFAP is primarily expressed by retinal astrocytes, and is therefore detectable only in the RNFL and ganglion cell layer (GCL), while it is absent in Müller cells. In animal and human models of DM, GFAP is hyper-expressed by Müller cells, whereas its expression decreases to null in astrocytes [15, 31, 32, 40]. Barber et al. [43] demonstrated the increase in GFAP production only in Müller cells, and its reduced expression by astrocytes (preceding the increase in GFAP expression in Müller cells) in diabetic mice. The same authors noted that a remarkable reduction of GFAP in astrocytes disappears after the administration of insulin. The increase in GFAP concentration is considered a common marker for reactive gliosis and an early sensor for retinal stress [32, 44]. Vujosevic et al. [42] detected that at early stages of DM, in diabetics without DR, there is no significant change in GFAP versus controls, whereas in diabetics with DR, there is a significant increase in GFAP. The increase of GFAP in AH may be the consequence of macroglial cell activation, namely Müller cells activation [45–49]. The GFAP increase in AH, secondary to a significant activation of Müller cells, may be therefore a later biomarker of Müller cell activation. Different experimental studies have confirmed this hypothesis, suggesting that the glial activation may be responsible for the establishment of functional and metabolic imbalances of the retina causing both neuronal and microvascular damages [45, 46, 50, 51].

In normal conditions, fluids that accumulate inside the neuroretina and in the subretinal space are redirected into the blood via transcellular transport osmotically coupled with the flow of various molecules, especially ions, at the level of the RPE and Müller cells. AQPs facilitate transcellular water flow: AQP1 in RPE and AQP4 mostly in Müller cells (besides astrocytes). Müller cells regulate the flow of potassium released by active neurons, which if present in excess in the extracellular space may induce neuronal excitability. Recently, Vujosevic et al. [42] detected that AQP4 was significantly increased in AH of diabetic patients, even in those without clinical signs of retinopathy, versus healthy subjects. In diabetic patients with retinopathy, AQP4 was approximately 25-fold increased versus healthy subjects. Moreover, when diabetic patients with and without DR were compared, there was a 4-fold increase in those with DR. AQP4 is a channel protein, which allows the flow of free water through the cell membrane [52]. In the retina, AQP4 is normally expressed by Müller cells and astrocytes [53, 54]. Due to its ability to transport free water and its functional pairing with K+ channels, AQP4 maintains an osmotic balance between the intra- and the extra-cellular matrices, thus guaranteeing optimal cell functioning [55]. Different histological studies have been done regarding the variation in AQP4 expression in the retina during DM [40, 56–59]. Zhang et al. [56] and Cui et al. [57] have recently provided evidence, in the rat retina, that there is an increase in AQP4 during DM, specifically in Müller cells and astrocytes. Since AQP4 is expressed in the retina, selectively in the retinal glial cells, it is possible to consider this molecule as an early and effective marker of retinal Müller cell alteration during the course of DM, even without clinical signs of DR, as astrocyte loss had already occurred (experimental studies in diabetic rat retina show a significant loss of astrocytes as soon as 4 weeks after streptozotocin-induced diabetes) [15].

Moreover, Vujosevic et al. [42] detected a significant increase in AH AQP1 in diabetic patients with retinopathy compared both to diabetics without DR (approximately 1.4-fold increase) and healthy subjects (approximately 2-fold increase). Similar to AQP4, the function of AQP1 is also involved in the regulation of the transcellular flow of free water [55]. Several histological studies analyzed the AQP1 expression changes, both in animal and human tissues, during the course of DM [41, 59–61]. AQP1 gene expression was upregulated in the retinas of diabetic rats [62]. AQP1 was present, additionally, in the inner retinal layers (whereas in control tissues, it is normally expressed in the outer retina by photoreceptors and amacrine cells), in particular in Müller cells, and the substitution of AQP4 with AQP1 in retinal surface vessels was found, entailing an increase in its production in streptozotocin-induced diabetic rats [53]. Perivascular AQP4 expression was reported to be reduced in the superficial vessel plexus and not altered around the deep vessels in the inner nuclear layer [53]. Such a switch in the localization of AQP1 and AQP4 suggests that the glial-cell mediated water transport in the retina is altered, especially at the superficial layer plexus [41, 53]. Different expressions of AQP1 during DM have been demonstrated on histological specimens.

Since no increase in AQP1 was found in diabetic patients without DR compared to controls, it has been hypothesized that such an increase can be detected only when the retinal damage is clinically evident, and may be a sign of glial cell modification subsequent to those previously mentioned [42]. AQP1 could, therefore, become a useful marker of glial activation, capable of indicating the progression of retinal damage during the course of DM.

Glial activation detected during the course of DM is also confirmed by clinical studies with OCT analysis of retinal layer thickness. In a recent study, a significant increase in the thickness of the inner nuclear layer (mostly comprising the nuclei of bipolar and Müller cells) has been described in patients with non-proliferative DR [23]. The increase in thickness in inner nuclear layer may represent a clinical sign of Müller cell activation due to hypertrophy of these cells [23].

In conclusion, Müller cells are particularly susceptible to diabetes-induced damage and are recognized today as key elements in the onset and progression of DR. Müller cells and astrocytes, besides supporting retinal synaptic activity, maintain the integrity of blood-retinal barrier and regulate the vasoconstriction related to neuronal activity. They react, however, in different ways with regard to hyperglycemic damage: while Müller cells undergo gliosis, functional activation, and cell proliferation (with consequent relative increase of their number, even though there is a moderate increase in cell apoptosis), few studies have analyzed the alterations of astrocytes, though it seems that there is a significant loss and a functional alteration of these cells, prior to the events relative to Müller cells [15]. Reactive gliosis of Müller cells includes both cytoprotective and cytotoxic effects with respect to retinal neurons: mostly in the initial stages of DM, it is neuroprotective and may be interpreted as an effort to limit the extension of tissue damage; later in the course of DM, it contributes to neurodegeneration and prevents tissue restoration and normal neuroregeneration [31].

Retinal Microglial Cell Activation

One of the first signs of inflammation in DM is the activation of retinal microglia cells (RMC) [63]. Activated RMC release cytotoxic substances responsible for the recruitment of leukocytes, blood-retinal barrier breakdown, and direct glial dysfunction and neuronal cell death [64]. An increasing body of scientific evidence has documented that cytokines and chemokines (chemotactic cytokines) specifically released by activated RMC include colony stimulating factors: macrophage-colony-stimulating factor (M-CSF) and granulocyte M-CSF (GM-CSF), interleukin (IL)-1 α/β, IL-3, IL-6, IL-8, IL-10, IL-12, IL-15, IL-18, tumor necrosis factor (TNF-α), interferon gamma (IFN-γ), and IFN-γ-induced protein (IP)-10, transforming growth factor-β (TGF-β), VEGF, lymphotoxin, macrophage inflammatory protein 1 (MIP-1), MIP-2, MIP-3, monocyte chemotactic protein (MCP)-1, regulated and normal T cell expressed and secreted (RANTES), MMPs, and other reactive oxygen species (glutamate, proteases, leukotrienes) [63–69].

Different studies have evaluated changes in concentrations of inflammatory and angiogenic cytokines in the AH or vitreous of diabetic patients, focusing mostly on DME or proliferative DR [70–75]. Recently, the specific cytokine profile (secreted by RMC) of AH samples collected from diabetic patients without or with early DR and compared to non-diabetic subjects has been analyzed to evaluate early intraocular inflammatory biomarkers of RMC activation. A general increase of RMC-related inflammatory cytokines in the AH was detected even in diabetics without DR and with mild DR versus non-diabetic subjects. In particular, in diabetic patients without DR, IFN-γ, IL-1α, IL-3, and MCP-2 were significantly increased compared to non-diabetic controls. IFN-γ was increased approximately 3-fold, while MCP-2 was increased more than 10-fold. In diabetics with mild DR, IFN-γ was increased when compared to non-diabetic subjects, similar to diabetics without DR. IP-10 was increased approximately 3-fold, IL-10 increased approximately 5-fold, only in diabetics with mild DR versus non-diabetic subjects, whereas, RANTES, GM-CSF and sTNF-RII were increased only in the DR group compared to both non-diabetic subjects and diabetics without DR. MIP-1β was significantly increased, whereas IL-3 was significantly decreased in patients with DR versus diabetic patients without DR. IL-1β, released by activated microglial cells, is considered a trigger of the neuroinflammatory cascade in DM [76, 77]. IL-1β and TNF-α increase the caspase 3 activity, thus inducing endothelial cell damage. Therefore, the release of inflammatory mediators and neurotransmitters may contribute to early neuronal cell death in the retina in DM [78]. MCP-2 was increased even in diabetic patients without clinical signs of DR. MCP-2 is a monocyte chemotactic factor, and higher levels of this chemokine suggest an early inflammatory response [79, 80]. MIP-1, IL-1, and IL-3 have a role in angiogenesis, as established in experimental ischemic mouse models [63, 72, 81, 82]. In humans, the plasma level of IL-3 was not associated with DR [83]. GM-CSF is an important regulator of macrophage, granulocyte, and dendritic cell behavior and function [84]. A decrease in a specific chemokine, fractalkine, secreted by microglial cells, induces neurotoxicity and an increase in inflammatory IL-1β and IFN-γ in DR, thus inducing a modulation of RMC function and morphological abnormalities [85, 86].

Although some evidences suggest that proteins in vitreous samples may be different from those in aqueous samples, Funatsu et al. [90] found that levels of VEGF and IL-6 were highly correlated between AH and vitreous and also with the severity of DR [87]. Recently, there has been an increased interest in the AH cytokine determination [88–92]. The cytokine profile in AH samples from diabetic patients in other studies is variable, although this may be partly due to differing limits of detection of the various methods used for protein analysis [84]. Different studies reported that IL-6 is commonly increased in the AH of patients with DM, irrespective of the presence of DR [89, 91–93]. Data concerning TNF-α are controversial, as some reported an increase while Cheung et al. [84] reported a decrease in TNF-α in diabetic patients with DR versus controls [63, 69]. In diabetics with DR, commonly increased inflammatory mediators include IP-10, MCP-1, IL-8, ICAM-1, and TGF-β [13, 23, 24]. In diabetic patients with DR versus non-diabetic controls, IL-10, IL-12, and IFN-γ were decreased [84]. The results from the recent studies show that investigation of inflammatory processes in the diabetic eye using AH samples is a feasible approach, and confirmation of the robustness of aqueous sampling in terms of achieved results is important as it is less invasive than vitreous sampling. Although both AH and vitreous sampling are invasive techniques, AH sampling has a very limited risk to the intraocular tissues. As a consequence, use of AH sampling may be justified to characterize the intraocular phenotype in diabetic eyes.

The early RMC involvement in animal models and humans with DR has been demonstrated by histopathologic and morphological studies. In a rat model of DM, RMC density was increased, and changes in cellular morphology indicated that the microglia were activated [93]. In human histopathologic and clinical studies, an increase in the number of microglia cells (or cells aggregate) in the retina was reported. Zeng et al. [94] showed, on histopathology, a moderate increase in the number of perivascular RMC in all retinal layers in background DR. Vujosevic et al. [23] showed, in a clinical study using SD-OCT, that eyes with DM had an increased number of hyperreflective spots (HRS) compared to controls, in inner and outer retina, and this number increases with DR progression. The HRS were believed to correspond to aggregates of activated microglia which migrate from inner to outer retina [23]. These authors reported that HRS are initially present in the same retinal location (inner retinal layers) where microglia are usually resident. Moreover, with the progression of retinopathy, HRS appear in the middle and outer retina, mimicking the migration of microglial cells in the outer retina (Fig. 1). Thus, the HRS may represent a sign of microglial activation [23]. Coscas et al. [95, 96] were the first to report

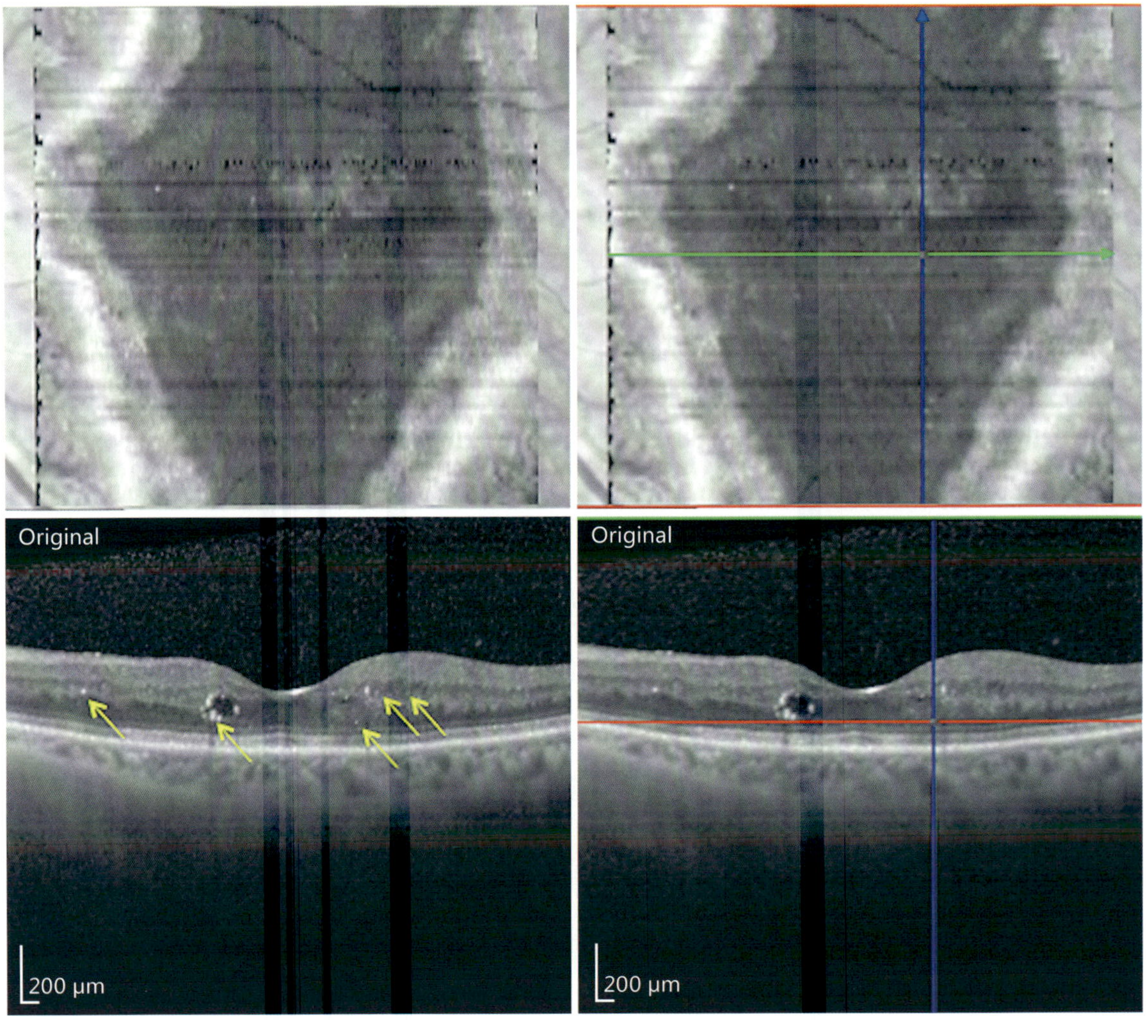

Fig. 1. Hyper-reflective spots (HRSs) seen on the en-face map (top) and on the corresponding linear 0° scan. Yellow arrows indicate some HRSs visualized on OCT linear scan. One of the HRSs is indicated by the crossing red and blue lines on the optical coherence tomography scan and by the blue and green lines on the en-face map. En-face image allows distinguishing HRS from vessels or other structures.

the presence of HRS on SD OCT, as small in size, punctiform hyper-reflective elements, suggesting that they may represent aggregates of activated microglia cells. The same authors, while discussing the management of retinal vein occlusions, also described the presence of HRS, demonstrating a reduction of their number after treatment and thus reinforcing the hypothesis that HRS represent activated microglia cells [95]. Recently, Turgut and Yildirim [97] analyzed the presence of HRS in several patients affected by maculopathies, excluding those with DME or retinal vein occlusions. It is interesting that these authors avoided cases with hard exudates; still, they found HRS, once again confirming that inflammatory cells may be responsible for intraretinal HRS [97]. Murakami et al. [98] reported the presence of HRS in the outer retinal layers, sometimes in association with serous retinal detachments in DME. The localization of these foci suggests that the pathophysiology of retinal fluid accumulation may be investigated at the interface between photoreceptors and retinal pigment epithelium. Uji et al. [99] also demonstrated that the presence of HRS in the outer retina is closely associated with a disruption of the external limiting membrane and photoreceptor layers on SD-OCT, also correlated with decreased visual acuity. HRS in the outer retinal layers on SD-OCT images may thus represent a marker of visual disturbance and are associated with foveal photoreceptor damage. New interesting information to clarify the nature of these HRS comes from the en face OCT of the macular region. This multi-slice technique allows a precise localization (along the C axis) of tiny lesions, and thus the HRS are precisely localized in the retinal layers and may be correlated to fundus findings. En face technique may facilitate the definition of where these HRS are located, and allow one to differentiate them from other hyperreflective structures (mainly intraretinal capillary plexus and small hard exudates).

Recently, it has been shown that HRS decrease after both dexamethasone and ranibizumab treatment in DME patients [100–102]. Whereas it is well known that steroids (and in particular intravitreal dexamethasone) are anti-inflammatory by definition, even anti-VEGF agents have an anti-activated microglia action, in addition to an anti-angiogenic one [103, 104]. Moreover, it has also been demonstrated that VEGF induces chemotaxis and proliferation of microglial cells [103]. Therefore, both drugs significantly decrease the HRS number, reducing microglia-related retinal "inflammatory" condition.

In conclusion, there is a growing body of scientific evidence that activated RMC play an important rule in the development of DR. Further clinical investigation into the role of microglia in DR is therefore warranted, as treatments that target microglial cells may reduce the release of several pro-inflammatory cytokines, as well as suppress microglial activation, proliferation, and migration, and may protect against microglia-mediated neurotoxicity.

Conclusion

An increasing body of evidence suggests that DR and DME are more than a pure microvascular complication of DM. Retinal neurodegeneration and inflammation occur in human diabetes eyes even before the development of clinical signs of DR. Retinal neural cell loss has been demonstrated in vivo as thinning of retinal nerve fiber and GCLs. Moreover, retinal microglial and retinal macroglial activation, histologically documented in the past, is now recognized as the key element in the onset and progression of DR. Understanding the upstream factors in the pathogenesis of DR and DME will lead to a more targeted therapy.

Acknowledgments

The contribution of the GB Bietti Foundation, IRCCS, has been supported by the Ministry of Health and Fondazione Roma.

References

1 Das A, McGuire PG, Rangasamy S: Diabetic macular edema: pathophysiology and novel therapeutic targets. Ophthalmology 2015;122:1375–1394.

2 Aiello LP; DCCT/EDIC Research Group: Diabetic retinopathy and other ocular findings in the diabetes control and complications trial/epidemiology of diabetes interventions and complications study. Diabetes Care 2014;37:17–23.

3 Anderson JM, Van Itallie CM: Tight junctions and the molecular basis for regulation of paracellular permeability. Am J Physiol 1995;269(4 pt 1):G467–G475.

4 Antonetti DA, Barber AJ, Khin S, Lieth E, Tarbell JM, Gardner TW: Vascular permeability in experimental diabetes is associated with reduced endothelial occludin content: vascular endothelial growth factor decreases occludin in retinal endothelial cells. Penn State Retina Research Group. Diabetes 1998;47:1953–1959.
5 Barber AJ: A new view of diabetic retinopathy: a neurodegenerative disease of the eye. Prog Neuropsychopharmacol Biol Psychiatry 2003;27:283–290.
6 Simó R, Hernández C; European Consortium for the Early Treatment of Diabetic Retinopathy (EUROCONDOR): Neurodegeneration in the diabetic eye: new insights and therapeutic perspectives. Trends Endocrinol Metab 2014;25:23–33.
7 Villarroel M, Ciudin A, Hernández C, Simó R: Neurodegeneration: an early event of diabetic retinopathy. World J Diabetes 2010;1:57–64.
8 Antonetti DA, Klein R, Gardner TW: Diabetic retinopathy. N Engl J Med 2012;366:1227–1239.
9 Barber AJ, Gardner TW, Abcouwer SF: The significance of vascular and neural apoptosis to the pathology of diabetic retinopathy. Invest Ophthalmol Vis Sci 2011;52:1156–1163.
10 Bresnick GH: Diabetic retinopathy viewed as a neurosensory disorder. Arch Ophthalmol 1986;104:989–990.
11 Gastinger MJ, Singh RS, Barber AJ: Loss of cholinergic and dopaminergic amacrine cells in streptozotocin-diabetic rat and Ins2Akita-diabetic mouse retinas. Invest Ophthalmol Vis Sci 2006;47:3143–3150.
12 Hammes HP, Federoff HJ, Brownlee M: Nerve growth factor prevents both neuroretinal programmed cell death and capillary pathology in experimental diabetes. Mol Med 1995;1:527–534.
13 Kerrigan LA, Zack DJ, Quigley HA, Smith SD, Pease ME: TUNEL-positive ganglion cells in human primary open-angle glaucoma. Arch Ophthalmol 1997;115:1031–1035.
14 Kim SY, Johnson MA, McLeod DS, Alexander T, Otsuji T, Steidl SM, Hansen BC, Lutty GA: Retinopathy in monkeys with spontaneous type 2 diabetes. Invest Ophthalmol Vis Sci 2004;45:4543–4553.
15 Ly A, Yee P, Vessey KA, Phipps JA, Jobling AI, Fletcher EL: Early inner retinal astrocyte dysfunction during diabetes and development of hypoxia, retinal stress, and neuronal functional loss. Invest Ophthalmol Vis Sci 2011;52:9316–9326.
16 Biallosterski C, Van Velthoven ME, Michels RP, Schlingemann RO, DeVries JH, Verbraak FD: Decreased optical coherence tomography-measured pericentral retinal thickness in patients with diabetes mellitus type 1 with minimal diabetic retinopathy. Br J Ophthalmol 2007;91:1135–1138.
17 Browning DJ, Fraser CM, Clark S: The relationship of macular thickness to clinically graded diabetic retinopathy severity in eyes without clinically detected diabetic macular edema. Ophthalmology 2008;115:533–539.e2.
18 Nilsson M, Von Wendt G, Wanger P, Martin L: Early detection of macular changes in patients with diabetes using Rarebit Fovea Test and optical coherence tomography. Br J Ophthalmol 2007;91:1596–1598.
19 Oshitari T, Hanawa K, Adachi-Usami E: Changes of macular and RNFL thicknesses measured by Stratus OCT in patients with early stage diabetes. Eye (Lond) 2009;23:884–889.
20 Van Dijk HW, Verbraak FD, Kok PH, Garvin MK, Sonka M, Lee K, Devries JH, Michels RP, van Velthoven ME, Schlingemann RO, Abràmoff MD: Decreased retinal ganglion cell layer thickness in patients with type 1 diabetes. Invest Ophthalmol Vis Sci 2010;51:3660–3665.
21 Van Dijk HW, Kok PH, Garvin M, Sonka M, Devries JH, Michels RP, van Velthoven ME, Schlingemann RO, Verbraak FD, Abràmoff MD: Selective loss of inner retinal layer thickness in type 1 diabetic patients with minimal diabetic retinopathy. Invest Ophthalmol Vis Sci 2009;50:3404–3409.
22 Cabrera Fernandez D, Somfai GM, Tátrai E, Ranganathan S, Yee DC, Ferencz M, Smiddy WE: Potentiality of intraretinal layer segmentation to locally detect early retinal changes in patients with diabetes mellitus using optical coherence tomography. Invest Ophthalmol Vis Sci 2008;49:2751.
23 Vujosevic S, Bini S, Midena G, Berton M, Pilotto E, Midena E: Hyperreflective intraretinal spots in diabetics without and with nonproliferative diabetic retinopathy: an in vivo study using spectral domain OCT. J Diabetes Res 2013;2013:491835.
24 Cabrera DeBuc D, Somfai GM: Early detection of retinal thickness changes in diabetes using optical coherence tomography. Med Sci Monit 2010;16:MT15–MT21.
25 Lopes de Faria JM, Russ H, Costa VP: Retinal nerve fibre layer loss in patients with type 1 diabetes mellitus without retinopathy. Br J Ophthalmol 2002;86:725–728.
26 Takahashi H, Goto T, Shoji T, Tanito M, Park M, Chihara E: Diabetes-associated retinal nerve fiber damage evaluated with scanning laser polarimetry. Am J Ophthalmol 2006;142:88–94.
27 Sugimoto M, Sasoh M, Ido M, Wakitani Y, Takahashi C, Uji Y: Detection of early diabetic change with optical coherence tomography in type 2 diabetes mellitus patients without retinopathy. Ophthalmologica 2005;219:379–385.
28 Peng PH, Lin HS, Lin S: Nerve fibre layer thinning in patients with preclinical retinopathy. Can J Ophthalmol 2009;44:417–422.
29 Lonneville YH, Ozdek SC, Onol M, Yetkin I, Gürelik G, Hasanreisoğlu B: The effect of blood glucose regulation on retinal nerve fiber layer thickness in diabetic patients. Ophthalmologica 2003;217:347–350.
30 Villarroel M, Ciudin A, Hernández C, Simó R: Neurodegeneration: an early event of diabetic retinopathy. World J Diabetes 2010;1:57–64.
31 Bringmann A, Iandiev I, Pannicke T, Wurm A, Hollborn M, Wiedemann P, Osborne NN, Reichenbach A: Cellular signaling and factors involved in Müller cell gliosis: neuroprotective and detrimental effects. Prog Retin Eye Res 2009;28:423–451.
32 Bringmann A, Wiedemann P: Müller glial cells in retinal disease. Ophthalmologica 2012;227:1–19.
33 Joussen AM, Poulaki V, Le ML, Koizumi K, Esser C, Janicki H, Schraermeyer U, Kociok N, Fauser S, Kirchhof B, Kern TS, Adamis AP: A central role for inflammation in the pathogenesis of diabetic retinopathy. FASEB J 2004;18:1450–1452.

34 Ibrahim AS, El-Remessy AB, Matragoon S, Zhang W, Patel Y, Khan S, Al-Gayyar MM, El-Shishtawy MM, Liou GI: Retinal microglial activation and inflammation induced by amadori-glycated albumin in a rat model of diabetes. Diabetes 2011;60:1122–1133.
35 Midena E, Segato T, Giuliano M, Zucchetto M: Macular recovery function (nyctometry) in diabetics without and with early retinopathy. Br J Ophthalmol 1990;74:106–108.
36 Midena E, Vujosevic S: Visual psychophysics in diabetic retinopathy; in Tink JT, Barnstable CJ, Gardner TW (eds): Visual Disfunction in Diabetes. New York, Springer, 2012, pp 69–105.
37 Kern TS, Barber AJ: Retinal ganglion cells in diabetes. J Physiol 2008;586: 4401–4408.
38 Newman EA: Müller cells and the retinal pigment epithelium; in Albert DM, Jakobiec FA (eds): Principles and Practice of Ophthalmology. Philadelphia, W.B. Saunders Company, 1994, 398–419.
39 Bringmann A, Pannicke T, Grosche J, Francke M, Wiedemann P, Skatchkov SN, Osborne NN, Reichenbach A: Müller cells in the healthy and diseased retina. Prog Retin Eye Res 2006;25:397–424.
40 Curtis T, Hamilton R, Yong PH, McVicar CM, Berner A, Pringle R, Uchida K, Nagai R, Brockbank S, Stitt AW: Müller glial dysfunction during diabetic retinopathy in rats is linked to accumulation of advanced glycation end-products and advanced lipoxidation end-products. Diabetologia 2011;54:690–698.
41 Fukuda M, Nakanishi Y, Fuse M, Yokoi N, Hamada Y, Fukagawa M, Negi A, Nakamura M: Altered expression of aquaporins 1 and 4 coincides with neurodegenerative events in retinas of spontaneously diabetic Torii rats. Exp Eye Res 2010;90:17–25.
42 Vujosevic S, Micera A, Bini S, Berton M, Esposito G, Midena E: Aqueous humor biomarkers of Müller Cell activation in diabetic eyes. Invest Ophthalmol Vis Sci 2015;56:3913–3918.
43 Barber AJ, Antonetti DA, Gardner TW: Altered expression of retinal occludin and glial fibrillary acidic protein in experimental diabetes. Invest Ophthalmol Vis Sci 2000;41:3561–3568.
44 Sarthy V: Focus on Molecules: glial fibrillary acidic protein (GFAP). Exp Eye Res 2007;84:381–382.
45 Carrasco E, Hernández C, Miralles A, Huguet P, Farrés J, Simó R: Lower somatostatin expression is an early event in diabetic retinopathy and is associated with retinal neurodegeneration. Diabetes Care 2007;30:2902–2908.
46 Carrasco E, Hernández C, De Torres I, Farrés J, Simó R: Lowered cortistatin expression is an early event in the human diabetic retina and is associated with apoptosis and glial activation. Mol Vis 2008;14:1496–1502.
47 Lieth E, Barber AJ, Xu B, Dice C, Ratz MJ, Tanase D, Strother JM: Glial reactivity and impaired glutamate metabolism in short-term experimental diabetic retinopathy. Penn State Retina Research Group. Diabetes 1998;47:815–820.
48 Mizutani M, Gerhardinger C, Lorenzi M: Müller cell changes in human diabetic retinopathy. Diabetes 1998;47:445–449.
49 Abu-El-Asrar AM, Dralands L, Missotten L, Al-Jadaan IA, Geboes K: Expression of apoptosis markers in the retinas of human subjects with diabetes. Invest Ophthalmol Vis Sci 2004;45:2760–2766.
50 Van Dijk HW, Verbraak FD, Kok PH, Stehouwer M, Garvin MK, Sonka M, DeVries JH, Schlingemann RO, Abràmoff MD: Early neurodegeneration in the retina of type 2 diabetic patients. Invest Ophthalmol Vis Sci 2012;53: 2715–2719.
51 Gardner TW, Antonetti DA, Barber AJ, LaNoue KF, Levison SW: Diabetic retinopathy: more than meets the eye. Surv Ophthalmol 2002;47(suppl 2):S253–S262.
52 Huber VJ, Tsujita M, Nakada T: Aquaporins in drug discovery and pharmacotherapy. Mol Aspects Med 2012;33:691–703.
53 Iandiev I, Pannicke T, Reichenbach A, Wiedemann P, Bringmann A: Diabetes alters the localization of glial aquaporins in rat retina. Neurosci Lett 2007;421: 132–136.
54 Iandiev I, Pannicke T, Hollborn M, Wiedemann P, Reichenbach A, Grimm C, Remé CE, Bringmann A: Localization of glial aquaporin-4 and Kir4.1 in the light-injured murine retina. Neurosci Lett 2008;434:317–321.
55 Castle NA: Aquaporins as targets for drug discovery. Drug Discov Today 2005;10:485–493.
56 Zhang Y, Xu G, Ling Q, Da C: Expression of aquaporin 4 and Kir4.1 in diabetic rat retina: treatment with minocycline. J Int Med Res 2011;39:464–479.
57 Cui B, Sun JH, Xiang FF, Liu L, Li WJ: Aquaporin 4 knockdown exacerbates streptozotocin-induced diabetic retinopathy through aggravating inflammatory response. Exp Eye Res 2012;98:37–43.
58 Gerhardinger C, Costa MB, Coulombe MC, Toth I, Hoehn T, Grosu P: Expression of acute-phase response proteins in retinal Müller cells in diabetes. Invest Ophthalmol Vis Sci 2005;46:349–357.
59 Fukuda M, Naka M, Mizokami J, Negi A, Nakamura M: Diabetes induces expression of aquaporin-0 in the retinal nerve fibers of spontaneously diabetic Torii rats. Exp Eye Res 2011;92:195–201.
60 Hollborn M, Dukic-Stefanovic S, Pannicke T, Ulbricht E, Reichenbach A, Wiedemann P, Bringmann A, Kohen L: Expression of aquaporins in the retina of diabetic rats. Curr Eye Res 2011;36: 850–856.
61 Qin Y, Fan J, Ye X, Xu G, Liu W, Da C: High salt loading alters the expression and localization of glial aquaporins in rat retina. Exp Eye Res 2009;89:88–94.
62 Gerhardinger C, Costa MB, Coulombe MC, Toth I, Hoehn T, Grosu P: Expression of acute-phase response proteins in retinal Müller cells in diabetes. Invest Ophthalmol Vis Sci 2005:46:349–357.
63 Grigsby JG, Cardona SM, Pouw CE, Muniz A, Mendiola AS, Tsin AT, Allen DM, Cardona AE: The role of microglia in diabetic retinopathy. J Ophthalmol 2014;2014:705783.
64 Yang LP, Sun HL, Wu LM, Guo XJ, Dou HL, Tso MO, Zhao L, Li SM: Baicalein reduces inflammatory process in a rodent model of diabetic retinopathy. Invest Ophthalmol Vis Sci 2009;50:2319–2327.
65 Martinez-Moczygemba M, Huston DP: Biology of common beta receptor-signaling cytokines: IL-3, IL-5, and GM-CSF. J Allergy Clin Immunol 2003;112: 653–665.
66 Maurer M, von Stebut E: Macrophage inflammatory protein-1. Int J Biochem Cell Biol 2004;36:1882–1886.
67 Kremlev SG, Roberts RL, Palmer C: Differential expression of chemokines and chemokine receptors during microglial activation and inhibition. J Neuroimmunol 2004;149:1–9.
68 Langmann T: Microglia activation in retinal degeneration. J Leukoc Biol 2007; 81:1345–1351.

69 Hanisch UK, Kettenmann H: Microglia: active sensor and versatile effector cells in the normal and pathologic brain. Nat Neurosci 2007;10:1387–1394.
70 Sohn HJ, Han DH, Kim IT, Oh IK, Kim KH, Lee DY, Nam DH: Changes in aqueous concentrations of various cytokines after intravitreal triamcinolone versus bevacizumab for diabetic macular edema. Am J Ophthalmol 2011;152:686–694.
71 Adamiec-Mroczek J, Oficjalska-Mlynczak J, Misiuk-Hojlo M: Roles of endothelin-1 and selected proinflammatory cytokines in the pathogenesis of proliferative diabetic retinopathy: analysis of vitreous samples. Cytokine 2010;49: 269–274.
72 Demircan N, Safran BG, Soylu M, Ozcan AA, Sizmaz S: Determination of vitreous interleukin-1 (IL-1) and tumour necrosis factor (TNF) levels in proliferative diabetic retinopathy. Eye (Lond) 2006; 20:1366–1369.
73 El-Asrar AM, Nawaz MI, Kangave D, Geboes K, Ola MS, Ahmad S, Al-Shabrawey M: High-mobility group box-1 and biomarkers of inflammation in the vitreous from patients with proliferative diabetic retinopathy. Mol Vis 2011;17: 1829–1838.
74 Funatsu H, Noma H, Mimura T, Eguchi S, Hori S: Association of vitreous inflammatory factors with diabetic macular edema. Ophthalmology 2009;116: 73–79.
75 Funatsu H, Yamashita H, Sakata K, Noma H, Mimura T, Suzuki M, Eguchi S, Hori S: Vitreous levels of vascular endothelial growth factor and intercellular adhesion molecule 1 are related to diabetic macular edema. Ophthalmology 2005;112:806–816.
76 Liu Y, Biarnés Costa M, Gerhardinger C: IL-1β is upregulated in the diabetic retina and retinal vessels: cell-specific effect of high glucose and IL-1β autostimulation. PLoS One 2012;7:e36949.
77 Rothwell NJ, Luheshi GN: Interleukin 1 in the brain: biology, pathology and therapeutic target. Trends Neurosci 2000;23:618–625.
78 Pereira Tde O, da Costa GN, Santiago AR, Ambrósio AF, dos Santos PF: High glucose enhances intracellular Ca2+ responses triggered by purinergic stimulation in retinal neurons and microglia. Brain Res 2010;1316:129–138.
79 Oh IK, Kim SW, Oh J, Lee TS, Huh K: Inflammatory and angiogenic factors in the aqueous humor and the relationship to diabetic retinopathy. Curr Eye Res 2010;35:1116–1127.
80 Vujosevic S, Micera A, Bini S, Berton M, Esposito G, Midena E: Proteome analysis of retinal glia cells-related inflammatory cytokines in the aqueous humour of diabetic patients. Acta Ophthalmol 2016;94:56–64.
81 Krady JK, Basu A, Allen CM, Xu Y, LaNoue KF, Gardner TW, Levison SW: Minocycline reduces proinflammatory cytokine expression, microglial activation, and caspase-3 activation in a rodent model of diabetic retinopathy. Diabetes 2005;54:1559–1565.
82 Yoshida S, Yoshida A, Ishibashi T, Elner SG, Elner VM: Role of MCP-1 and MIP-1alpha in retinal neovascularization during postischemic inflammation in a mouse model of retinal neovascularization. J Leukoc Biol 2003;73:137–144.
83 Hang H, Yuan S, Yang Q, Yuan D, Liu Q: Multiplex bead array assay of plasma cytokines in type 2 diabetes mellitus with diabetic retinopathy. Mol Vis 2014; 20:1137–1145. eCollection 2014.
84 Cheung CM, Vania M, Ang M, Chee SP, Li J: Comparison of aqueous humor cytokine and chemokine levels in diabetic patients with and without retinopathy. Mol Vis 2012;18:830–837.
85 Cardona AE, Pioro EP, Sasse ME, Kostenko V, Cardona SM, Dijkstra IM, Huang D, Kidd G, Dombrowski S, Dutta R, Lee JC, Cook DN, Jung S, Lira SA, Littman DR, Ransohoff RM: Control of microglial neurotoxicity by the fractalkine receptor. Nat Neurosci 2006;9:917–924.
86 Garcia JA, Pino PA, Mizutani M, Cardona SM, Charo IF, Ransohoff RM, Forsthuber TG, Cardona AE: Regulation of adaptive immunity by the fractalkine receptor during autoimmune inflammation. J Immunol 2013;191:1063–1072.
87 Ecker SM, Hines JC, Pfahler SM, Glaser BM: Aqueous cytokine and growth factor levels do not reliably reflect those levels found in the vitreous. Mol Vis 2011;17:2856–2863.
88 Sohn HJ, Han DH, Kim IT, Oh IK, Kim KH, Lee DY, Nam DH: Changes in aqueous concentrations of various cytokines after intravitreal triamcinolone versus bevacizumab for diabetic macular edema. Am J Ophthalmol 2011;152:686–694.
89 Funatsu H, Yamashita H, Noma H, Mimura T, Yamashita T, Hori S: Increased levels of vascular endothelial growth factor and interleukin-6 in the aqueous humor of diabetics with macular edema. Am J Ophthalmol 2002;133: 70–77.
90 Funatsu H, Yamashita H, Noma H, Mimura T, Nakamura S, Sakata K, Hori S: Aqueous humor levels of cytokines are related to vitreous levels and progression of diabetic retinopathy in diabetic patients. Graefes Arch Clin Exp Ophthalmol 2005;243:3–8.
91 Jonas JB, Jonas RA, Neumaier M, Findeisen P: Cytokine concentration in aqueous humor of eyes with diabetic macular edema. Retina 2012;32:2150–2157.
92 Oh IK, Kim SW, Oh J, Lee TS, Huh K: Inflammatory and angiogenic factors in the aqueous humor and the relationship to diabetic retinopathy. Curr Eye Res 2010;35:1116–1127.
93 Zeng XX, Ng YK, Ling EA: Neuronal and microglial response in the retina of streptozotocin-induced diabetic rats. Vis Neurosci 2000;17:463–471.
94 Zeng HY, Green WR, Tso MO: Microglial activation in human diabetic retinopathy. Arch Ophthalmol 2008;126: 227–232.
95 Coscas G, De Benedetto U, Coscas F, Li Calzi CI, Vismara S, Roudot-Thoraval F, Bandello F, Souied E: Hyperreflective dots: a new spectral-domain optical coherence tomography entity for follow-up and prognosis in exudative age-related macular degeneration. Ophthalmologica 2013;229:32–37.
96 Coscas G, Coscas F, Vismara S, Zourdani A, Li Calzi CI: Clinical features and natural history of AMD; in Coscas G, Coscas F, Vismara S, Zourdani A, Li Calzi CI (eds): Optical Coherence Tomography in Age-Related Macular Degeneration. Heidelberg, Springer, 2009, pp 171–274.
97 Turgut B, Yildirim H: The causes of hyperreflective dots in optical coherence tomography excluding diabetic macular edema and retinal venous occlusion. Open Ophthalmol J 2015;9:36–40.
98 Murakami T, Yoshimura N: Structural changes in individual retinal layers in diabetic macular edema. J Diabetes Res 2013:920713.

99 Uji A, Murakami T, Nishijima K, Akagi T, Horii T, Arakawa N, Muraoka Y, Ellabban AA, Yoshimura N: Association between hyperreflective foci in the outer retina, status of photoreceptor layer, and visual acuity in diabetic macular edema. Am J Ophthalmol 2012;153:710–717.
100 Vujosevic S, Torresin T, Bini S, Convento E, Pilotto E, Parrozzani R, Midena E: Imaging retinal inflammatory biomarkers after intravitreal steroid and anti-VEGF treatment in diabetic macular oedema. Acta Ophthalmol 2016, Epub ahead of print.
101 Framme C, Schweizer P, Imesch M, Wolf S, Wolf-Schnurrbusch U: Behavior of SD-OCT-detected hyperreflective foci in the retina of anti-VEGF-treated patients with diabetic macular edema. Invest Ophthalmol Vis Sci 2012;53: 5814–5818.
102 Vujosevic S, Berton M, Bini S, Casciano M, Cavarzeran F, Midena E: Hyperreflective retinal spots and visual function after anti-vascular endothelial growth factor treatment in center-involving diabetic macular edema. Retina 2016;36:1298–1308.
103 Forstreuter F, Lucius R, Mentlein R: Vascular endothelial growth factor induces chemotaxis and proliferation of microglial cells. J Neuroimmunol 2002;132:93–98.
104 Ishida S, Usui T, Yamashiro K, Kaji Y, Ahmed E, Carrasquillo KG, Amano S, Hida T, Oguchi Y, Adamis AP: VEGF164 is proinflammatory in the diabetic retina. Invest Ophthalmol Vis Sci 2003;44:2155–2162.

Edoardo Midena
Department of Ophthalmology, University of Padova
Via Giustiniani 2
IT–35128 Padova (Italy)
E-Mail edoardo.midena@unipd.it

Bandello F, Zarbin MA, Lattanzio R, Zucchiatti I (eds): Management of Diabetic Retinopathy.
Dev Ophthalmol. Basel, Karger, 2017, vol 60, pp 28–37 (DOI: 10.1159/000459723)

Emerging Issues for Optical Coherence Tomography

Luisa Pierro • Alessandro Rabiolo

Department of Ophthalmology, University Vita-Salute, IRCCS San Raffaele, Milan, Italy

Abstract

Almost 25 years after its introduction, optical coherence tomography (OCT) is still a crucial test in the evaluation of patients affected by diabetic retinopathy. In this chapter, the authors provide an extensive overview of the posterior segment pathological changes induced by diabetes, characterized using OCT. OCT plays a key role in diabetic macular edema (DME) as it assesses related retinal changes both in a qualitative (i.e., DME pattern, presence and aspects of cysts, fluid localization, integrity, and reflectivity of retinal layers) and quantitative (i.e., macula volume, central and sectorial retinal thickness) way, and it is therefore essential for diagnosis, characterization, and follow-up of DME. Diabetic macular ischemia is associated with retinal structural changes which can be investigated using OCT, although its diagnosis relies mostly on fluorescein angiography. Beyond DME and macular ischemia, OCT permits the individuation of many other lesions occurring in the setting of both non-proliferative (i.e., hyperreflective spots, micropseudocysts, hard exudates, microaneurysm, cotton-wool spots) and proliferative (i.e., neovascularization, vitreoschisis, tractional retinal detachment, hemorrhage) retinopathies. OCT provides precious information on several structures, including vitreo-retinal interface, retinal nerve fiber layers, ganglion cell complex, and choroid.

Optical coherence tomography (OCT) is a non-invasive diagnostic tool, crucial in the evaluation of patients affected by diabetic retinopathy (DR). Although its main application relies on diabetic macular edema (DME), OCT provides precious information on several structures, including vitreo-retinal interface, retinal nerve fiber layers (RNFL), ganglion cell complex (GCC), and choroid. OCT nomenclature adopted in this chapter adheres to the consensus document published by the International Nomenclature for OCT Panel [1], and is displayed in Figure 1.

DME is caused by the disruption of inner blood-retinal barrier and, thus, intraretinal fluid accumulation. Three different patterns of DME may be appreciated (alone or mixed): cystoid (Fig. 2a), characterized by the presence of discrete pseudocysts into retinal layers; intraretinal (Fig. 2b), seen as swelling of retinal tissue; serous retinal detachment (Fig. 2c), defined as subretinal fluid accumulation [2]. In case of cystoid DME, cysts may be distinguished according to (i) retinal layer involved (e.g., outer nuclear layer [ONL], inner nuclear layer [INL], inner plexiform layer [IPL]); (ii) location (i.e., foveal, parafoveal); (iii) size (i.e., small [<100 μm], medium [100 to <220 μm], large [>220 μm]); (iv) reflectivity, which ranges from

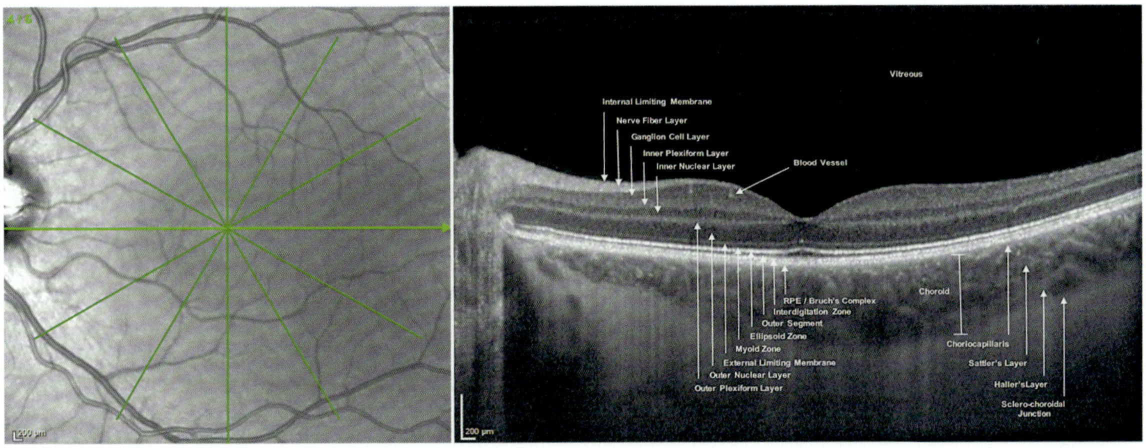

Fig. 1. Nomenclature of optical coherence tomography (OCT) structures proposed by the International Nomenclature for Optical Coherence Tomography Panel. RPE, retinal pigment epithelium.

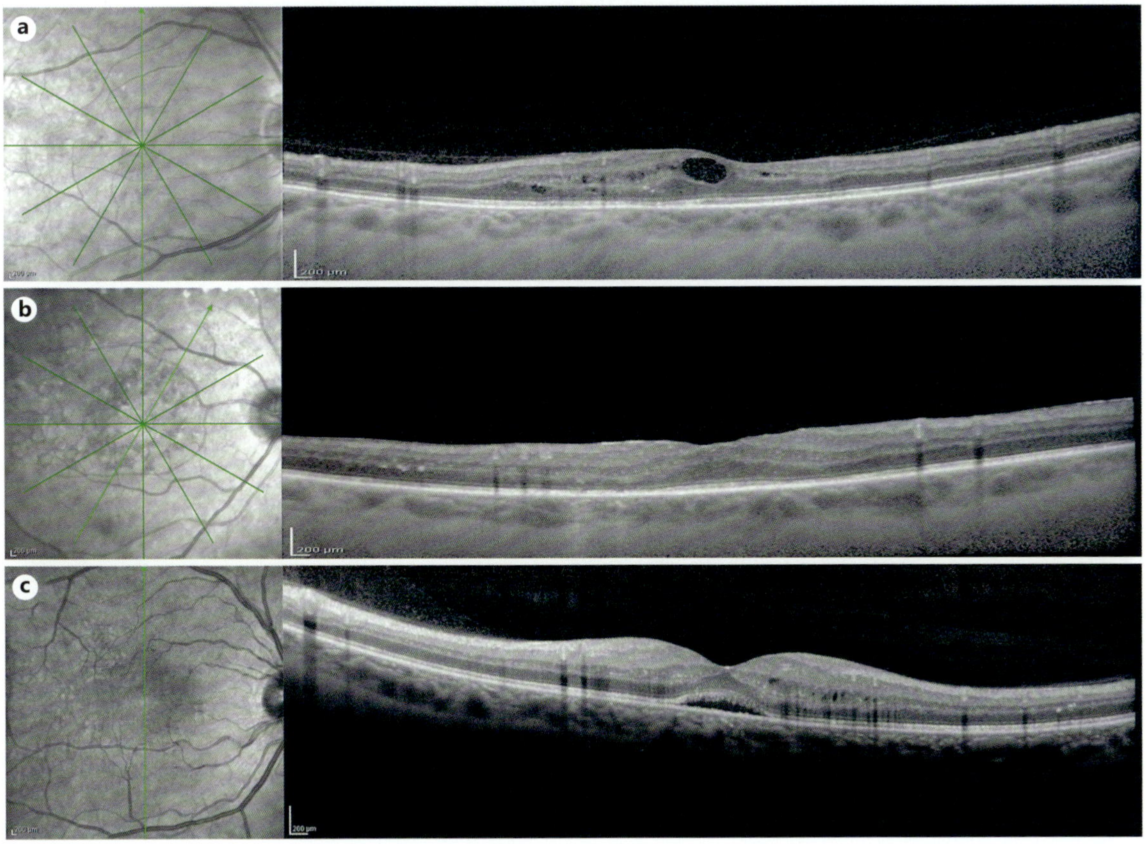

Fig. 2. Different patterns of diabetic macular edema at optical coherence tomography. **a** Cystoid macular edema with multiple small pseudocysts localized in inner and outer nuclear layers and large cyst deforming foveal profile. **b** Intraretinal macular edema with swelling of retinal tissue, note thickening of internal limiting membrane. **c** Subfoveal serous retinal detachment associated with small pseudocysts in inner layer.

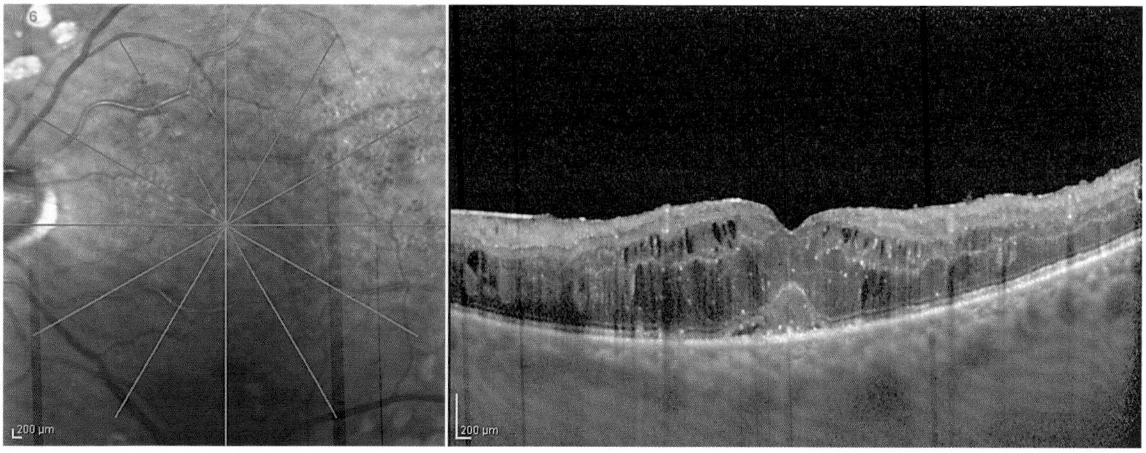

Fig. 3. Left eye of a patient affected by diabetic macular edema. Intraretinal cysts with various degrees of reflectivity are found. Several small hyperreflective spots smaller than hard exudates lining pseudocysts and microaneurysms wall, the outer border of external limiting membrane, the posterior border of inner segment and the outer border of retinal pigment epithelium are also noticeable.

weak to high depending on the properties of the material stored into the cyst (Fig. 3). In a recent study correlating DME morphology to microperimetric function, large ONL cysts and serous retinal detachment were associated with the worst reduction of retinal sensitivity; conversely, small ONL cysts had no effect on the retinal function [3].

Vitreous is a protagonist in DME pathogenesis and vitreo-macular interface disease may be responsible for tractional DME. Posterior vitreous detachment (PVD) is less frequent in diabetic patients [4]; on the contrary, PVD can result in spontaneous DME resolution [5]. OCT allows to stage the PVD, and eyes with DME were found to have higher prevalence of perifoveal PVD with foveolar attachment (stage 1) [6].

In addition, OCT allows visualization of epiretinal membrane, which is more common in eyes with DR and can cause tractional DME [7]. Vitrectomy performed in patients with tractional DME disclosed anatomic and functional improvements in the majority of eyes [8]. Figure 4 shows a case of tractional DME improved after *pars plana* vitrectomy with posterior hyaloid and inner limiting membrane (ILM) peeling.

OCT assesses retinal changes, both in a qualitative (i.e., DME pattern, presence and aspects of cysts, fluid localization, integrity, and reflectivity of retinal layers) and quantitative (i.e., macular volume, central retinal thickness [CRT], and sectorial retinal thickness) way, and it is therefore essential for diagnosis, characterization and follow-up of DME.

CRT permits quantification of the degree of macular edema, and it is extensively used both in trials and clinical practice for the follow-up and the evaluation of treatment response. Although CRT correlates with visual function, integrity of retinal layers is the main prognostic factor linked to visual acuity and response to treatment [2, 9]. Specifically, the disruption of ellipsoid zone (EZ), external limiting membrane (ELM), and outer segment layer are the best predictors of visual function, reflecting loss of photoreceptor integrity [10–12].

It has been recently demonstrated that inflammation and activation of glial cells are the main characters in the pathophysiology of DME [13]. Vitreous and aqueous humor of patients affected by DME exhibited a higher concentration of in-

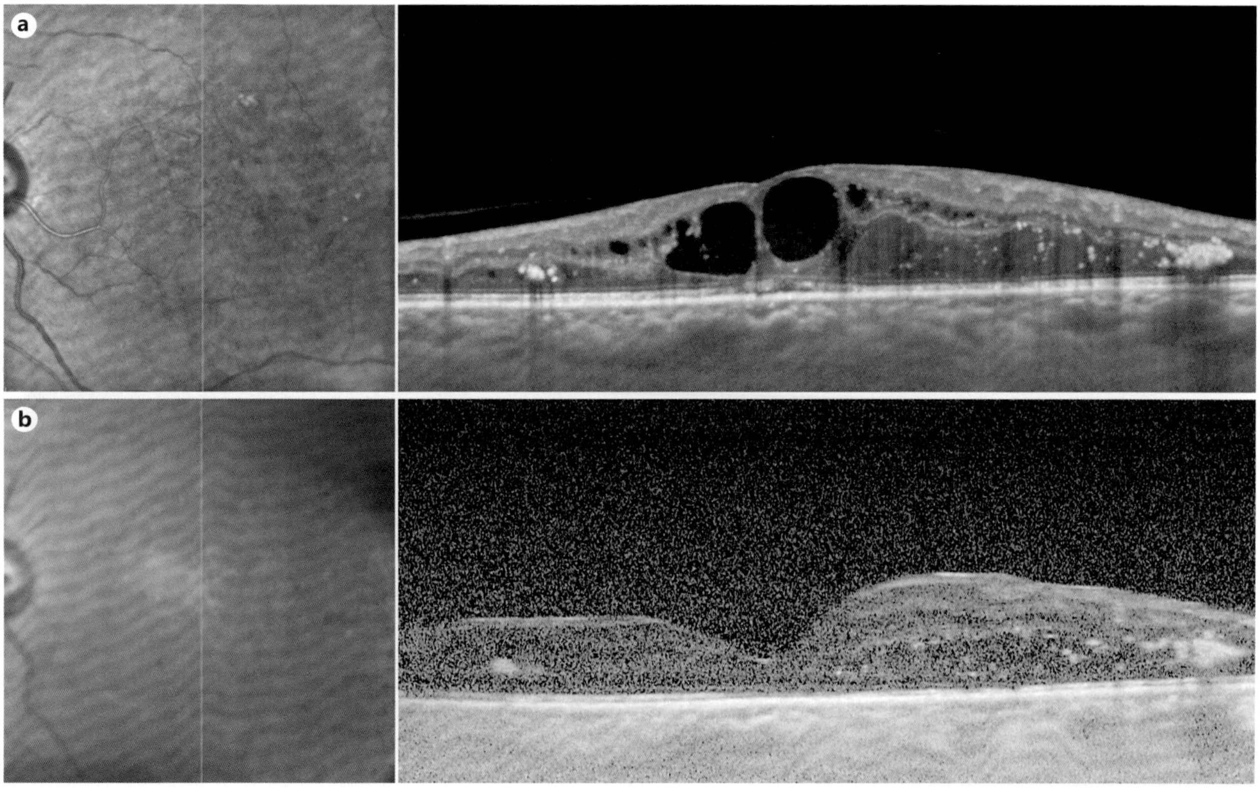

Fig. 4. Optical coherence tomography of the left eye of a diabetic patient with diabetic macular edema (**a**) markedly improved after *pars plana* vitrectomy with posterior hyaloid and ILM peeling (**b**).

flammatory factors (e.g., ICAM-1, MCP-1, vascular endothelial growth factor [VEGF], interleukins-6, -8, -1β) and their level was positively correlated to CRT [14, 15]. OCT evaluates in a non-invasive fashion retinal biomarkers inflammation, including hyperreflective spots (HRS), serous retinal detachment, and increased foveal fundus autofluorescence. Firstly described in the setting of DR, HRS are an OCT finding and are not detectable at fundus examination [16]. HRS (Fig. 3) are defined as hyperreflective foci smaller than hard exudates lining pseudocysts and microaneurysms wall, the outer border of ELM, the posterior border of inner segment in case of foveal detachment and the outer border of retina pigmented epithelium (RPE) [16]. HRS have also been identified in diabetic patients without retinopathy and in other retinal diseases, including age-related macular degeneration, retinal vessel occlusion, central serous chorioretinopathy, uveitis, macular telangiectasia, and radiation macular edema [17–22]. It has been hypothesized that HRS represent retinal microexudation of extravasated proteins, lipoproteins, and lipid-filled macrophages and they could be precursors of hard exudates; otherwise they may represent a sign of microglial activation [13]. It has been recently proposed that HRS ≤30 μm, reflectivity similar to nerve fiber layer, and absence of back shadowing may represent activated microglial cells; HRS >30 μm, reflectivity similar to RPE/Bruch's membrane complex, presence of back shadowing, and location in the outer retina may represent hard exudate; HRS >30 μm, presence of back

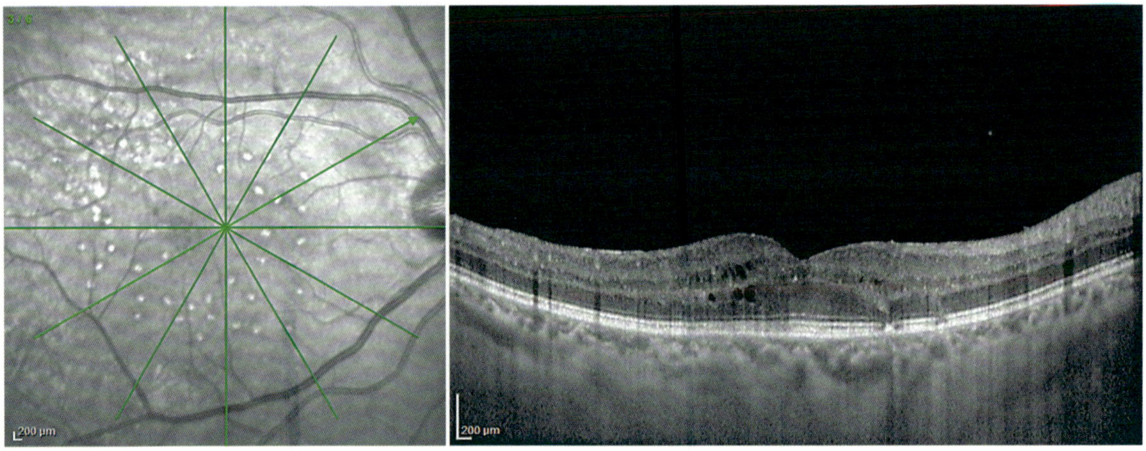

Fig. 5. Right eye of the patient affected by diabetic macular edema. On infrared image (left), several round hyperreflective spots secondary to laser photocoagulation, corresponding to focal interruption and irregularity of retina pigmented epithelium, cone outer segment tip line, outer nuclear and plexiform layers at optical coherence tomography (right).

shadowing, and location in the inner retina may represent microaneurysms [23].

Since it is associated with ELM and EZ disruptions, the presence of HRS in the outer retina reflects photoreceptor damage and, thus, patients with HRS have a decreased VA and poorer prognosis after vitrectomy for DME [24, 25]. HRS are dynamic structures undergoing morphological, numerical, and topographic changes following treatments (e.g., anti-VEGF, focal macular photocoagulation) [26–28]. Among patients with DME, those with serous subretinal detachment have the worst visual prognosis after therapy and this seems to be related to the interruption of ELM and EZ zones [29]. ELM disruption with subsequent microglial cell attraction has been hypothesized, and this could explain the higher concentration of intravitreal inflammatory cytokines in eyes with subretinal detachment [30]. Different patterns of increased foveal fundus autofluorescence have been reported in DME and this could be explained by the accumulation of oxidative products induced by activated microglial cells [31–33].

Therapy of DME is mainly based on focal/grid laser photocoagulation and intravitreal injections (i.e., anti-VEGF, steroids), and OCT allows us to observe the anatomical response to treatment. Laser spots can be visualized as focal interruption and irregularity of RPE, cone outer segment tip line, ONL and, sometimes, OPL (Fig. 5) [34].

Almost 55% of patients with DME also exhibit diabetic macular ischemia, which is a cause of visual impairment [35]. Although diabetic macular ischemia is a fluoroangiographic entity defined as enlargement of the foveal avascular zone, OCT may reveal associated structural changes including macular atrophy (Fig. 6), shortening of the photoreceptor outer segment, EZ disruption and disorganization of retinal inner layers (DRIL) [36, 37].

Beyond DME and macular ischemia, OCT allows the individuation of several other lesions occurring in the setting of non-proliferative (i.e., HRS, micropseudocysts, hard exudates, microaneurysm, cotton-wool spots) and proliferative (i.e., neovascularization [NV], vitreoschisis, tractional retinal detachment, hemorrhage) DR. Micropseudocysts are small hyporeflective areas (≈50 μm) with no funduscopic correspondent [38]; hard exudates (Fig. 7) are highly hyperreflective

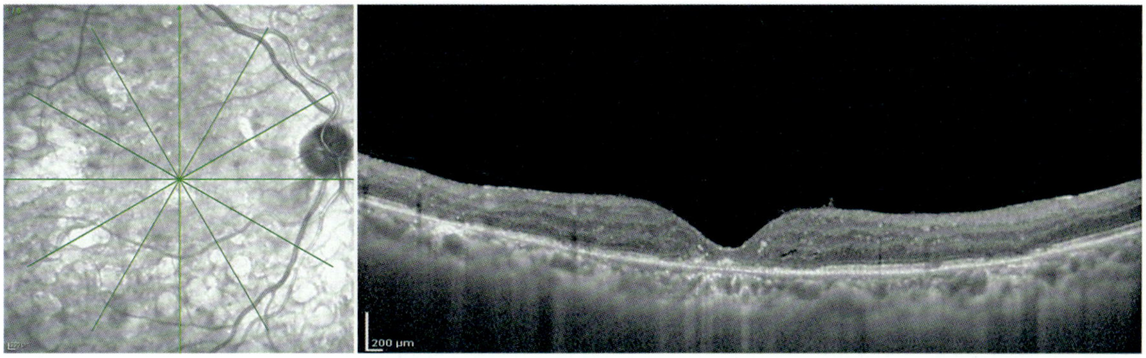

Fig. 6. Right eye of a patient affected by diabetic retinopathy. Optical coherence tomography reveals foveal thinning with disruption of outer retinal layers with light backscattering indicating foveal atrophy. Focal interruptions of retinal pigment epithelium, photoreceptors and outer limiting membrane corresponding to laser burns are also appreciable.

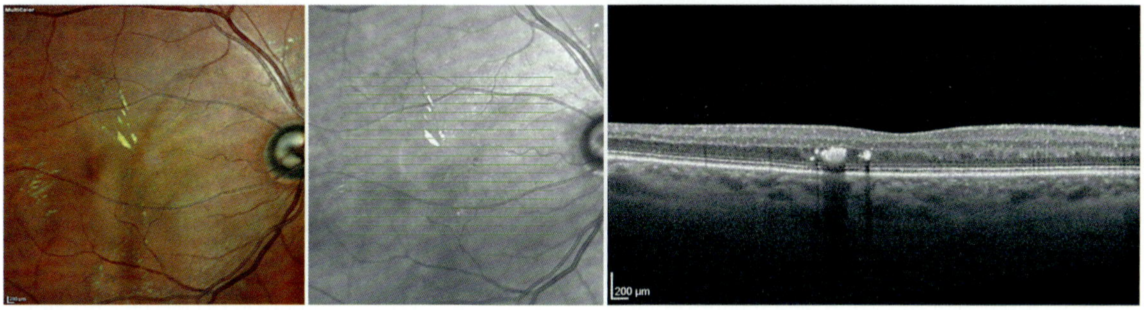

Fig. 7. Hard exudates are visible as intraretinal hyperreflective structures at multicolor (left), infrared (middle), and optical coherence tomography (right).

intraretinal structures made of extravasated lipids and proteins. Microaneurysm are round- or oval-shaped hyperreflective lesions ranging from 14 to 200 μm in diameter and mainly located in OPL, although they can also be found in INL, IPL, ganglion cell layer, and RNFL; microaneurysm can be encircled by a highly hyperreflective capsular structure (ring sign) which can be continuous, interrupted or absent (complete, partial, and absent ring sign, respectively) and, sometimes, by outer hyporeflective cuff corresponding to perilesional fluid [39]. Moreover, internal reflectance of microaneurysm may be either homogenous or heterogeneous with HRS, especially if the ring sign is present or absent, respectively [39]. Cotton-wool spots (Fig. 8) well-delimited hyperreflective areas in the inner retina in their acute stage, after their clinical resolution usually in 4–12 weeks, they are still visible at OCT as areas of residual hyperreflectance (hyperreflective sign) [40]. NVs (Fig. 9) are seen as hyperreflective structures on retinal surface adherent to ILM. NVs appearance varies according to their stage, being small and homogenous in early stages and bulky, heterogeneous, tenaciously attached or even incorporated into the posterior hyaloid in advanced stages [41]. NV in regression appears as a homogenous hyperreflective structure which is broadly adherent to the posterior vitreous surface [41]. By generating tractional forces, active or regressive NV can lead

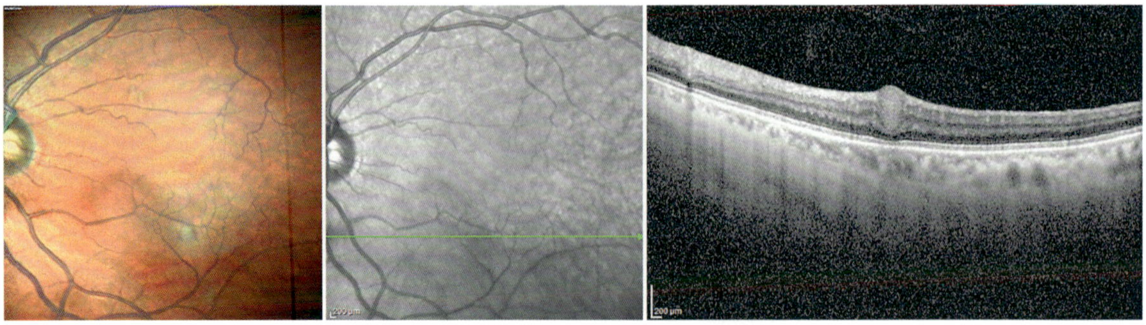

Fig. 8. Multicolor (left), infrared (middle), and optical coherence tomography (OCT; right) of a cotton-wool spot. At OCT, cotton-wool spot is seen as a well-delimited hyperreflective area in the inner retinal layers.

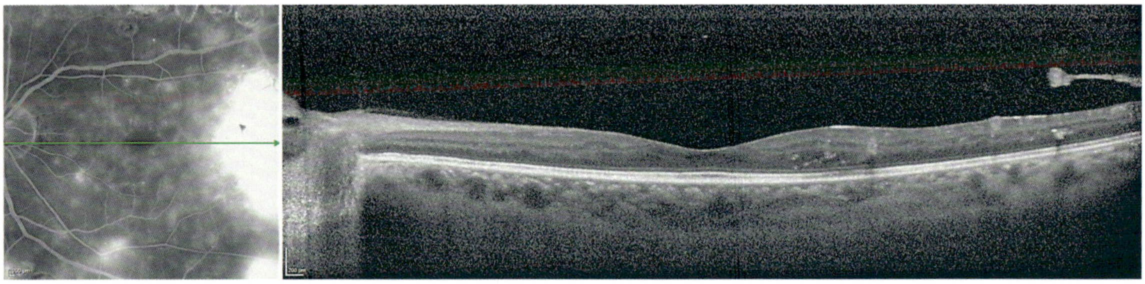

Fig. 9. Proliferative diabetic retinopathy. Fluorescein angiography (left) discloses the disruption of blood-retinal barrier in the foveal area and highly hyperfluorescent lesion temporally to fovea corresponding to epiretinal neovascularization (NV). At optical coherence tomography (right), NV appears a hyperreflective structure on the retina surface.

to intravitreal or preretinal hemorrhages seen as mild vitreal hyperreflectivity and hyperreflective material filling the gap between posterior hyaloid and retinal surface, respectively [41]. Vitreoschisis appears as a bilaminar hyperreflectance corresponding to the boundaries of inner and outer vitreous layers; tractional retinal detachment is concave in shape and often associated with retinoschisis, vitreo-neovascular adhesions, and disorganization of inner and outer retinal layers [41].

Recently, evidences indicate that retinal ganglion cells death may occur in patients with diabetes, and neurodegeneration seems to play a key role in DR pathogenesis. By means of OCT, reduction of RNFL and GCC thickness has been demonstrated in patients with diabetes even before the onset of microvascular lesions [42–44].

Choroidal thickness (CT) changes in diabetic patients without DR is still under debate and available studies showed contradictory results (i.e., choroidal thickening, thinning or no changes) [45–49]. Conversely, choroidal thinning has been extensively reported in patients with DR, although correlation with disease severity remains uncertain [50]. Most of the evidence points toward a reduction of CT in eyes with DME, even if contradictory results have been reported [46–48, 51]. CT undergoes modifications following treatment. In the short-term period, panretinal photocoagulation induces choroidal thickening due to choroidal engorgement and effusion;

subsequently, CT decreases in the long-term period [52–54]. Although contradicted by some studies, it is widely accepted that anti-VEGF agents cause a decrease in CT [55–57]. The role of CT to predict treatment response is still under debate: thicker choroid at baseline seems to correlate with good treatment response; on the contrary, variation of CT is not linked to therapeutic outcomes [50]. Variation in CT can be due to modification of vasculature, stroma or both. Choroidal vascular index, defined as the ratio between luminal and total choroidal areas after binarization, disclosed a reduction in choroidal vasculature in patients with DM [58]. Thanks to its better definition of Sattler's and Haller's layers, swept source-OCT allowed to identified in diabetic eyes choroidal abnormalities going beyond CT, including unvisualized vessels in Sattler's layer, focal narrowing of choroidal vessels in Haller's layer, and vascular stumps (choroidal vessel termination in superficial and middle portion of Haller's layer) [59]. Interestingly, vascular stumps correlated to DR severity, VA, CMT, and CT [59].

References

1 Staurenghi G, Sadda S, Chakravarthy U, Spaide RF; International Nomenclature for Optical Coherence Tomography (IN · OCT) Panel: Proposed lexicon for anatomic landmarks in normal posterior segment spectral-domain optical coherence tomography: the IN*OCT consensus. Ophthalmology 2014;121: 1572–1578.

2 Otani T, Kishi S, Maruyama Y: Patterns of diabetic macular edema with optical coherence tomography. Am J Ophthalmol 1999;127:688–693.

3 Deak GG, Bolz M, Ritter M, Prager S, Benesch T, Schmidt-Erfurth U, et al: A systematic correlation between morphology and functional alterations in diabetic macular edema. Invest Ophthalmol Vis Sci 2010;51:6710–6714.

4 Nasrallah FP, Jalkh AE, Van Coppenolle F, Kado M, Trempe CL, McMeel JW, et al: The role of the vitreous in diabetic macular edema. Ophthalmology 1988; 95:1335–1339.

5 Hikichi T, Fujio N, Akiba J, Azuma Y, Takahashi M, Yoshida A: Association between the short-term natural history of diabetic macular edema and the vitreomacular relationship in type II diabetes mellitus. Ophthalmology 1997;104: 473–478.

6 Gaucher D, Tadayoni R, Erginay A, Haouchine B, Gaudric A, Massin P: Optical coherence tomography assessment of the vitreoretinal relationship in diabetic macular edema. Am J Ophthalmol 2005; 139:807–813.

7 Meuer SM, Myers CE, Klein BE, Swift MK, Huang Y, Gangaputra S, et al: The epidemiology of vitreoretinal interface abnormalities as detected by spectral-domain optical coherence tomography: the beaver dam eye study. Ophthalmology 2015;122:787–795.

8 Diabetic Retinopathy Clinical Research Network Writing Committee, Haller JA, Qin H, Apte RS, Beck RR, Bressler NM, et al: Vitrectomy outcomes in eyes with diabetic macular edema and vitreomacular traction. Ophthalmology 2010;117: 1087–1093.e3.

9 Murakami T, Yoshimura N: Structural changes in individual retinal layers in diabetic macular edema. J Diabetes Res 2013;2013:920713.

10 Alasil T, Keane PA, Updike JF, Dustin L, Ouyang Y, Walsh AC, et al: Relationship between optical coherence tomography retinal parameters and visual acuity in diabetic macular edema. Ophthalmology 2010;117:2379–2386.

11 Maheshwary AS, Oster SF, Yuson RM, Cheng L, Mojana F, Freeman WR: The association between percent disruption of the photoreceptor inner segment-outer segment junction and visual acuity in diabetic macular edema. Am J Ophthalmol 2010;150:63–67.e1.

12 Shin HJ, Lee SH, Chung H, Kim HC: Association between photoreceptor integrity and visual outcome in diabetic macular edema. Graefes Arch Clin Exp Ophthalmol 2012;250:61–70.

13 Midena E, Bini S: Multimodal retinal imaging of diabetic macular edema: toward new paradigms of pathophysiology. Graefes Arch Clin Exp Ophthalmol 2016;254:1661–1668.

14 Dong N, Xu B, Chu L, Tang X: Study of 27 aqueous humor cytokines in type 2 diabetic patients with or without macular edema. PLoS One 2015;10:e0125329.

15 Funatsu H, Noma H, Mimura T, Eguchi S, Hori S: Association of vitreous inflammatory factors with diabetic macular edema. Ophthalmology 2009;116: 73–79.

16 Bolz M, Schmidt-Erfurth U, Deak G, Mylonas G, Kriechbaum K, Scholda C, et al: Optical coherence tomographic hyperreflective foci: a morphologic sign of lipid extravasation in diabetic macular edema. Ophthalmology 2009;116:914–920.

17 De Benedetto U, Sacconi R, Pierro L, Lattanzio R, Bandello F: Optical coherence tomographic hyperreflective foci in early stages of diabetic retinopathy. Retina 2015;35:449–453.

18 Fong AH, Li KK, Wong D: Choroidal evaluation using enhanced depth imaging spectral-domain optical coherence tomography in Vogt-Koyanagi-Harada disease. Retina 2011;31:502–509.

19 Frizziero L, Parrozzani R, Midena G, Miglionico G, Vujosevic S, Pilotto E, et al: Hyperreflective intraretinal spots in radiation macular edema on spectral domain optical coherence tomography. Retina 2016;36:1664–1669.

20 Gaudric A, Ducos de Lahitte G, Cohen SY, Massin P, Haouchine B: Optical coherence tomography in group 2A idiopathic juxtafoveolar retinal telangiectasis. Arch Ophthalmol 2006;124:1410–1419.

21 Kon Y, Iida T, Maruko I, Saito M: The optical coherence tomography-ophthalmoscope for examination of central serous chorioretinopathy with precipitates. Retina 2008;28:864–869.

22 Vujosevic S, Bini S, Midena G, Berton M, Pilotto E, Midena E: Hyperreflective intraretinal spots in diabetics without and with nonproliferative diabetic retinopathy: an in vivo study using spectral domain OCT. J Diabetes Res 2013;2013:491835.

23 Vujosevic S, Bini S, Torresin T, Berton M, Midena G, Parrozzani R, et al: Hyperreflective retinal spots in normal and diabetic eyes: B-scan and en face spectral domain optical coherence tomography evaluation. Retina 2016, Epub ahead of print.

24 Nishijima K, Murakami T, Hirashima T, Uji A, Akagi T, Horii T, et al: Hyperreflective foci in outer retina predictive of photoreceptor damage and poor vision after vitrectomy for diabetic macular edema. Retina 2014;34:732–740.

25 Uji A, Murakami T, Nishijima K, Akagi T, Horii T, Arakawa N, et al: Association between hyperreflective foci in the outer retina, status of photoreceptor layer, and visual acuity in diabetic macular edema. Am J Ophthalmol 2012;153:710–717.e1.

26 Deak GG, Bolz M, Kriechbaum K, Prager S, Mylonas G, Scholda C, et al: Effect of retinal photocoagulation on intraretinal lipid exudates in diabetic macular edema documented by optical coherence tomography. Ophthalmology 2010;117:773–779.

27 Pemp B, Deak G, Prager S, Mitsch C, Lammer J, Schmidinger G, et al: Distribution of intraretinal exudates in diabetic macular edema during anti-vascular endothelial growth factor therapy observed by spectral domain optical coherence tomography and fundus photography. Retina 2014;34:2407–2415.

28 Vujosevic S, Berton M, Bini S, Casciano M, Cavarzeran F, Midena E: Hyperreflective retinal spots and visual function after anti-vascular endothelial growth factor treatment in center-involving diabetic macular edema. Retina 2016;36:1298–1308.

29 Seo KH, Yu SY, Kim M, Kwak HW: Visual and morphologic outcomes of intravitreal ranibizumab for diabetic macular edema based on optical coherence tomography patterns. Retina 2016;36:588–595.

30 Sonoda S, Sakamoto T, Yamashita T, Shirasawa M, Otsuka H, Sonoda Y: Retinal morphologic changes and concentrations of cytokines in eyes with diabetic macular edema. Retina 2014;34:741–748.

31 Pece A, Isola V, Holz F, Milani P, Brancato R: Autofluorescence imaging of cystoid macular edema in diabetic retinopathy. Ophthalmologica 2010;224:230–235.

32 Vujosevic S, Casciano M, Pilotto E, Boccassini B, Varano M, Midena E: Diabetic macular edema: fundus autofluorescence and functional correlations. Invest Ophthalmol Vis Sci 2011;52:442–448.

33 Xu H, Chen M, Manivannan A, Lois N, Forrester JV: Age-dependent accumulation of lipofuscin in perivascular and subretinal microglia in experimental mice. Aging Cell 2008;7:58–68.

34 Cole ED, Novais EA, Louzada RN, Moult EM, Lee BK, Witkin AJ, et al: Visualization of changes in the choriocapillaris, choroidal vessels, and retinal morphology after focal laser photocoagulation using OCT angiography. Invest Ophthalmol Vis Sci 2016;57:OCT356–OCT361.

35 Sim DA, Keane PA, Zarranz-Ventura J, Fung S, Powner MB, Platteau E, et al: The effects of macular ischemia on visual acuity in diabetic retinopathy. Invest Ophthalmol Vis Sci 2013;54:2353–2360.

36 Lee DH, Kim JT, Jung DW, Joe SG, Yoon YH: The relationship between foveal ischemia and spectral-domain optical coherence tomography findings in ischemic diabetic macular edema. Invest Ophthalmol Vis Sci 2013;54:1080–1085.

37 Nicholson L, Ramu J, Triantafyllopoulou I, Patrao NV, Comyn O, Hykin P, et al: Diagnostic accuracy of disorganization of the retinal inner layers in detecting macular capillary non-perfusion in diabetic retinopathy. Clin Exp Ophthalmol 2015;43:735–741.

38 Tremolada G, Pierro L, de Benedetto U, Margari S, Gagliardi M, Maestranzi G, et al: Macular micropseudocysts in early stages of diabetic retinopathy. Retina 2011;31:1352–1358.

39 Horii T, Murakami T, Nishijima K, Sakamoto A, Ota M, Yoshimura N: Optical coherence tomographic characteristics of microaneurysms in diabetic retinopathy. Am J Ophthalmol 2010;150:840–848.

40 Kozak I, Bartsch DU, Cheng L, Freeman WR: Hyperreflective sign in resolved cotton wool spots using high-resolution optical coherence tomography and optical coherence tomography ophthalmoscopy. Ophthalmology 2007;114:537–543.

41 Muqit MM, Stanga PE: Fourier-domain optical coherence tomography evaluation of retinal and optic nerve head neovascularisation in proliferative diabetic retinopathy. Br J Ophthalmol 2014;98:65–72.

42 Carpineto P, Toto L, Aloia R, Ciciarelli V, Borrelli E, Vitacolonna E, et al: Neuroretinal alterations in the early stages of diabetic retinopathy in patients with type 2 diabetes mellitus. Eye (Lond) 2016;30:673–679.

43 Ng DS, Chiang PP, Tan G, Cheung CG, Cheng CY, Cheung CY, et al: Retinal ganglion cell neuronal damage in diabetes and diabetic retinopathy. Clin Exp Ophthalmol 2016;44:243–250.

44 Vujosevic S, Midena E: Retinal layers changes in human preclinical and early clinical diabetic retinopathy support early retinal neuronal and Muller cells alterations. J Diabetes Res 2013;2013:905058.

45 Kim JT, Lee DH, Joe SG, Kim JG, Yoon YH: Changes in choroidal thickness in relation to the severity of retinopathy and macular edema in type 2 diabetic patients. Invest Ophthalmol Vis Sci 2013;54:3378–3384.

46 Querques G, Lattanzio R, Querques L, Del Turco C, Forte R, Pierro L, et al: Enhanced depth imaging optical coherence tomography in type 2 diabetes. Invest Ophthalmol Vis Sci 2012;53:6017–6024.

47 Unsal E, Eltutar K, Zirtiloglu S, Dincer N, Ozdogan Erkul S, Gungel H: Choroidal thickness in patients with diabetic retinopathy. Clin Ophthalmol 2014;8:637–642.

48 Vujosevic S, Martini F, Cavarzeran F, Pilotto E, Midena E: Macular and peripapillary choroidal thickness in diabetic patients. Retina 2012;32:1781–1790.

49 Xu J, Xu L, Du KF, Shao L, Chen CX, Zhou JQ, et al: Subfoveal choroidal thickness in diabetes and diabetic retinopathy. Ophthalmology 2013;120:2023–2028.

50 Campos A, Campos EJ, Martins J, Ambrosio AF, Silva R: Viewing the choroid: where we stand, challenges and contradictions in diabetic retinopathy and diabetic macular oedema. Acta Ophthalmol 2016, Epub ahead of print.
51 Regatieri CV, Branchini L, Carmody J, Fujimoto JG, Duker JS: Choroidal thickness in patients with diabetic retinopathy analyzed by spectral-domain optical coherence tomography. Retina 2012;32: 563–568.
52 Cho GE, Cho HY, Kim YT: Change in subfoveal choroidal thickness after argon laser panretinal photocoagulation. Int J Ophthalmol 2013;6:505–509.
53 Okamoto M, Matsuura T, Ogata N: Effects of panretinal photocoagulation on choroidal thickness and choroidal blood flow in patients with severe nonproliferative diabetic retinopathy. Retina 2016;36:805–811.
54 Zhang Z, Meng X, Wu Z, Zou W, Zhang J, Zhu D, et al: Changes in choroidal thickness after panretinal photocoagulation for diabetic retinopathy: a 12-week longitudinal study. Invest Ophthalmol Vis Sci 2015;56:2631–2638.
55 Lains I, Figueira J, Santos AR, Baltar A, Costa M, Nunes S, et al: Choroidal thickness in diabetic retinopathy: the influence of antiangiogenic therapy. Retina 2014;34:1199–1207.
56 Lee SH, Kim J, Chung H, Kim HC: Changes of choroidal thickness after treatment for diabetic retinopathy. Curr Eye Res 2014;39:736–744.
57 Rayess N, Rahimy E, Ying GS, Bagheri N, Ho AC, Regillo CD, et al: Baseline choroidal thickness as a predictor for response to anti-vascular endothelial growth factor therapy in diabetic macular edema. Am J Ophthalmol 2015;159: 85–91.e1–e3.
58 Tan KA, Laude A, Yip V, Loo E, Wong EP, Agrawal R: Choroidal vascularity index – a novel optical coherence tomography parameter for disease monitoring in diabetes mellitus? Acta Ophthalmol 2016;94:e612–e616.
59 Murakami T, Uji A, Suzuma K, Dodo Y, Yoshitake S, Ghashut R, et al: In vivo choroidal vascular lesions in diabetes on swept-source optical coherence tomography. PLoS One 2016;11:e0160317.

Luisa Pierro
Department of Ophthalmology, IRCCS Ospedale San Raffaele
University Vita-Salute San Raffaele
Via Olgettina 60, IT–20132 Milan (Italy)
E-Mail pierro.luisa@hsr.it

Bandello F, Zarbin MA, Lattanzio R, Zucchiatti I (eds): Management of Diabetic Retinopathy.
Dev Ophthalmol. Basel, Karger, 2017, vol 60, pp 38–49 (DOI: 10.1159/000459688)

Optical Coherence Tomography Angiography in Diabetic Maculopathy

Gabriel Coscas[a, b] • Marco Lupidi[b, c] • Florence Coscas[a, b]

[a]Hôpital de Créteil. Département d'Ophtalmologie de Créteil, Université Paris XII, Val de Marne, [b]Centre d'Exploration Ophtalmologique de l'Odéon, Paris, France; [c]Department of Biomedical and Surgical Sciences, Section of Ophtalmology, "S. Maria della Misericordia" Hospital, University of Perugia, Perugia, Italy

Abstract

Fluorescein angiography (FA) and indocyanine green angiography have provided information about the normal retinal and choroidal anatomy, nearly comparable to histological findings. These tests have been fundamental in the evaluation of all retinal and choroidal vascular diseases and have allowed clinicians to define and diagnose several pathological conditions. FA became the "gold standard" in retinal imaging due to the capacity to visualize the retinal capillary bed and its changes, both in the macular area and in the periphery. Although the fluorescence of the injected dye enabled improved visualization of retinal capillaries, not all the different layers of the retinal capillary network could be visualized in this bi-dimensional examination, mainly because of the light scattering phenomenon. By calculating the difference between static and non-static tissues, optical coherence tomography angiography (OCT-A) allows a depth-resolved visualization of the retinal and choroidal microvasculature. Given that the main moving elements in the ocular fundus are contained in blood vessels, determining a vascular decorrelation signal enables visualization of the 3-dimensional retinal and choroidal vascular networks without the intravenous dye injection, reducing therefore the risk of potential adverse events. Since OCT-A is perfectly co-registered with its structural OCT, both morphological findings, such as macular edema, and functional ones, like capillary drop-out, may be clearly evaluated on a single dye-free examination. Proficient detection of the different findings in diabetic maculopathy on OCT-A can result in a rapid analysis of the examination, and in the capacity to distinguish truly decorrelated structures (perfused vessels) from artifacts. Moreover, a complete morpho-functional assessment may help in determining both the origin and the clinical activity of a given vascular disease.

Introduction

Optical coherence tomography angiography (OCT-A) is a new method of non-invasive examination, which allows the visualization of the entire retinal and choroidal vasculature, thanks to a novel technique of conventional OCT imaging analysis.

This diagnostic approach is rapidly spreading among the largest part of Ophthalmologists. It is a new step forward in OCT technology, which will allow each clinician to easily have a snapshot of the vessels and retinal capillaries and/or choroidal vasculature.

Definition and Principles of OCT-A

This imaging modality is coupled with traditional OCT images, which can highlight lesions of outer retinal layers and fluid accumulations. In this way, both functional and morphological information are obtained with a single examination.

OCT-A is a new "instant imaging": since it is easy, quick and non-invasive, it seems very promising for all retinal and choroidal vascular diseases, particularly in diabetes.

Both components of diabetic maculopathy: macular edema (ME) and macular ischemia, associated with diverse diabetic changes, such as microaneurysms, capillary non- perfusion, and ischemia within the retina, ultimately lead to neovascularization and/or ME, both of which can severely compromise the visual function.

Imaging Techniques

Fluorescein angiography (FA), the imaging method of choice ("Gold standard") for the analysis of vascular and capillary beds, has been in use for the past 50 years now.

OCT, and in particular the Spectral Domain OCT SD-OCT), has recently entered the field of retinal imaging in clinical daily routine. Since 20 years, the OCT has tremendously developed as a non-invasive imaging method and medical diagnostic, a real «Optical Biopsy» of retinal microstructures.

The OCT-A is a new revolutionary technique that allows a clear, depth-resolved visualization of the retinal 10 and choroidal microvasculature [1].

OCT-A is based on the concept that in a static eye, the only moving structure in the eye fundus are blood cells, flowing in the vessels. By calculating the decorrelation of signal amplitude from repeated consecutive B-scans at the same section, a contrast between static and non-static tissues is generated. This will determine a vascular decorrelation signal that enables visualization of 3-dimensional retinal and choroidal vasculature, of a variable intensity signal according to the speed of blood flow [2, 3].

Technical Aspects

The automated layer segmentation provides a fast way to evidence the presence of a decorrelation signal, due to perfused vascular structures, in any OCT-angiogram.

This automated segmentation is based on different levels of reflectivity, which are mainly visible on conventional OCT B-scan (Fig. 1).

"Spectralis OCT2" Device

The "Spectralis OCT2" device (Spectralis, Heidelberg Engineering, Heidelberg, Germany) is a prototype able to acquire 85,000 A-scans per second, with a resolution of 7 μm axially and 14 μm laterally, and a bandwidth of 50 nm. An amplitude decorrelation algorithm developed by Heidelberg Engineering (Heidelberg, Germany) is applicable to a volume scan, on a 15 × 5° or 15 × 10°area (4.3 × 1.5 or 4.3 × 2.9 mm), which is composed of a variable number of B-scans (ranging from 131 to 261, respectively) at a distance of 11 μm each (this value is very near to the limit of eye resolution).

C-Scan ("en-face") Visualization of OCT-A

The C-scan ("en-face") visualization of this OCT-A is automatically derived from OCT B-scan angiograms. The Automated Real-Time (ART) mode, which helps the effective discrimination between image "noise" and true signals from real tissue structures, associated with the limited distance between 2 consecutive B-scans (11 μm) allows the best high-resolution C-scan angiogram. The prototype device, using the ART mode, allows

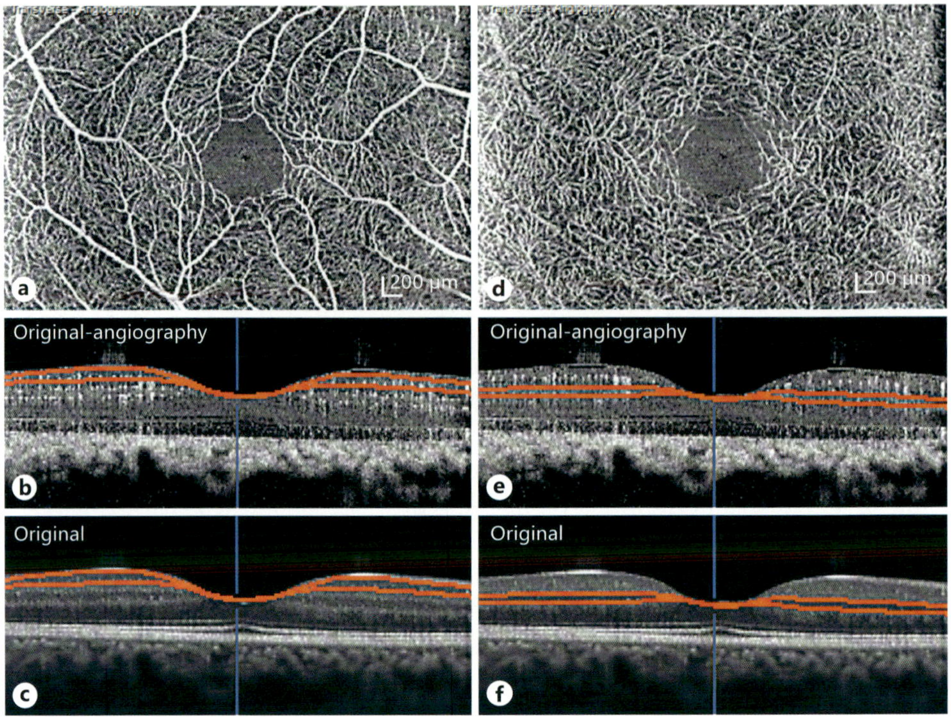

Fig. 1. Automated segmentation on optical coherence tomography-angiography (OCT-A). **a** Superficial capillary plexus (SCP) shown in C-scan OCT-A visualization. This vascular layer is typically identified at the level of the ganglion cell layer in macular area. **b, c** The B-scans show, both in OCT-A (**b**) and conventional OCT (**c**), the exact level where the C-scan (**a**) is taken. **d** Deep capillary plexus (SCP) shown in C-scan OCT-A visualization. This vascular layer is typically identified at the level of the inner nuclear layer. **e**, **f**. The B-scans show, both in OCT-A (**e**) and conventional OCT (**f**), the exact level where the C-scan (**a**) is taken.

varying the number of frames per scan, to average the image, increase the quality of each single B-scan, and improve the signal-to-noise ratio.

Macular OCT-A: Superficial and Deep Capillary Plexuses

The major advantage of OCT-A is the capability to resolve the vascular layers of the retina with a tri-dimensional (3D) approach. In diabetic maculopathy, macular ischemia and enlargement of the FAZ can differentially affect the superficial capillary plexus (SCP) and the deep capillary plexus (DCP) [4].

Moreover, the disorganization of the retinal inner layers [5] and para-central acute middle maculopathy [6], both commonly occur in diabetic retinopathy (RD). They are likely manifestations of ischemia at the level of the SCP and DCP, respectively.

Retinal Microvasculopathy

Different degrees of macular involvement can be observed in case of RD, and their 3D analysis is useful in determining the corresponding impairment of the superficial and deep capillary plexuses during the evolution from the incipient form to severe proliferative or non-proliferative disease (Fig. 2, 3).

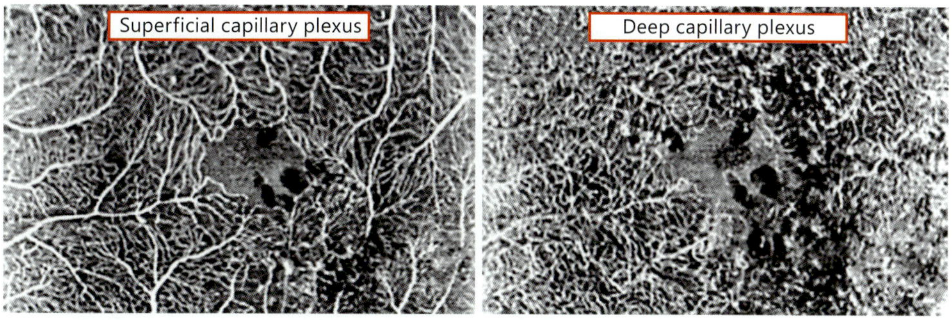

Fig. 2. Diabetic patient with mild non-proliferative diabetic maculopathy. Superficial capillary plexus (SCP) on optical coherence tomography angiography (OCT-A): the SCP and the perifoveal vascular arcade appear mildly rarefied. A few perifoveal areas of non-perfusion are visible: in these areas, the vascular network seems rarefied. Microaneurysms and tiny cystoid spaces are also appreciable. Deep capillary plexus (DCP) on OCT-A: a few focal vessel dilations and microaneurysms are detectable. Small cystoid spaces are present at the border of the scanned area.

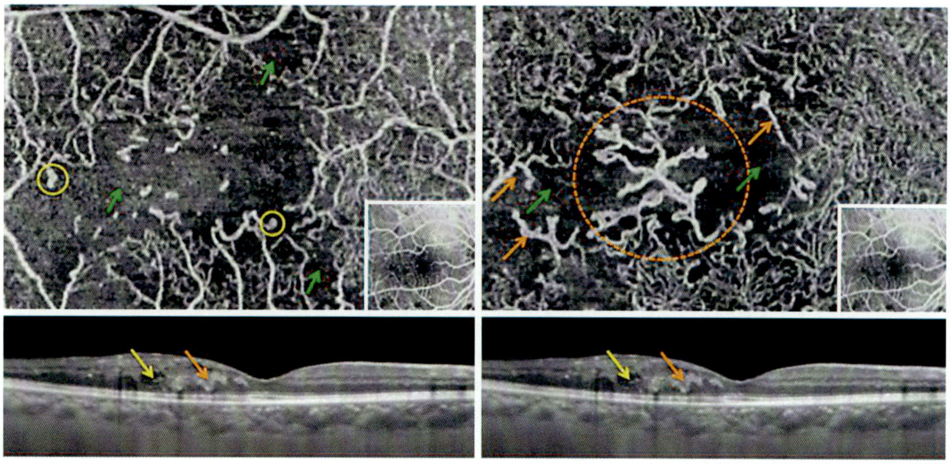

Fig. 3. Diabetic patient with severe non-proliferative diabetic maculopathy. Superficial capillary plexus (SCP) on optical coherence tomography angiography (OCT-A): extensive area of non-perfusion. An extensive area of non-perfusion involves the central part of the figure including the foveal avascular zone. In this area, vessels are dilated and microaneurysms are also visible. Cystoid spaces and intraretinal microvascular abnormality (IRMA; hyperreflective intraretinal lesions involving the inner and outer retinal layers are visible on structural OCT). Deep capillary plexus (DCP) on OCT-A: large central area of capillary dropout. The large central area of capillary dropout shows the presence of a large intraretinal hyperintense structure, which is related to the presence of an IRMA. Several focally dilated capillaries are also appreciable at the borders of the non-perfused area.

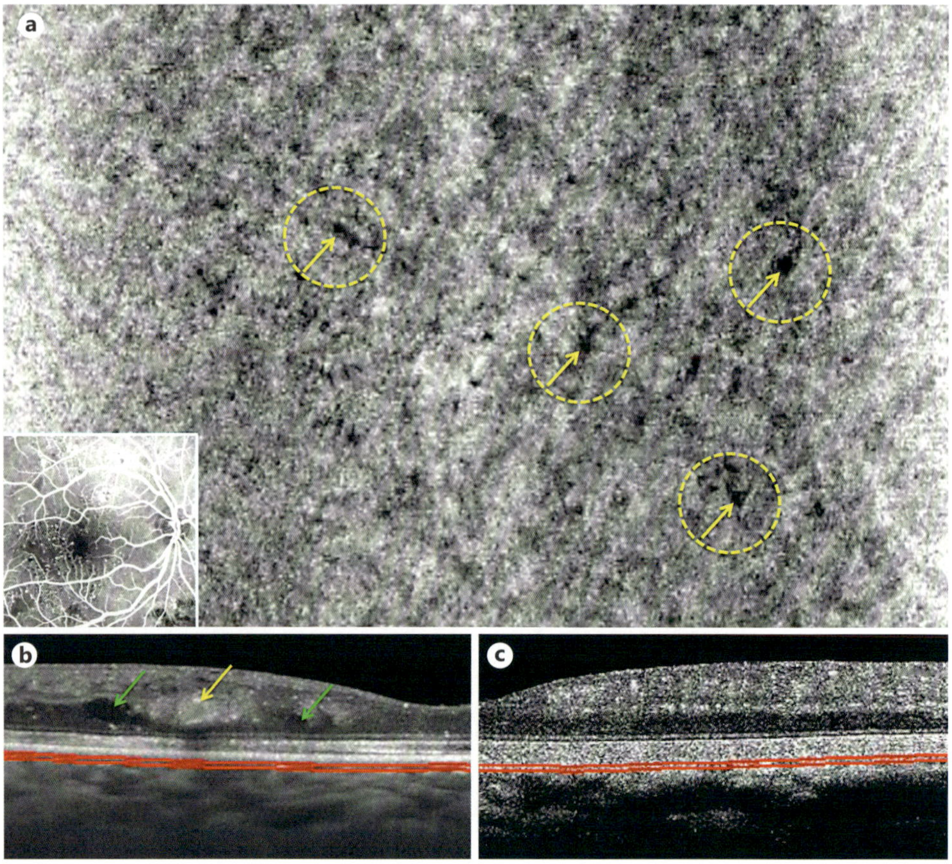

Fig. 4. Choriocapillaris on optical coherence tomography angiography (OCT-A) (patient with severe non-proliferative diabetic maculopathy). **a** C-scan OCT-angiogram (20-µm-thick): the choriocapillaris appears slightly rarefied in the macular area. Limited areas of flow void (yellow arrows with dashed yellow circle) are visible, probably due to small non-perfused areas. **b–c** The cross-sectional structural OCT and OCT-angiogram at the level of the choriocapillaris (red lines): severe impairment of the retina: an intraretinal abnormal hyperreflectivity (yellow arrow), probably due to IRMA and a few cystoid spaces (green arrows), are shown.

Choriocapillaris and Choroidal Assessment

Diabetic signs of choroidal vascular impairment are therefore evaluated principally at the level of choriocapillaris, since it is the unique structure clearly defined on OCT-A.

In the C-scan OCT-angiogram, the choriocapillaris may appear slightly rarefied in macular area. A few areas of "flow void" could be visible, probably due to small non-perfused areas. This process could result in a direct damage of the outer retinal layers and photoreceptors, which obtain the oxygen supply and nourishments from choriocapillaris circulation (Fig. 4).

Diabetic ME

The most common cause of visual impairment among diabetic patients is diabetic ME (DME), accounting for about three-fourths of cases of visual loss. The diagnosis of ME is mainly clinical, based on

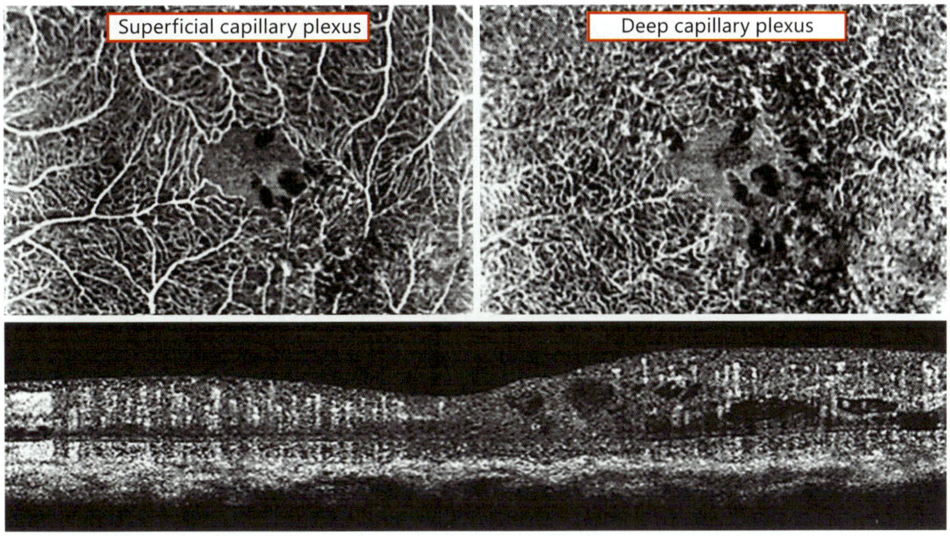

Fig. 5. Diabetic macular edema (Mild NPDR): C-scan of the superficial capillary plexus. The enlargement of the foveal avascular zone (FAZ) is associated with focal capillary dilations and small areas of capillary non-perfusion. The presence of large, roundish, hypointense lesions is due to cystoid spaces in the perifoveal area. Smaller black cystoid lesions are also visible in the extra-foveal area. Deep capillary plexus (DCP): the OCT-A, taken at the level of the inner nuclear layer, clearly shows the DCP. A diffuse reduction of the vascularity is visible, coupled with an enlargement of the FAZ, focal capillary dilations, and areas of capillary non-perfusion. Numerous hypointense lesions (cystoid spaces) are appreciable in the macular area.

biomicroscopy, FA, and OCT: conventionally, DME is defined as retinal thickening and/or presence of hard exudates. SD-OCT can visualize small cystoid spaces within 1 disc diameter of the center of the macula and frequently a serous retinal detachment.

DME may appear on OCT-A as Hypo-intense or Grayish intraretinal spaces (Fig. 5) and focal hyper-intense clumps (Fig. 6).

Focal Hyperintense Clumps

On C-scan OCT-angiograms of a patient with diabetic maculopathy often shows highly decorrelated roundish or fusiform structures, which are generally interpreted as microaneurysms or intra retinal microvascular abnormalities.

This focal hyper-intense signal may unfortunately be related also to non-decorrelated lesions such as hard exudates (Fig. 6).

DME: Different Degrees of Macular Involvement

Case 1: Moderate non-proliferative RD with focal MEME (Fig. 7).

Case 2: Moderate non-proliferative RD with ME (Fig. 8).

Case 3: Severe non-proliferative RD with cystoid ME (Fig. 9).

Diabetic Macular Ischemia

Diabetic macular ischemia is an important cause of severe visual impairment in patients with RD.

Moderate Macular Ischemia

Moderate macular ischemia (MMI) is characterized by the enlargement of the foveal avascular zone, by the disruption of the perifoveal capillary

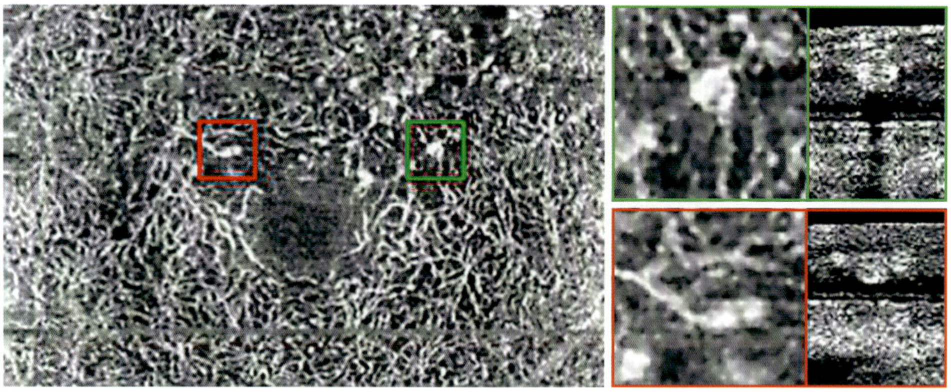

Fig. 6. Diabetic Macular Edema: optical coherence tomography angiography (OCT-A) C-scan of the deep capillary plexus (DCP). The OCT-angiogram taken at the level of the inner nuclear layer clearly shows the DCP. The fusiform hyperintense structure (red square) shows the typical appearance of a microaneurysm. The roundish hyperintense lesion (green box), although similar to the previous one, is due to the focal accumulation of hard exudates. These assume this aspect of OCT-A because, as hyperreflective structures, they are able to reflect the refracted signal coming from the perfused (decorrelated) vessels above. The latter are hyperreflective structures on structural OCT and hyper-intense ones on OCT-angiography. The B-scan OCT-angiogram (top) shows 2 decorrelated intraretinal structures. One of these does not show any additional finding above or below the lesion itself, while the second one is associated with a dark back shadowing. This phenomenon is linked to the high reflectivity of the hard exudates. The corresponding structural B-scan (bottom) highlights the difference in reflectivity of the two intraretinal lesions (microaneurysm versus hard exudates).

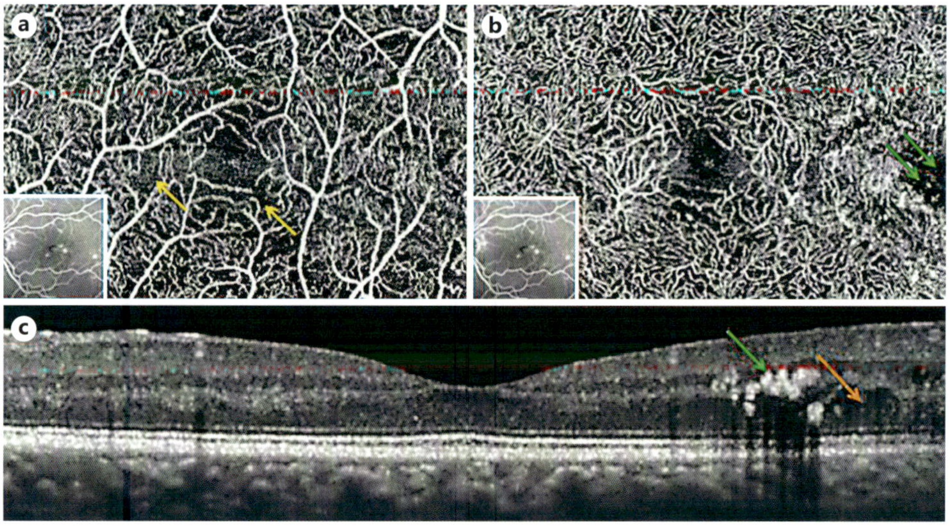

Fig. 7. Mild non-proliferative diabetic retinopathy with focal macular edema. **a** The optical coherence tomography (OCT)-angiogram shows a rarefied superficial capillary plexus with numerous perifoveal areas of non-perfusion. **b** At the level of the deep capillary plexus, several roundish, hypointense lesions (green arrows) are visible: these are due to cystoid spaces and hard exudates in the extra-foveal area. **c** The structural B-scan OCT highlights the presence of hyperreflective intraretinal lesions (hard exudates, green arrow) and extra-foveal cystoid spaces (orange arrow).

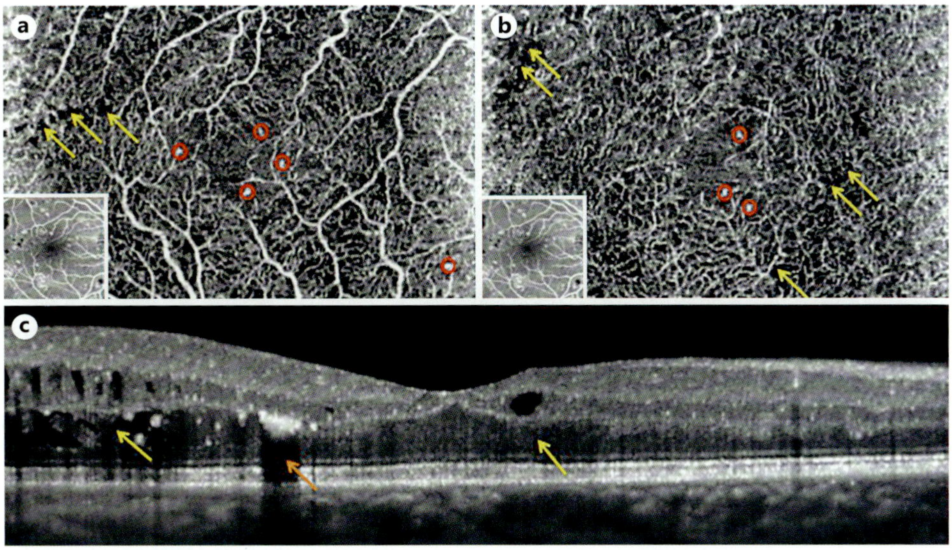

Fig. 8. Moderate non-proliferative diabetic retinopathy with macular edema. **a** The superficial capillary plexus (SCP) shows numerous hyperintense structures, probably due to microaneurysms (red circles) and some hypointense intraretinal spaces (yellow arrows). **b** At the level of the deep capillary plexus (DCP), microaneurysms are still visible (red circles). The number of cystoid spaces (hypointense intraretinal structures, yellow arrows) is substantially higher than SCP. **c** The structural B-scan OCT highlights the presence of hyperreflective intraretinal lesions (hard exudates, orange arrow) and cystoid spaces (yellow arrows).

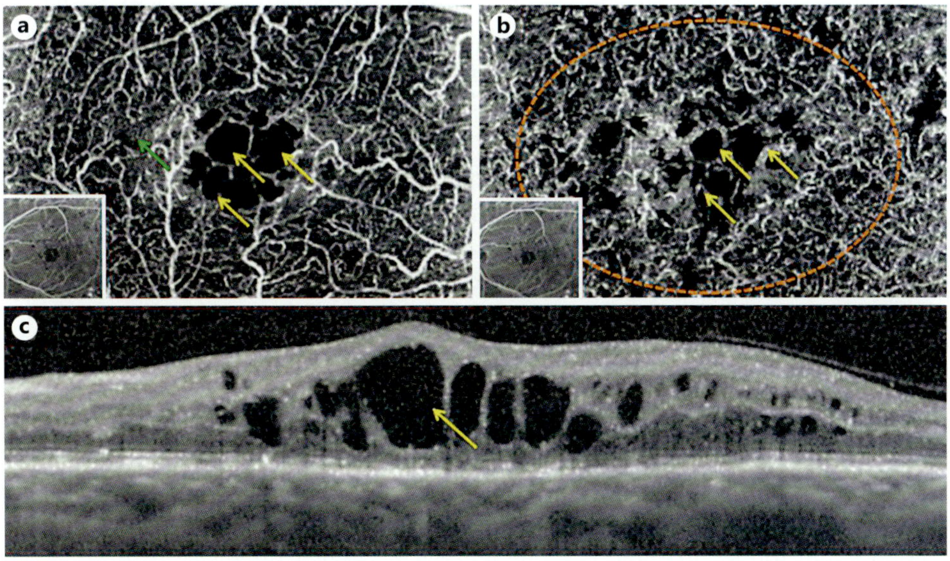

Fig. 9. Severe non-proliferative diabetic retinopathy with cystoid macular edema. **a** The superficial capillary plexus (SCP) shows focal vessel dilations, variably sized non-perfused areas (green arrow) and numerous hypointense roundish structures due to intraretinal cystoid spaces (yellow arrows). **b** The deep capillary plexus (DCP) appears rarefied (orange dashed line). Numerous cystoid spaces (hypointense intraretinal structures, yellow arrows) are also appreciable. **c** The structural B-scan OCT highlights the presence of an extensive intraretinal exudation (yellow arrows).

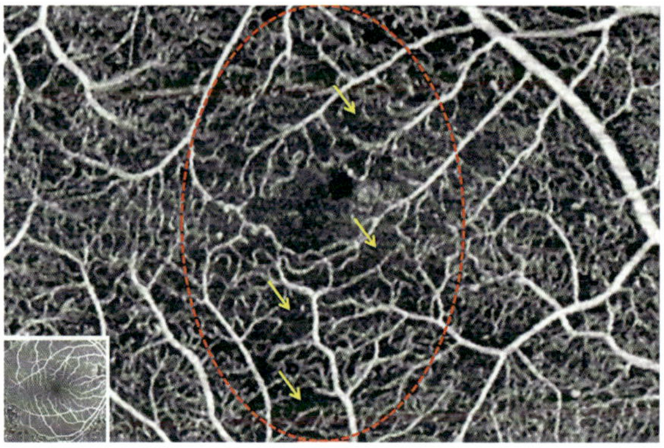

Fig. 10. Optical coherence tomography angiography (OCT-A) C-scan of a diabetic patient with moderate macular ischemia (MMI). The OCT-A shows several areas of flow absence (yellow arrows) in a diffusely rarefied superficial capillary network. These flow-void areas and the contiguous vascular abnormalities such as microaneurysms, venous beading and focal vessel dilations are related to a more severe stage of diabetic retinopathy.

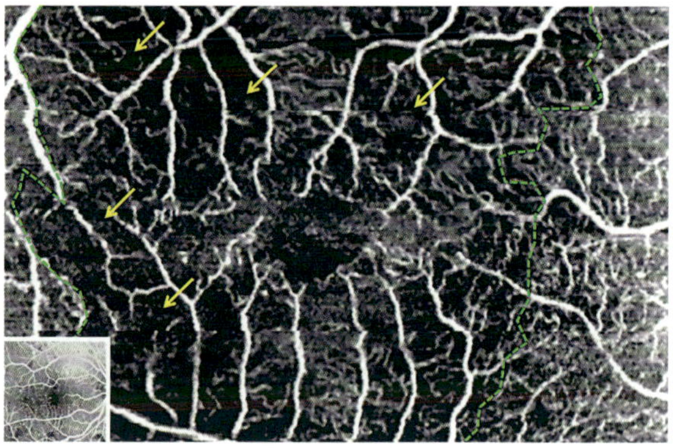

Fig. 11. Optical coherence tomography angiography (OCT-A) C-scan of a diabetic patient with severe macular ischemia (MMI). The OCT-A shows large areas of flow absence (yellow arrows) in a diffusely rarefied superficial capillary network (green dashed lines). These flow-void areas are related to the severe stage of non-proliferative diabetic retinopathy or proliferative diabetic retinopathy.

arcade, and by retinal capillary loss in other, non-contiguous areas of the macula (capillary dropout) [7] (Fig. 10).

Severe Macular Ischemia
Severe macular ischemia is the late stage of diabetic macular impairment, where confluent areas without any decorrelation signal largely involve the scanned area (Fig. 11). Capillaries are rare and the only decorrelation signal in large areas is the one belonging to large retinal vessels. These findings are related to late stages of non-proliferative RD or to proliferative RD.

Follow-Up after Treatment

The recent introduction of OCT-A might allow a non-invasive functional assessment of diabetic maculopathy. This achievement, coupled with structural OCT, could result in a comprehensive morpho-functional examination of the status of the disease and its response to treatment.

Here, we follow some cases of diabetic maculopathy, assessed with both OCT-A and structural OCT, before and after anti-VEGF treatment. This analysis is performed to evaluate the potential outcome of the intravitreal treatment on intraretinal (or sub-retinal) exudation and on vascular perfusion, but it is not based on the indications or the results of different treatments (Fig. 12, 13).

Quantitative Image Analysis

Automated quantification of macular diseases could translate the theoretical usefulness of OCT-A into "clinical practice." Therefore an automated algorithm, which analyzes OCT-A images, can detect and quantify macular vascular impairment in RD. The authors have recently developed an Automated, Custom-built Software (AngiOCTool™), able to provide a quantitative assessment of vascular perfusion in macular area [8, 9] (Fig. 14).

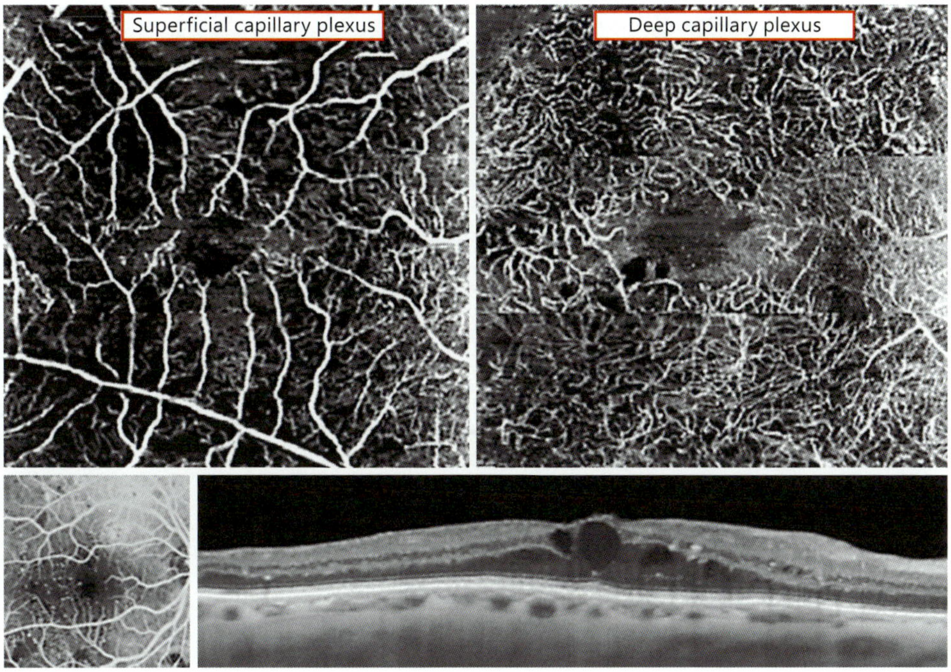

Fig. 12. Optical coherence tomography angiography (OCT-A-15 × 10°) C-scan and structural OCT of a 56 years-old patient with Diabetic Maculopathy before a single intravitreal injection of VEGF-Trap. The superficial capillary plexus (SCP; top left image) shows large areas of flow absence in a diffusely rarefied vascular network. The deep capillary plexus (DCP; top right image) appears impaired as well, with focal vascular dilations and areas of absence of signal coming from decorrelated structures. These flow-void areas are generally related to severe stages of non-proliferative diabetic retinopathy or proliferative diabetic retinopathy. Reference fluorescein angiography (bottom left image). Structural OCT (bottom image) shows the presence diabetic macular edema. Cystoid spaces mainly involve the inner and outer nuclear layers. Some hyperreflective clumps are also appreciable.

The image analysis provides several quantitative parameters:

- FAZ metrics (perimeter, surface, major axis, orientation),
- Total Vascular Surface,
- Total Avascular Surface.

Quantitative data may be achieved within a circular area of 2,000 μm diameter, centered on FAZ. This approach has been already validated on healthy subjects, and it is an ongoing application in case of different retinal vascular diseases.

Conclusions

RD remains the leading cause of legal blindness in working age populations in industrialized countries. DME and non-perfusions of macular capillary bed will directly alter the central vision. The development of modern imagery such as OCT has enabled the evaluation of the earliest stages of DME, including the sub-clinical ones. The recent introduction of OCT-A may allow non-invasive functional evaluation of diabetic maculopathy.

13

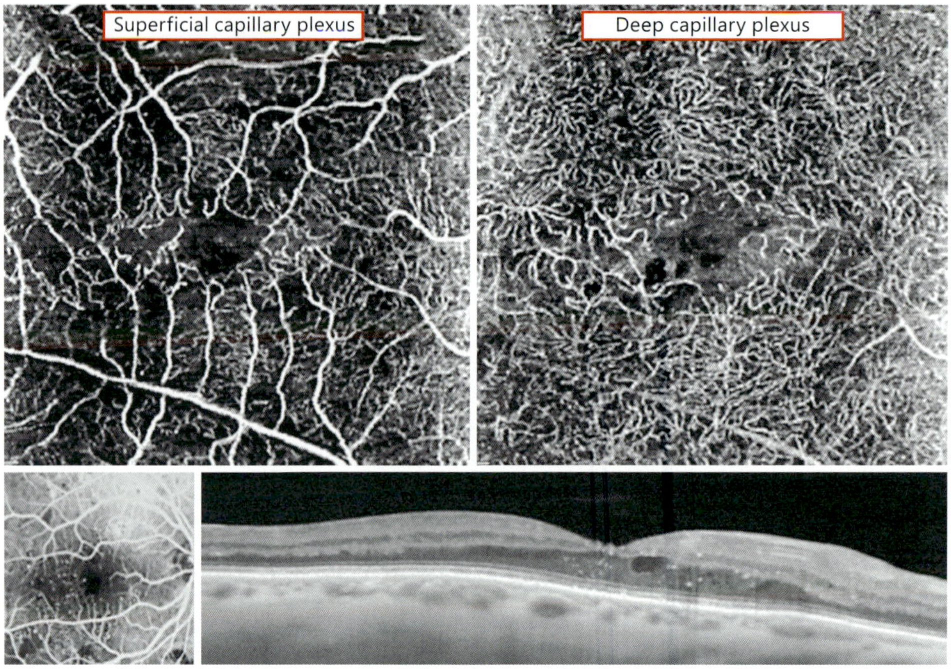

14

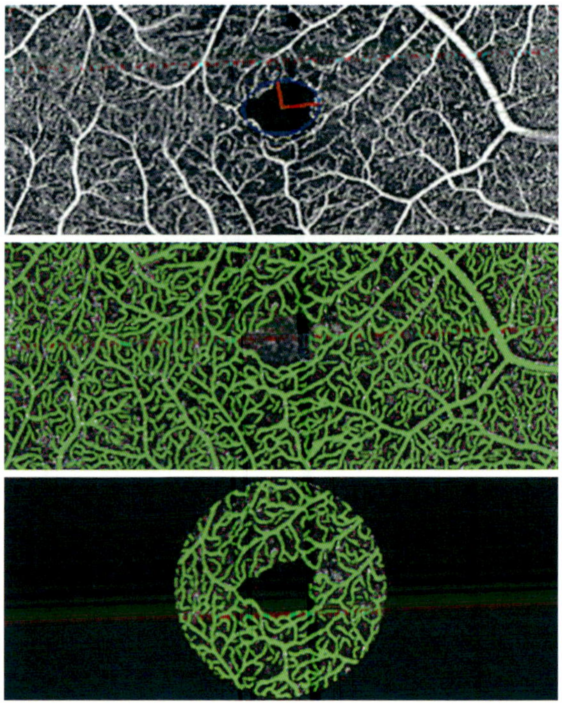

Fig. 13. Optical coherence tomography angiography (OCT-A) C-scan and structural OCT of a 56-year-old patient with Diabetic Maculopathy 1 month after a single intravitreal injection of VEGF-Trap. The superficial capillary plexus (SCP; top left image) appears less rarefied, due to the substantial reduction of the capillary dropout. The deep capillary plexus (DCP; top right image), showing severe impairment of vascular architecture in the perifoveal area, seems to be slightly improved. On OCT-A, a more homogeneous signal comes from perfused structures, either in SCP or in DCP; structural OCT confirms an evident decrease of intraretinal exudation. Some residual cystoid spaces are seen, but foveal depression is almost maintained.

Fig. 14. Total vascular surface assessment. Top – The foveal avascular zone (FAZ) is automatically detected in case of SCP by outlining a contour along the vascular rim of the perifoveal capillary arcade or in case of DCP: by connecting decorrelated pixels at the border of a central non-flow area. FAZ perimeter, axes (red lines), surface (equivalent circular surface, blue line) are computed. Middle – Vessels' detection was both based on the exact identification of each decorrelated pixel and on the trajectory taken by contiguous decorrelated pixels. This process allowed to render the vessel thickness and to obtain, with a vector representation, the shape of perfused structures. Bottom – Quantitative data are achieved within a circular area of 2,000 μm diameter, centered on the FAZ, to reduce potential artifacts and because of the relevance of this area in terms of the visual function.

References

1 Yau JW, Rogers SL, Kawasaki R, et al: Global prevalence and major risk factors of diabetic retinopathy. Diabetes Care 2012;35:556–564.

2 Spaide RF, Klancnik JM Jr, Cooney MJ: Retinal vascular layers imaged by fluorescein angiography and optical coherence tomography angiography. JAMA Ophthalmol 2015;133:45–50.

3 Jia Y, Bailey ST, Wilson DJ, et al: Quantitative optical coherence tomography angiography of choroidal neovascularization in age-related macular degeneration. Ophthalmology 2014;121:1435–1444.

4 Yu PK, Balaratnasingam C, Cringle SJ, McAllister IL, Provis J, Yu DY: Microstructure and network organization of the microvasculature in the human macula. Invest Ophthalmol Vis Sci 2010; 51:6735–6743.

5 Ishibazawa A, Nagaoka T, Takahashi A, et al: Optical coherence tomography angiography in diabetic retinopathy: a prospective Pilot study. Am J Ophthalmol 2015;160:35–44.e1.

6 Nemiroff J, Kuehlewein L, Rahimy E, et al: Assessing deep retinal capillary ischemia in paracentral acute middle maculopathy by optical coherence tomography angiography. Am J Ophthalmol 2016;162:121–132.e1.

7 Bradley PD, Sim DA, Keane PA, et al: The evaluation of diabetic macular ischemia using optical coherence tomography angiography. Invest Ophthalmol Vis Sci 2016;57:625–631.

8 Lupidi M, Coscas F, Cagini C, Fiore T, Spaccini E, Fruttini D, Coscas G: Automated quantitative analysis of retinal microvasculature in normal eyes on optical coherence tomography angiography. Am J Ophthalmol 2016;169:9–23.

9 Coscas G, Lupidi M, Coscas F: Atlas d'OCT-Angiographie dans la Maculopathie diabétique Européenne d'Edition, Paris, 2016, p 152.

Gabriel Coscas
Hôpital de Créteil, Département d'Ophtalmologie de Créteil
Université Paris XII, Val de Marne-France
Centre d'Exploration Ophtalmologique de l'Odéon
F–75006 Paris (France)
E-Mail gabriel.coscas@gmail.com

Bandello F, Zarbin MA, Lattanzio R, Zucchiatti I (eds): Management of Diabetic Retinopathy.
Dev Ophthalmol. Basel, Karger, 2017, vol 60, pp 50–55 (DOI: 10.1159/000459689)

Emerging Issues for Ultra-Wide Field Angiography

Alessandro Rabiolo[a] · Luigi Antonio De Vitis[a] · Riccardo Sacconi[a, b] · Adriano Carnevali[a, c] · Lea Querques[a] · Francesco Bandello[a] · Giuseppe Querques[a]

[a]Department of Ophthalmology, University Vita-Salute, IRCCS San Raffaele, Milan, [b]Eye Clinic, Department of Neurological and Movement Sciences, University of Verona, Verona, and [c]Department of Ophthalmology, University of "Magna Graecia," Catanzaro, Italy

Abstract

Fluorescein angiography (FA) is a useful test in patients affected by diabetic retinopathy (DR) to evaluate the blood-retinal barrier integrity and the presence of non-perfused areas, vascular leakage, microvascular abnormalities, and neovascularization. The peripheral retina is involved in most DR lesions, and, thus, its proper visualization is crucial for the screening, diagnosis, monitoring, treatment, and prognosis of DR. To expand the field of view, wide-field and ultra-wide-field imaging have been developed, allowing images up to 200° of retinal surface in one single photo. In this chapter, emerging issues concerning ultra-wide-field FA in DR are illustrated.

Fluorescein angiography (FA) is a useful test in patients suffering from diabetic retinopathy (DR) to evaluate the blood-retinal barrier (BRB) integrity and the presence of non-perfused areas, vascular leakage, microvascular abnormalities, and neovascularization (NV). The peripheral retina is involved in most DR lesions, and, thus, its proper visualization is crucial for the screening, diagnosis, monitoring, treatment, and prognosis of DR [1]. Traditional angiograms, however, visualize only 30–50° degrees of retinal surface at once. Wide-field and ultra-wide-field FA (UWFA) systems have been developed to enlarge the surface of peripheral retina evaluated. Specifically, 3 different approaches have been applied.

- Photomontage of traditional angiograms (e.g., 7 standard field [7SF] and 2 field protocols exploring 75° and 45°, respectively) [2].
- Implementation of standard fundus camera or confocal selective laser ophthalmoscope (cSLO) with additional lenses (e.g., Staurenghi lens [150°] [3], Spectralis ultra-wide field lens [105°] [4]).

- *Ad-hoc* equipment (i.e., Pomerantzeff camera [148°] [5], Panoret [100°] [6], Retcam [130°] [7], Optos [200°] [8]).

However, most of these instruments have not been applied in daily clinical practice due to several limitations including need for mydriasis, technical skill of the photographer, patient collaboration, limited resolution, need for clear media, and contact lens application.

Optos Camera

Optos ultra-wide field camera (Optos, PLC, Scotland) has been developed to overcome those pitfalls. It is a cSLO instrument assembled with an ellipsoid mirror with 2 focal points, which explore 82% of human retina (200°) in a single photo with no need for mydriasis or contact lens. Field of view can be further widened by merging images taken using different steering positions, as recently described [9]. Optos camera displays twice the retinal surface of standard digital acquisition systems [8]; moreover, it is able to explore a wider retinal area compared to Heidelberg Spectralis ultra-wide field lens, especially in nasal and temporal quadrants [4].

The Optos device was initially approved by US Food and Drug Administration as a fundus camera in 1999 and commercialized in 2000. At the beginning, it was equipped with 2 scanning diode lasers: a green (532 nm) one for the retina and inner retinal pigment epithelium (RPE) and a red (633 nm) one for the outer RPE and choroid. A pseudocolor ultra-wide field retinography was obtained from the combination of these 2 channels. UWFA using the Optos camera was reported 4 years later by Friberg and Forrester [10], who introduced a blue 488 nm wavelength laser (to excite intravenously injected sodium fluorescein) to the standard hardware unit. Optos UWFA device was introduced in the market in 2007, and since then, it has been applied to the study of many retinal diseases, including DR.

Ultra-Wide Field in DR

In patients affected by DR, UWFA can provide several advantages over traditional FA, both in a clinical and research setting, including: the visualization of wider retinal surface; identification of peripheral retinal lesions; individuation of novel angiographic features; quantification of peripheral retinal ischemia through a numeric ischemic index (ISI); correlation of ISI with diabetic macular edema (DME), diabetic macular ischemia (DMI), recurrence of post-vitrectomy diabetic vitreous hemorrhage (PVDVH), or oxygen saturation of retinal arteries; changes in ISI following different treatments (i.e., anti-vascular endothelial growth factor [VEGF], intravitreal steroids); and UWFA-guided targeted retinal photocoagulation (TRP).

It has been demonstrated that compared to standard systems, UWFA explores a wider area of both retinal surface (8.7 ± 1.6 vs. 3.4 ± 0.76 disc diameter, $p < 0.001$) and retinal ischemia (16.9 ± 15 vs. 3.4 ± 4.26 sectors, $p < 0.05$), even with a loss in image quality [8]. Wessel et al. [11] compared UWFA to the gold standard 7SF, and they found that UWFA revealed 3.2 times more total retinal surface, 3.9 times more non-perfusion, 1.9 times more NV, and 3.8 times more laser PRP. Interestingly, 10% of the unaffected eye with 7SF presented some degree of DR at UWFA. According to these findings, UWFA is able to upgrade assessment of DR severity, and it may even outline signs of retinopathy in patients judged normal using conventional techniques. UWFA and simulated 7SF are compared in Figure 1.

In a retrospective study by Oliver and Schwartz [12], UWFA allowed the identification of a novel angiographic sign associated with DR, named peripheral vascular leakage (PVL). PVL was defined as the late leakage of dye from retinal veins and arteries, and it could reflect loss of BRB integrity in the setting of active DR. Since PVL correlated with peripheral ischemia, macular leakage, and NV, as shown in Figure 2, it has been

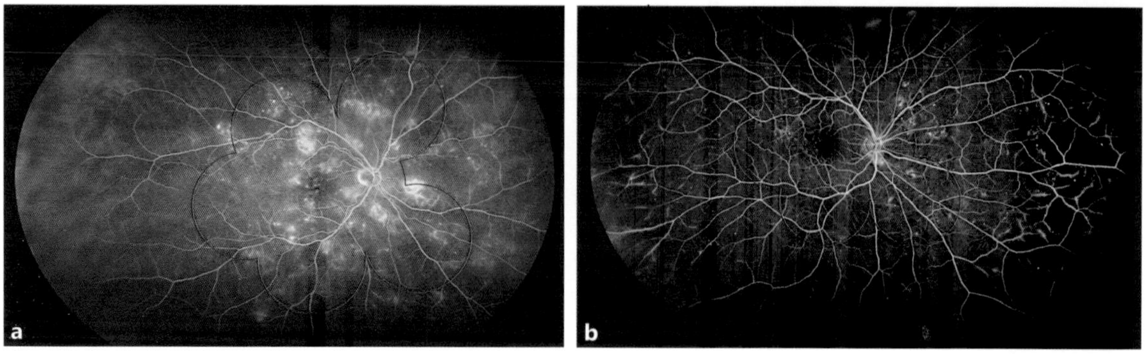

Fig. 1. Simulated 7 standard field (7SF) on ultra-wide field fluorescein angiography (UWFA). The overly of the 7SF border is outlined in red. **a** Right eye of a 48-year-old female patient with moderate diabetic retinopathy. Most of the retinal pathology is detected with both 7SF and UWFA. **b** Right eye of a 64-year-old, female patient affected by mild diabetic retinopathy. Microaneurysms are uniformly distributed between 7SF and UWFA; conversely, retinal ischemia and intra-retinal microvascular abnormalities are located outside 7SF boundaries.

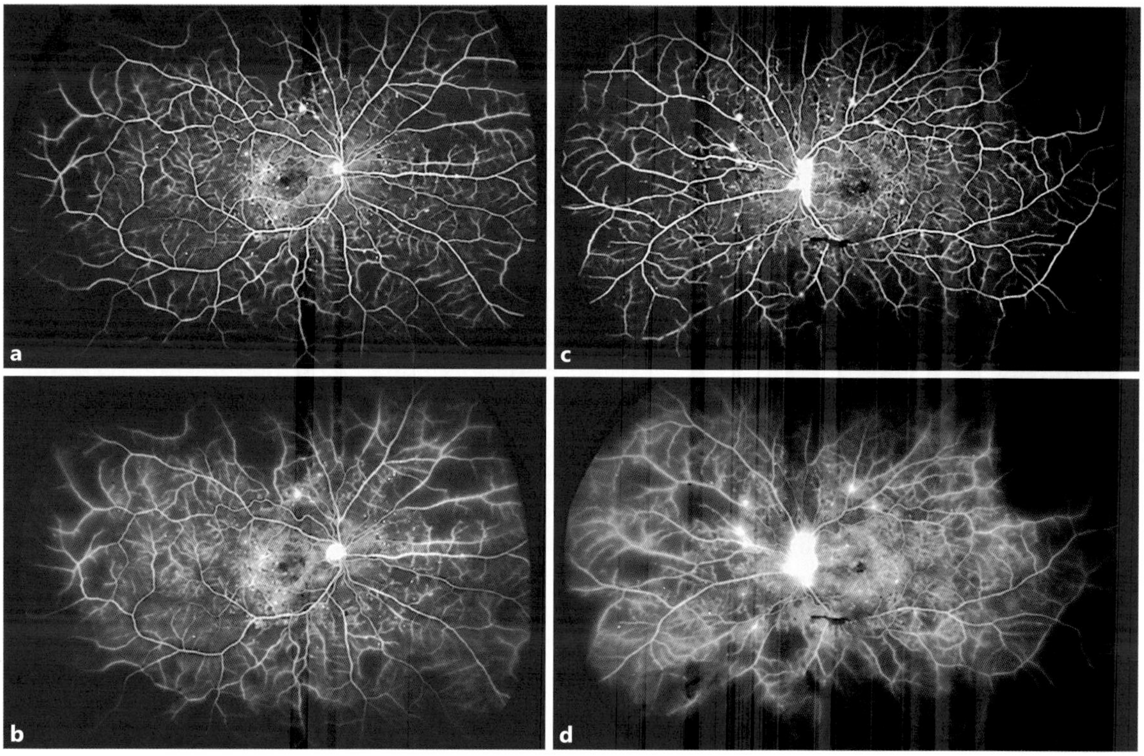

Fig. 2. Ultra-wide field fluorescein angiography (UWFA) of a 48-year-old male patient affected by proliferative diabetic retinopathy. **a**, **b** Early (01:02) and late (04:00) phases of the right eye, respectively. **c**, **d** Early (00:42) and late (05: 31) phases of the left eye, respectively. In early phases, UWFA reveals in both eyes hyperfluorescent dots suggestive of microaneurysms, and broad peripheral and mid peripheral areas of capillary non-perfusion. In late angiographic frames, UWFA discloses in both eyes peripheral perivascular and macular dye leakage, suggestive of blood-retina barrier disruption, and intense hyperfluorescence of the optic disc and retinal surface, indicative of epiretinal neovascularization. In the left eye, the presence of vitreous hemorrhage next to the inferior temporal arcade is observed.

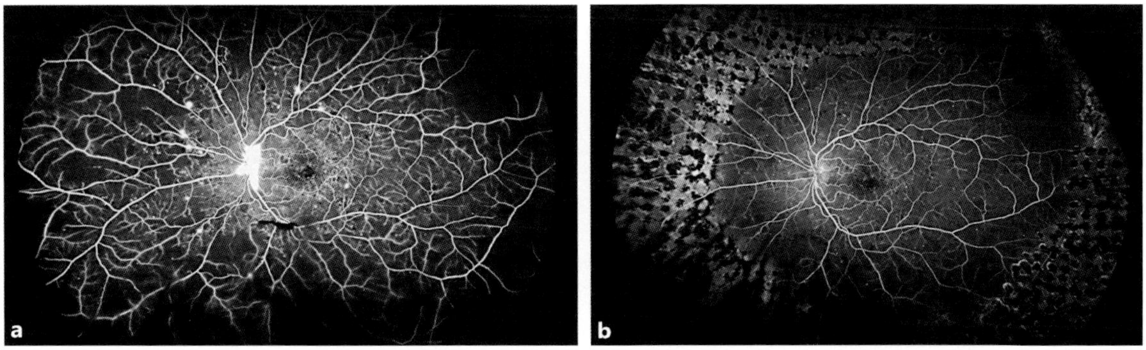

Fig. 3. Ultra-wide field fluorescein angiography of the left eye of the same patient of Figure 2 before (**a**) and 6 (**b**) months after targeted retinal photocoagulation. Following the photocoagulation of ischemic areas, sustained regression of proliferative vessels and no late macular leakage indicative of blood-retina barrier disruption are evident.

hypothesized that ischemic retina upregulates VEGF production through a hypoxia-induced mechanism, which, in turn, could cause NV growth and BRB disruption both in macular and peripheral areas leading to macular leakage and PVL, respectively. In the same study, however, peripheral ischemia was associated with NV but not with DME. Nevertheless, the link between DME and capillary non-perfusion was found by other studies where retinal ischemia was quantitatively assessed by means of ISI, which is defined as the percentage of non-perfusion over the total retinal area. Specifically, Wessel at al. [13] reported a positive association between ISI and DME and, moreover, ISI was an independent risk factor for DME. In a study by Patel et al. [14], recalcitrant DME was worse in patients with higher DR grade and ISI.

Since both peripheral ischemia and DMI could share a common pathogenesis, that is, capillary non-perfusion, their correlation was investigated. Sim et al. [15] disclosed a positive correlation between peripheral ischemia and DMI assessed by means of ISI and foveal avascular zone (FAZ) area at UWFA, respectively. Another study, exploring the correlation between peripheral ischemia and macular ischemia assessed using UWFA and optical coherence tomography angiography, confirmed the outcomes of the previous study, and demonstrated that ISI correlates also to FAZ area at superficial capillary plexus and to DR grade [16].

Since peripheral ischemia and PVL are correlated with NV, DME, and DMI, UWFA could help in identifying diabetic patients at high risk of developing those complications and, thus, could have an impact on the clinical management. Figure 3 shows a patient with broad confluent areas of peripheral ischemia associated with NV.

In a study by Kim et al. [17], eyes with recurrent PVDVH compared to non-PVDVH ones had a higher rate of peripheral non-perfusion, NV, and PVL, and this difference was not appreciated with 7SF. Moreover, peripheral ischemia was also associated with DR severity and predominantly peripheral lesions, defined as more than 50% of a specific DR lesion outside the 7SF. Guduru et al. [18] demonstrated that peripheral ischemia is not only correlated with the DR grade but also with the oxygen saturation of retinal arteries.

Little is known about the impact of intravitreal therapy on peripheral ischemia. Since VEGF is a survival factor for endothelial cells, it has been postulated that anti-VEGF could worsen retinal non-perfusion by neutralizing VEGF, and this

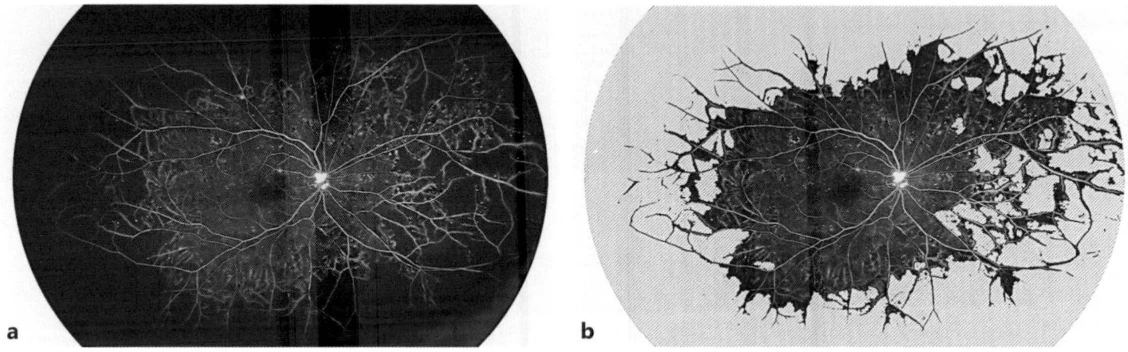

Fig. 4. Ultra-wide field fluorescein angiography (UWFA) of the right eye of a 76-year-old female patient affected by proliferative diabetic retinopathy. **a** UWFA discloses broad peripheral ischemia, disç hyperfluorescence suggestive of proliferative vessels, microaneurysms, and intra-retinal microvascular abnormalities. In panel **b**, retinal ischemia was substituted with a pattern.

hypothesis has been supported by several reports [19–21]. In a post-hoc analysis of RISE and RIDE trials, Campochiaro et al. [22] observed a positive effect of anti-VEGF therapy on posterior retinal non-perfusion evaluated using standard angiograms. No study is present in the current literature on the effect of intravitreal anti-VEGF on peripheral retina evaluated using UWFA. With regards to intravitreal steroid, dexamethasone implant seems to reduce peripheral ischemia at 2 months after injection (Querques G, personal communication).

Another emerging issue is the capability of UWFA to guide laser photocoagulation only to ischemic areas avoiding the destruction of perfused peripheral retina. This approach has been termed TRP and was developed to minimize the side effects related to standard PRP (i.e., visual acuity reduction, visual field constriction, DME onset/worsening, choroidal detachment, angle-closure glaucoma, decrease in color vision). Reddy et al. [23] were the first to explore this field, and they reported NV regression in 2 eyes treated by means of TRP with no PRP-related side effect. Subsequently, Muqit et al. [24, 25] prospectively confirmed on a larger sample that TRP and PRP have the same efficacy on NV regression, but the former causes higher reduction in CMT. Figure 4 shows the DR downgrade after TRP.

Conclusions

UWFA is an attractive examination in the diagnosis, staging, management, and therapy of DR. Most of our clinical knowledge, however, derives from high-quality clinical trials conducted prior to UWFA diffusion, and thus, it is based on standard angiographic protocols as 7SF. As previously described, UWFA adds a huge amount of information, especially concerning the peripheral retina, and the clinical utility of these data needs to be corroborated by high-quality clinical trials. To fill the gap, the DR Clinical Research Network protocol AA is currently investigating whether the assessment of the retinal far periphery using UWFA improves the ability to evaluate DR and predicts rates of DR worsening over time compared to 7SF [26]. To conclude, UWFA is going to remodel DR care. Recent studies revealed interesting observations; however, high-quality trials are warranted to corroborate preliminary findings and to translate them into the routine clinical practice.

References

1 Soliman AZ, Silva PS, Aiello LP, Sun JK: Ultra-wide field retinal imaging in detection, classification, and management of diabetic retinopathy. Semin Ophthalmol 2012;27:221–227.

2 Ghasemi Falavarjani K, Wang K, Khadamy J, Sadda SR: Ultra-wide-field imaging in diabetic retinopathy; an overview. J Curr Ophthalmol 2016;28:57–60.

3 Staurenghi G, Viola F, Mainster MA, Graham RD, Harrington PG: Scanning laser ophthalmoscopy and angiography with a wide-field contact lens system. Arch Ophthalmol 2005;123:244–252.

4 Witmer MT, Parlitsis G, Patel S, Kiss S: Comparison of ultra-widefield fluorescein angiography with the Heidelberg Spectralis(®) noncontact ultra-widefield module versus the Optos(®) Optomap(®). Clin Ophthalmol 2013;7:389–394.

5 Pomerantzeff O: Equator-plus camera. Invest Ophthalmol 1975;14:401–406.

6 Shields CL, Materin M, Shields JA: Panoramic imaging of the ocular fundus. Arch Ophthalmol 2003;121:1603–1607.

7 Azad R, Chandra P, Khan MA, Darswal A: Role of intravenous fluorescein angiography in early detection and regression of retinopathy of prematurity. J Pediatr Ophthalmol Strabismus 2008; 45:36–39.

8 Friberg TR, Gupta A, Yu J, Huang L, Suner I, Puliafito CA, et al: Ultrawide angle fluorescein angiographic imaging: a comparison to conventional digital acquisition systems. Ophthalmic Surg Lasers Imaging 2008;39:304–311.

9 Singer M, Sagong M, van Hemert J, Kuehlewein L, Bell D, Sadda SR: Ultra-widefield Imaging of the Peripheral Retinal Vasculature in Normal Subjects. Ophthalmology 2016;123:1053–1059.

10 Friberg TR, Forrester JV: Ultrawide angle (200°+) fluorescein angiography using a modified optos panoramic200TM imaging system. Invest Ophthalmol Vis Sci 2004;45:3001.

11 Wessel MM, Aaker GD, Parlitsis G, Cho M, D'Amico DJ, Kiss S: Ultra-wide-field angiography improves the detection and classification of diabetic retinopathy. Retina 2012;32:785–791.

12 Oliver SC, Schwartz SD: Peripheral vessel leakage (PVL): a new angiographic finding in diabetic retinopathy identified with ultra wide-field fluorescein angiography. Semin Ophthalmol 2010; 25:27–33.

13 Wessel MM, Nair N, Aaker GD, Ehrlich JR, D'Amico DJ, Kiss S: Peripheral retinal ischaemia, as evaluated by ultrawidefield fluorescein angiography, is associated with diabetic macular oedema. Br J Ophthalmol 2012;96:694–698.

14 Patel RD, Messner LV, Teitelbaum B, Michel KA, Hariprasad SM: Characterization of ischemic index using ultrawidefield fluorescein angiography in patients with focal and diffuse recalcitrant diabetic macular edema. Am J Ophthalmol 2013;155:1038–1044. e2.

15 Sim DA, Keane PA, Rajendram R, Karampelas M, Selvam S, Powner MB, et al: Patterns of peripheral retinal and central macula ischemia in diabetic retinopathy as evaluated by ultra-widefield fluorescein angiography. Am J Ophthalmol 2014;158:144–153.e1.

16 Corbelli E, Rabiolo A, Cicinelli MV, Querques L, Carnevali A, Querques G, et al: Assessment of Foveal Avascular Zone in Diabetic Retinopathy by Optical Coherence Tomography Angiography and Correlation Analysis with Perfusion Index. 16th Euretina Congress. Copenaghen, 2016.

17 Kim DY, Kim JG, Kim YJ, Joe SG, Lee JY: Ultra-widefield fluorescein angiographic findings in patients with recurrent vitreous hemorrhage after diabetic vitrectomy. Invest Ophthalmol Vis Sci 2014;55: 7040–7046.

18 Guduru A, Martz TG, Waters A, Kshirsagar AV, Garg S: Oxygen saturation of retinal vessels in all stages of diabetic retinopathy and correlation to ultra-wide field fluorescein angiography. Invest Ophthalmol Vis Sci 2016;57: 5278–5284.

19 Goel N, Kumar V, Ghosh B: Ischemic maculopathy following intravitreal bevacizumab for refractory diabetic macular edema. Int Ophthalmol 2011;31:39–42.

20 Sabet-Peyman EJ, Heussen FM, Thorne JE, Casparis H, Patel SJ, Do DV: Progression of macular ischemia following intravitreal bevacizumab. Ophthalmic Surg Lasers Imaging 2009;40:316–318.

21 Shimura M, Yasuda K: Macular ischaemia after intravitreal bevacizumab injection in patients with central retinal vein occlusion and a history of diabetes and vascular disease. Br J Ophthalmol 2010;94:381–383.

22 Campochiaro PA, Wykoff CC, Shapiro H, Rubio RG, Ehrlich JS: Neutralization of vascular endothelial growth factor slows progression of retinal nonperfusion in patients with diabetic macular edema. Ophthalmology 2014;121:1783–1789.

23 Reddy S, Hu A, Schwartz SD: Ultra wide field fluorescein angiography guided targeted retinal photocoagulation (TRP). Semin Ophthalmol 2009;24:9–14.

24 Muqit MM, Marcellino GR, Henson DB, Young LB, Patton N, Charles SJ, et al: Optos-guided pattern scan laser (Pascal)-targeted retinal photocoagulation in proliferative diabetic retinopathy. Acta Ophthalmol 2013;91:251–258.

25 Muqit MM, Young LB, McKenzie R, John B, Marcellino GR, Henson DB, et al: Pilot randomised clinical trial of Pascal TargETEd Retinal versus variable fluence PANretinal 20 ms laser in diabetic retinopathy: PETER PAN study. Br J Ophthalmol 2013;97:220–227.

26 Diabetic Retinopathy Clinical Research Network Study Group: Peripheral diabetic retinopathy (DR) lesions on ultrawide-field fundus images and risk of DR worsening over time. DRCRnet Web site. http://drcrnet.jaeb.org/Studies.aspx?RecID=239.

Giuseppe Querques
Department of Ophthalmology, IRCCS Ospedale San Raffaele
University Vita-Salute San Raffaele, Via Olgettina 60
IT–20132 Milan (Italy)
E-Mail giuseppe.querques@hotmail.it

Bandello F, Zarbin MA, Lattanzio R, Zucchiatti I (eds): Management of Diabetic Retinopathy.
Dev Ophthalmol. Basel, Karger, 2017, vol 60, pp 56–62 (DOI: 10.1159/000459690)

Emerging Simplified Retinal Imaging

Ashish Sharma

Department of Vitreoretina, Lotus Eye Hospital and Institute, Coimbatore, India

Abstract

Diabetic retinopathy (DR), a major microvascular complication of diabetes, has a significant impact on the world's health systems. Globally, the number of people with DR will grow from 126.6 million in 2010 to 191.0 million by 2030, and it is estimated that the number with vision-threatening diabetic retinopathy will increase from 37.3 million to 56.3 million if prompt action is not taken. Lack of early diagnosis and management is the leading cause of blindness in working-age populations The gap between demand and annual eye examinations has been a big challenge. Furthermore lack of availability of cost effective simplified retinal imaging tools has limited the diabetic retinopathy screening program in many parts of the world in last few decades. This has led to the development of innovative ideas and availability of cost effective simplified retinal imaging tools. In this chapter we will be describing some of the well known commercially available emerging simplified (Non Tabletop, Hand Held, Portable) retinal imaging tools that have potential to help in screening diabetic retinopathy with ease and without increasing financial burden.

MII Ret Cam

Make In India Retinal Camera (MII Ret Cam) is a fundus imaging device that works on the principle of indirect ophthalmoscopy. However, it works as a fundus camera due to its ability to capture fundus images and record them.

The device consists of a slot for a smartphone and 20 D lens with optional 28 D lens (Fig. 1). The device is specially designed for single-hand operation. This allows the other hand to be utilized either for indentation or to open the patient's eye lids [1]. The device has been designed to fit any smartphone, Android or IOS, provided the distance between cameras or flashlight is close.

MII Ret Cam Device needs a smartphone app (miiretcam app) while imaging. MII Ret Cam utilizes the smartphone light as an illumination source. MII Ret Cam app allows the smartphone flashlight to be ON even in still picture mode. Furthermore, it allows patient data storage which can be easily shared.

MII Ret Cam overcomes the imaging difficulties of traditional fundus cameras such as cost,

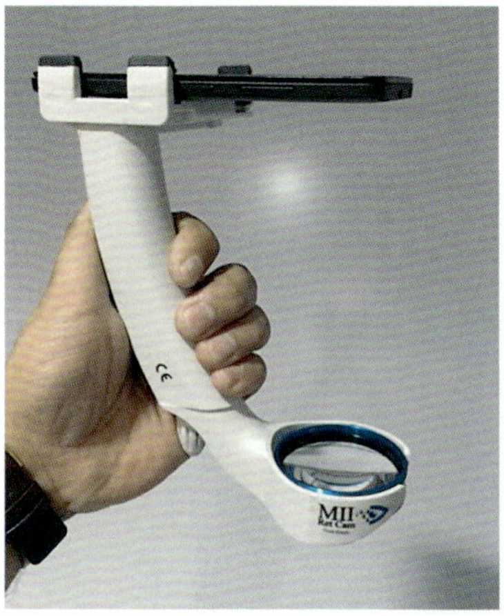

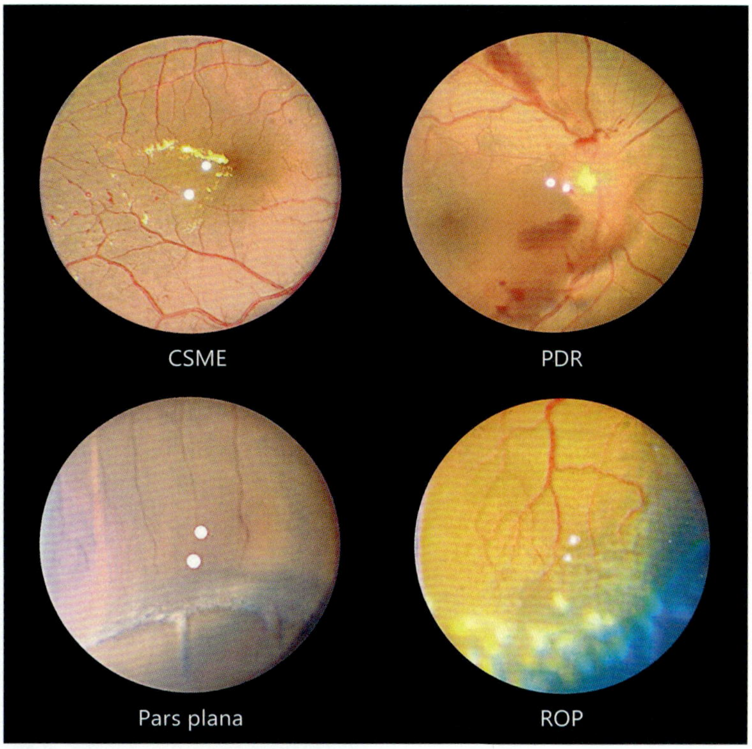

Fig. 1. MII Ret Cam fundus imaging device with smartphone and 20 D lens.

Fig. 2. Images captured with MII Ret Cam from central fundus up to ora serrata and pars plana. Further imaging capabilities in pediatric age group, including ROP.

portability, peripheral imaging, and pediatric imaging (Fig. 2). MII Ret Cam can also be utilized in diffuse light anterior segment imaging.

Advantages

Single-hand operation and light weight (150 g device weight).

Works on both Android and iPhones (MII Ret Cam iOS app has an inbuilt light intensity control).

Ability to capture peripheral retina images up to pars plana.

Ability to demonstrate retinopathy of prematurity and other pediatric retinal conditions.

Anterior segment imaging.

Limitations

Need dilation.

Approx cost – USD 350.

Information

www.miiretcam.com.

Paxos Scope

The Paxos Scope is another fundus imaging device that works on the principle of indirect ophthalmoscopy. It also works as a fundus camera due to its ability to capture fundus images and record them [2].

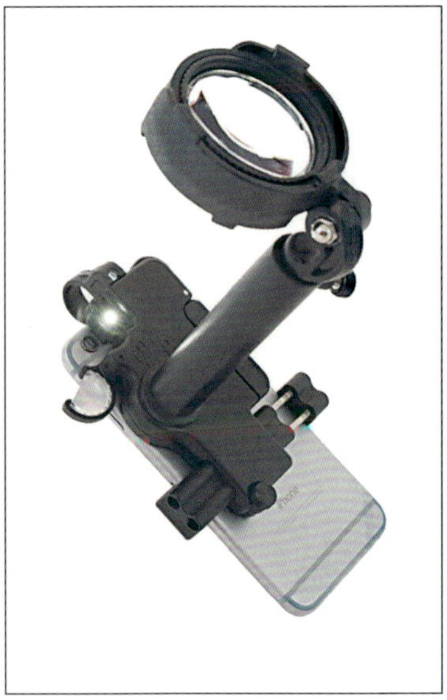

Fig. 3. Paxos Scope fundus imaging device with smartphone and 20 D lens.

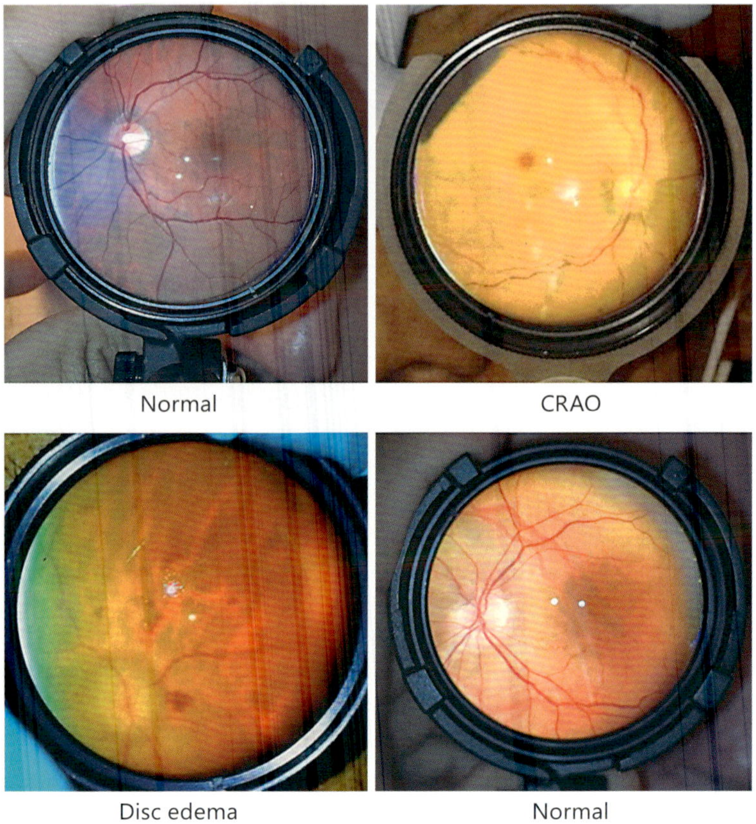

Fig. 4. Fundus images captured with Paxos Scope.

The device consists of a slot for a smartphone and 20 D lens with optional rings for other lenses (Fig. 3). The Paxos Scope uses external LED light as an illumination source with intensity control. Images are stored in the cloud.

The Paxos Scope overcomes imaging difficulties of traditional fundus cameras such as cost, portability etc. Apart from fundus imaging (Fig. 4), the Paxos Scope can also be utilized in diffuse light anterior segment imaging using the magnification lens inbuilt in the device.

Advantages

Light weight and portable.

Anterior segment imaging.

Limitations

Works with only iPhones.

Needs dilation.

Limitations for imaging retinal periphery.

Approx cost – subscription-based USD 79/month.

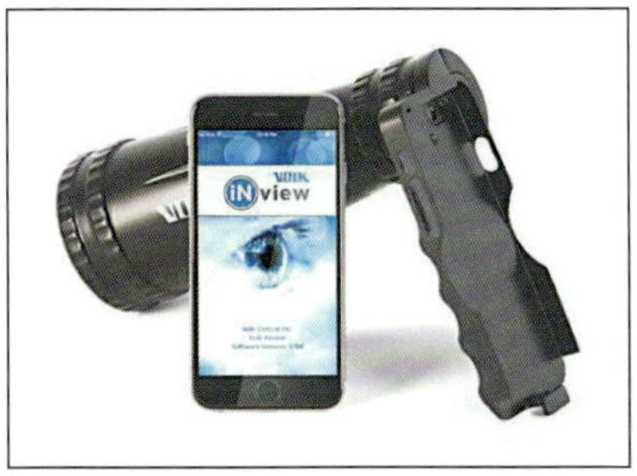

Fig. 5. Volk InView with adapter for iPhone.

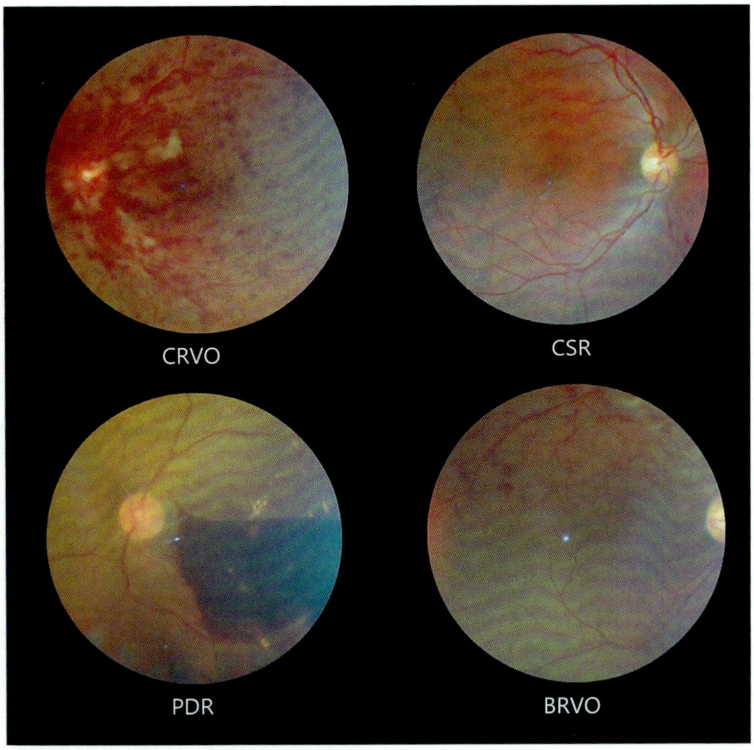

Fig. 6. Fundus images captured with Volk InView.

Information

https://www.digisight.net/ds/paxos-scope/.

Volk InView

Volk InView is a fundus imaging device that has an inbuilt condensing lens and an adapter for iPhone (Fig. 5). It is operated by 2 hands.

The Volk InView device needs a smartphone app (Volk InView) while imaging. Volk InView utilizes the smartphone light itself as an illumination source. Volk InView app allows the smartphone flashlight to be ON even in still picture mode and has an auto capture feature. Furthermore, it allows patient data storage in their cloud.

Volk InView overcomes imaging difficulties of traditional fundus cameras, such as cost, portability. It predominantly captures fundus images (Fig. 6).

Advantages

Light weight and portable.

Autocapture feature.

Limitations

Works only with iPhone 5, 6, 6s and ipod touch (Gen 6).

Needs dilation.

No anterior segment imaging.

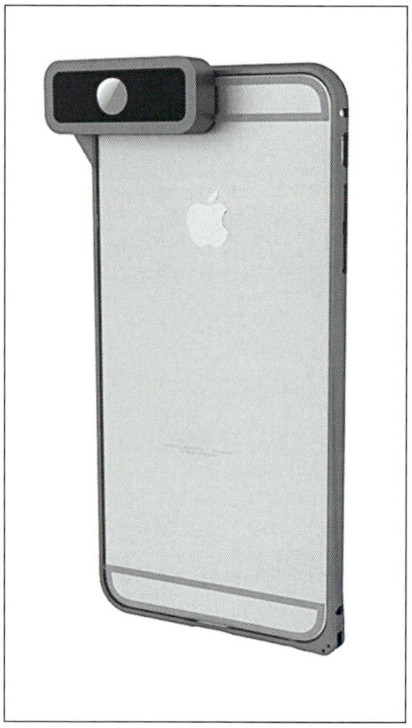

Fig. 7. D Eye device with smartphone.

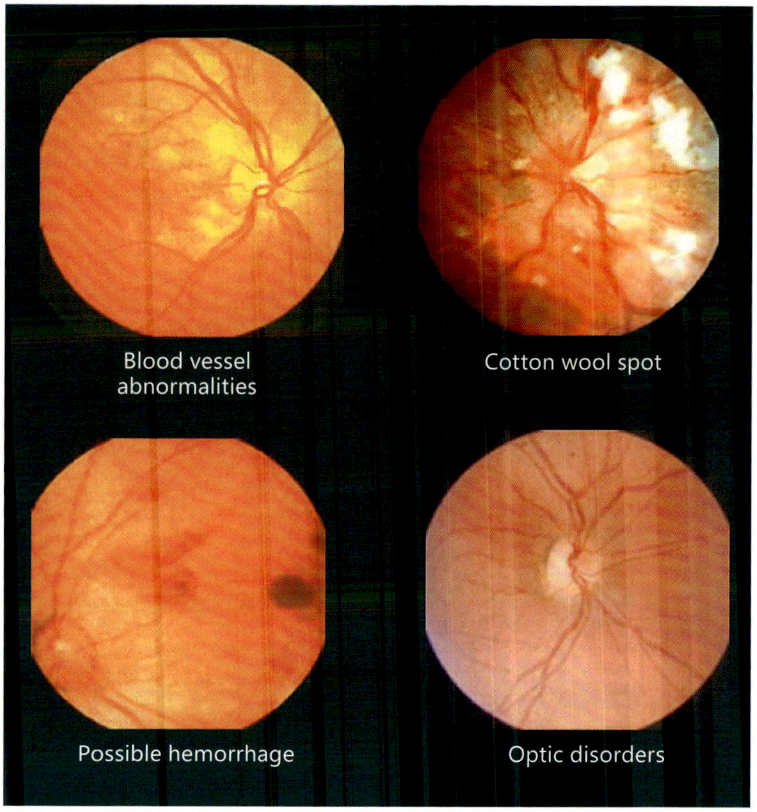

Fig. 8. Fundus images captured with D Eye.

Limitation to image retinal periphery.
Approx cost – USD 1,500.

Information

https://volk.com/index.php/volk-products/ophthalmic-cameras/volk-inview.htmlRef.

D-Eye

D-Eye is a fundus imaging device that is in the form of a small rectangular attachment having inbuilt optics (Fig. 7). The device needs to be attached magnetically to the smartphone camera. It is operated by one hand. It needs a bumper to be placed around the smartphone to fit the device [3].

D Eye utilizes the smartphone light itself as an illumination source.

D Eye overcomes imaging difficulties of traditional fundus cameras, such as cost, portability. It predominantly captures fundus images (Fig. 8).

Advantages

Light weight and portable.

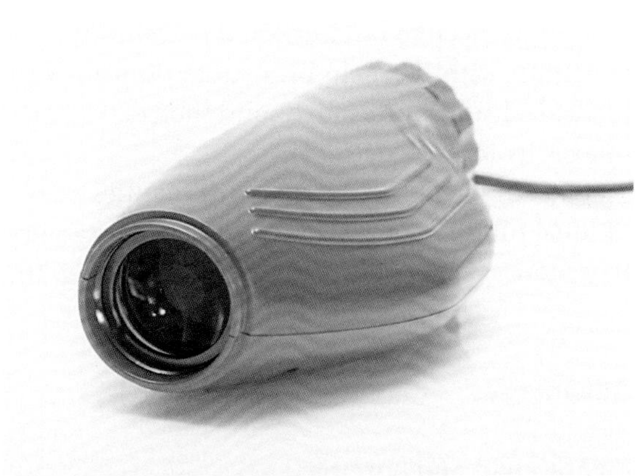

Fig. 9. Epicam device with connecting cable.

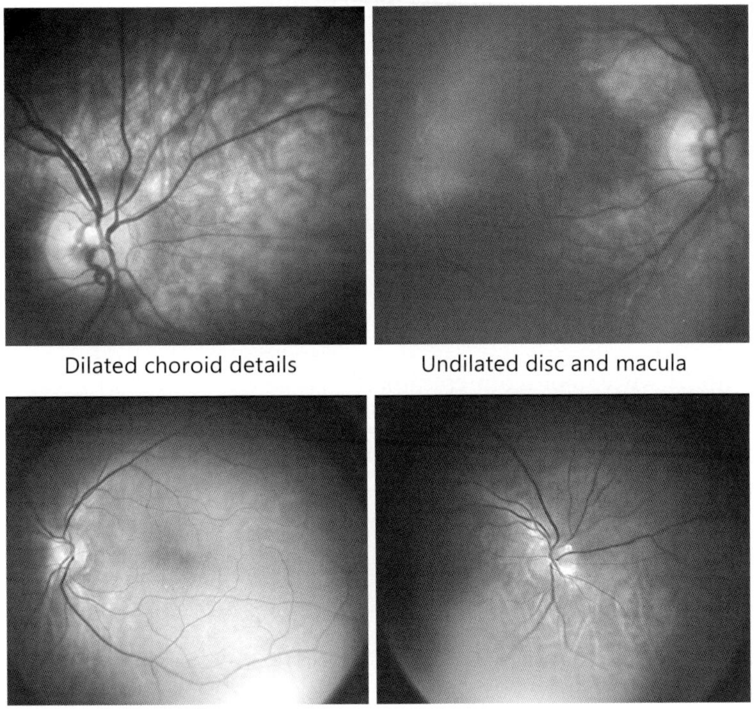

Dilated choroid details | Undilated disc and macula

Dilated disc and macula | Dilated optic disc

Fig. 10. Fundus images captured with Epicam.

Limitations

Works only with iPhone 5,5s 6, 6s, 6s Plus.

Very limited field of view (undilated- 6 degree; dilated- 20 degree).

Approx cost – USD 435.

Information

https://www.d-eyecare.com/en_US/product.

Epicam

Epicam is a fundus imaging device that is in the form of a tube having inbuilt optics (Fig. 9).

Epicam need to be connected to a smartphone or laptop with the help of a cable. Epicam captures black and white videos and then extracts the images from the videos [4].

Epicam overcomes imaging difficulties of traditional fundus cameras, such as cost, portability. It predominantly captures fundus images (Fig. 10).

Advantages

Light weight and portable.

Can be used in mid-dilated pupil (4 mm).

Limitations

Only black and white fundus images are captured.

Approx cost – USD 2,000.

Information

http://www.epipole.com/epicam/ef.

The above mentioned fundus imaging devices are smartphone-based and have revolutionized fundus imaging in the recent past in terms of simplicity. However, non-smartphone-based handheld fundus imaging devices are commercially available, manufactured by different companies. Here, we will mention the name of some of the most common fundus imaging devices. The major advantage of these devices over smartphone-based devices is that images can be achieved through an undilated pupil. However, cost effectiveness of these devices is poor, as they cost approximately 10–20 times more compared to smartphone-based devices mentioned above. Furthermore, the area of imaging is also much less compared to smartphone-based devices. Describing all the devices is beyond the scope of this chapter; hence, only brief information is provided.

1. VISUSCOT 100-ZEISS
2. SMARTSCOPE-OPTOMED
3. KOWA GENESIS D-KOWA
4. PICTOR PLUS-VOLK
5. BAUSCH FUNDUS CAMERA
6. HORUS SCOPE-JEDMED
7. VERSA CAM-NIDEK

Disclaimer

Dr. Ashish Sharma is the lead innovator of MII Ret Cam and has financial interest.

References

1 Sharma A, Subramaniam SD, Ramachandran KI, Lakshmikanthan C, Krishna S, Sundaramoorthy SK: Smartphone-based fundus camera device (MII Ret Cam) and technique with ability to image peripheral retina. Eur J Ophthalmol 2016;26:142–144.

2 Ludwig CA, Murthy SI, Pappuru RR, Jais A, Myung DJ, Chang RT: A novel smartphone ophthalmic imaging adapter: user feasibility studies in Hyderabad, India. Indian J Ophthalmol 2016;64:191–200.

3 Russo A, Morescalchi F, Costagliola C, Delcassi L, Semeraro F: A novel device to exploit the smartphone camera for fundus photography. J Ophthalmol 2015;2015:823139.

4 Watson S, Burgess F, Blaikie A: Remote Interpretation of Optic Nerve Head Cupping from Images Acquired Using A New Low Cost Retinal Camera (epiCam) Capable of Being Powered and Operated from an Android Based Mobile Phone. Presented at Scottish Ophthalmological Club, September 2016.

Dr. Ashish Sharma, MS
Department of Vitreoretina
Lotus Eye Hospital and Institute
Coimbatore, Tamil Nadu 641014 (India)
E-Mail drashish79@hotmail.com

Bandello F, Zarbin MA, Lattanzio R, Zucchiatti I (eds): Management of Diabetic Retinopathy.
Dev Ophthalmol. Basel, Karger, 2017, vol 60, pp 63–70 (DOI: 10.1159/000460496)

Intravitreal Ranibizumab in Diabetic Macular Edema: Long-Term Outcomes

Ilaria Zucchiatti • Francesco Bandello

Department of Ophthalmology, Vita-Salute University, Scientific Institute San Raffaele, Milan, Italy

Abstract

Intravitreal ranibizumab (RBZ) has been shown in multiple randomized clinical trials to be a valuable treatment for diabetic macular edema (DME), promoting a significant improvement in best-corrected visual acuity (BCVA) and in anatomic outcomes. Compared to sham (RISE and RIDE studies), RBZ rapidly and sustainably improved BCVA and decreased macular edema at 2 years, reducing the risk of further vision loss, with low rates of local or systemic side effects. Compared to macular laser photocoagulation (READ-2 study), RBZ provided a greater improvement in BCVA and regression in foveal thickness, but required a higher number of injections compared to patients treated with both RBZ and laser. In RESTORE trial, RBZ alone or combined with macular laser turned out to be superior to laser alone, without significant differences between the 2 RBZ groups. Compared to combined treatment (RBZ or triamcinolone associated with macular laser) or photocoagulation laser alone (Diabetic Retinopathy Clinical Research Network trial), RBZ with prompt or deferred laser was more effective than laser alone at 1-year follow-up. At 3 years, prompt laser was not better than deferring laser for 24 weeks or more. At 5 years, subjects treated with RBZ achieved better long-term visual outcomes than patients managed with triamcinolone or laser followed by very deferred RBZ. In conclusion, randomized clinical trials showed that RBZ was superior to laser in DME treatment, providing excellent long-term visual outcomes. Frequent injections were necessary in most of the patients to properly control DME and maximize the visual benefits.

Vascular endothelial growth factor (VEGF) has a crucial role in the development and progression of diabetic macular edema (DME). This homodimeric protein is implicated in vascular permeability and neovascularization, promoting vascular endothelial cell growth. Increased levels of VEGF have been identified in the anterior and vitreous chambers, correlating with DME severity [1, 2]. A number of clinical trials demonstrated that VEGF is an important therapeutic target for DME. Different classes of VEGF inhibitors are currently used, including ranibizumab (Lucentis®), bevacizumab (Avastin®), pegaptanib sodium (Macugen®), and aflibercept (Eylea®).

Ranibizumab (Lucentis®, Genentech, Inc., South San Francisco, CA, USA) is a humanized monoclonal antibody fragment designed to bind all active isoforms of VEGF-A and their biological degradation products [3]. Ranibizumab (RBZ) is currently approved in United States and European Union for the treatment of DME. Several randomized clinical trials have analyzed the effectiveness and safety of intravitreal RBZ alone or adjunctive to laser photocoagulation in DME treatment (Fig. 1, 2).

The READ-1 study published in 2006, the earliest results regarding intravitreal RBZ (0.5 mg) as a monotherapy compared to sham, showed in a few patients a significant reduction in central foveal thickness (CFT) and a meaningful improvement in best-corrected visual acuity (BCVA) [4].

In 2010, the RESOLVE study, a 12-month multicenter clinical trial, compared the effects of intravitreal RBZ (0.3 or 0.5 mg) to sham therapy [5]. Randomized patients underwent 3 monthly injections and were then retreated if needed, on a pro-re-nata (PRN) regimen. Rescue laser was offered according to protocol-defined criteria. After month-1, the subjects could receive a dose-doubling RBZ injection if they met the per-protocol-specified criteria. At 12 months, patients treated with RBZ experienced a significant improvement in BCVA (10.3 letter increase) compared to sham (1.4 letter decrease) and a meaningful reduction in central retinal thickness (CRT). Sixty percent of patients treated with RBZ experienced an increase of 10 or more letters, compared to 18% of placebo patients. In addition, intravitreal RBZ showed a safety profile consistent with previous studies.

In 2012, intravitreal RBZ (0.5 or 0.3 mg) was compared to sham injections in the RISE and RIDE studies [6]. Macular laser was considered as a rescue treatment according to defined criteria. At 24-month follow-up, patients treated with RBZ achieved a rapid and sustained improvement in vision and also a reduction in macular edema compared to sham. In the RIDE study, 33 and 45% of patients treated respectively with low and high RBZ dosing experienced a visual improvement of ≥15 letters compared to 12% of placebo subjects. In the RISE study, the percentage of patients that gained ≥15 letters was 45% in 0.3 mg RBZ group and 39% in 0.5 mg RBZ group versus 18% in the sham cohort. Low rates of local or systemic side effects were noted, consistent with prior RBZ studies. Moreover, patients treated with RBZ underwent fewer macular laser procedures compared to sham.

Recently, an analysis of data of RISE and RIDE studies evaluated the BCVA and retinal thickness outcomes of subjects with DME and delayed anatomic response after 3 RBZ injections over 24 months [7]. Patients included in the study were divided into 3 groups: immediate responders (patients treated with RBZ who showed more than 10% reduction in CFT after 3 injections), delayed responders (patients with a reduction of 10% or less), and sham-treated patients. The study revealed that 9–10% of RBZ-treated eyes were considered delayed responders. At 24 months, delayed responders turned out to have less CFT reduction but a similar number of letters gained from baseline and similar improvement in diabetic retinopathy (DR) severity compared to immediate responders. This analysis demonstrated that a small number of patients might be slow to respond anatomically, but they still could achieve vision improvement and DR improvement comparable to immediate responders with continued RBZ injections over 24 months of follow-up.

Fig. 1. A 68-year-old man with type-2 diabetes mellitus and poor glycemic control came for follow-up. Macular laser was performed 4 months earlier in the right eye. Nevertheless, the patient still complained of persistent metamorphopsia and low vision in the right eye; the best-corrected visual acuity was 20/63. **a** Ultra-wide-field fluorescein angiography of right eye showing a breakdown of the blood-retinal barrier, macular laser spots and localized areas of retinal ischemia. Autofluorescence (**b**) and color image (**c**) disclosed the presence of laser spots, retinal hemorrhages, hard exudates, and macular edema. **d** SD-OCT scan revealed macular edema with large intraretinal cysts and hard exudates.
(*For figure see next page.*)

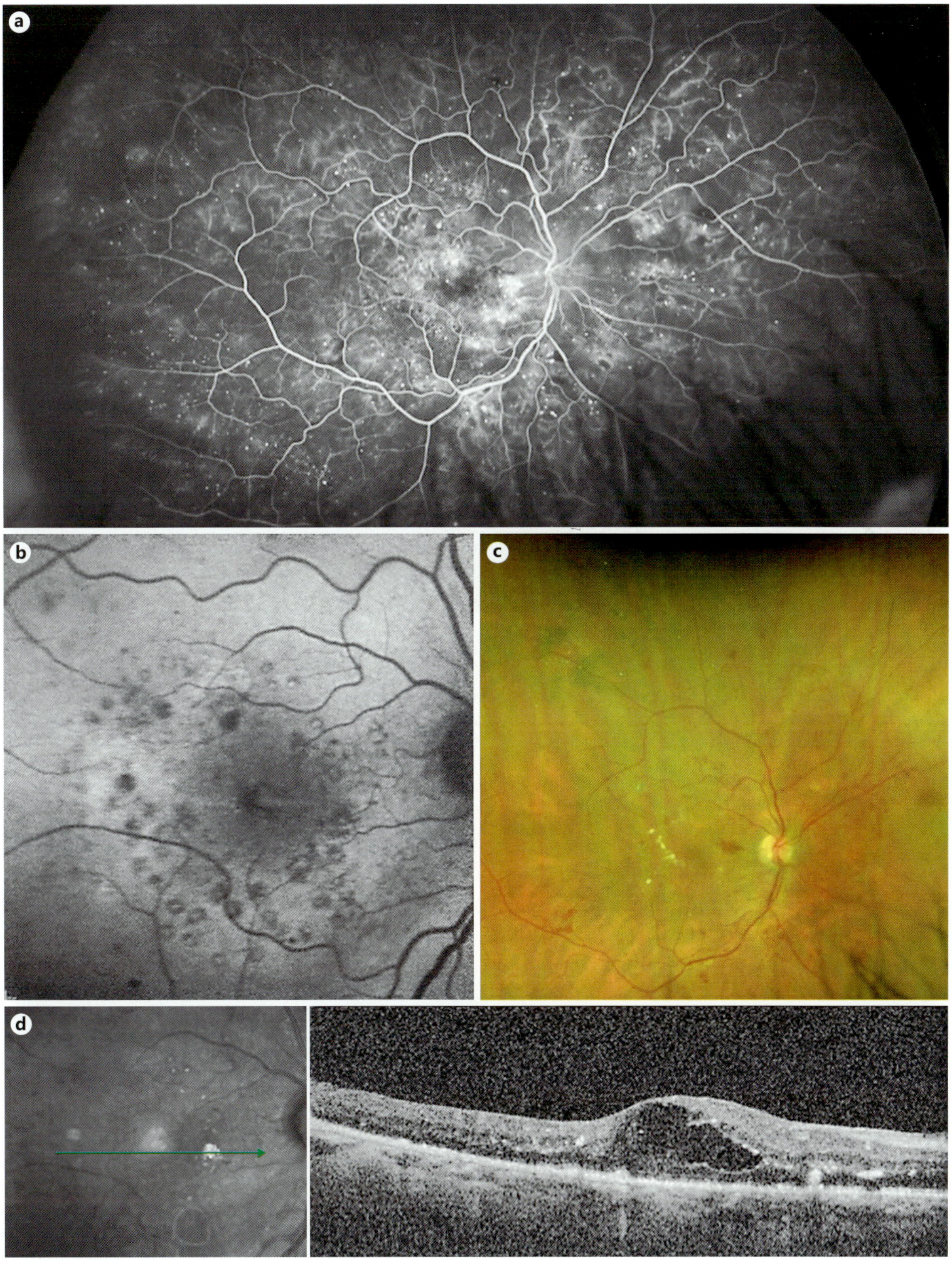

1

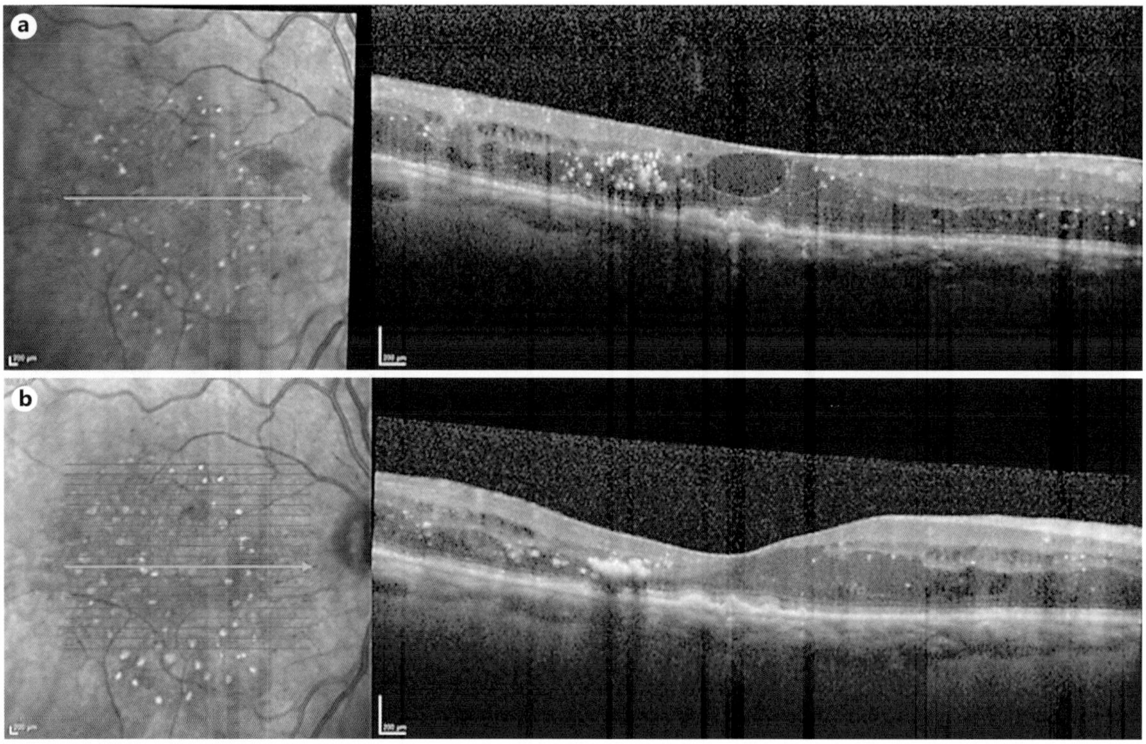

Fig. 2. Follow-up of the same patient of Figure 1 treated with intravitreal ranibizumab (RBZ) injections. **a** After 3 intravitreal injections of RBZ (loading phase), the best-corrected visual acuity (BCVA) showed a mild improvement to 20/50. SD-OCT examination revealed the persistence of macular edema with a large central intraretinal cyst and hard exudates. **b** At 9-month follow-up, after a total of 5 intravitreal injections, SD-OCT showed flattening of the retina with persistence of small intraretinal cysts and hard exudates. BCVA was 20/40.

Predictors of the frequency of RBZ injections for DME treatment in the open-label extension were identified [8]. Patients with less advanced disease at baseline received less frequent injections, responding better to RBZ.

The effect of RBZ on hard exudate resolution has been assessed in a recent exploratory analysis of RISE and RIDE studies, with RBZ-treated patients showing a greater reduction of hard exudates compared to sham controls [9]. The reabsorption of hard exudates was slower and more gradual than fluid resolution; nevertheless, the total area of hard exudates did not increase after treatment.

A recent post-hoc analysis of the RIDE and RISE trials evaluated the effects of systemic factors on vision changes from baseline in DME patients treated with RBZ [10]. The study revealed that the BCVA improvement with RBZ was not influenced by systemic factors, including diabetes medication history, serum glucose, glycosylated hemoglobin, blood pressure, body mass index, and renal function. This study suggested that the visual response to RBZ in DME was not influenced by systemic factors related to the management of diabetes.

The READ-2 randomized clinical trial compared RBZ with focal/grid laser photocoagulation or a combination of both in patients with DME [11, 12]. At 6 months (primary end-point), patients treated with intravitreal RBZ injections showed a significantly better outcome in BCVA

(+7.24 letters) than those treated with only macular laser photocoagulation (–0.43 letters) [5]. Patients included in the combination group did not achieve a statistically significant improvement in BCVA (+3.80 letters) compared to other groups. After the primary end-point, most subjects in all groups were treated only with RBZ. At 2 years, intravitreal RBZ continued to show positive effects in terms of BCVA gain or CFT reduction [12]. In addition, in the combination group, the amount of residual edema and the frequency of required injection were lower compared to other groups. The mean number of injections was 5.4, 4.4, and 2.9 in RBZ, laser, and combined groups, respectively during the 18 months following the primary end-point. The authors concluded that RBZ alone or with additional laser seemed to be more effective than macular laser alone. Later, the extended study [13] evaluated visual and anatomical outcomes at 3 years, analyzing also the need for prolonged frequent retreatment. Patients treated only with RBZ showed a further improvement in BCVA at month-36, compared to month-24 (10.3 vs. 7.2 letters) and an extra regression in CFT. The RBZ plus laser and the laser alone groups did not achieve a significant variation in terms of BCVA and CFT at year-3 compared to year-2. The mean number of injections was greater in the RBZ group (5.4) compared to laser alone (2.3 injections) and the RBZ + laser (3.3) groups, secondary to the more extensive laser therapy performed. Basically, the study showed that RBZ provided excellent long-term visual outcomes; however, frequent injections are required in most patients to properly control DME and maximize the visual benefits.

In 2011, in RESTORE trial, RBZ alone or combined with laser was compared to laser monotherapy in the treatment of DME [14]. Injections were administered for 3 months and then PRN; laser or sham laser was performed at baseline and then repeated, if needed. At 12 months, RBZ alone or combined with macular laser was superior to laser alone. Patients treated with RBZ alone or combined with laser gained almost 6 letters from baseline compared to laser monotherapy (+0.8 letters). Patients received a mean of 7 injections of RBZ or sham over 12 months. Basically, the study did not reveal significant differences between RBZ alone and RBZ + laser groups. The safety profile was similar to previous studies with RBZ.

The Diabetic Retinopathy Clinical Research Network (DRCR.net) evaluated with a large, multicenter, randomized trial (Protocol I) the effectiveness of RBZ (0.5 mg) versus triamcinolone (4 mg) combined with macular laser photocoagulation versus laser alone [15–17]. Subjects were randomized into 4 arms: sham injection + prompt laser, RBZ + prompt laser, RBZ + deferred (24 weeks or more after RBZ initiation) laser, and triamcinolone + prompt laser. At year-1, the study demonstrated that RBZ with prompt or deferred laser was more effective compared to laser alone [15]. The authors concluded that RBZ should be considered as a valuable treatment for patients with DME. Intravitreal triamcinolone + prompt laser at year-1 was more effective than laser alone even if the risk of intraocular pressure elevation was higher. The 2-year expanded trial confirmed these results, reinforcing the conclusion that RBZ could be considered for DME patients with similar characteristics to the enrolled subjects [16]. In the extended study, patients originally assigned to triamcinolone injections + prompt laser or sham injection + laser were considered for switching to intravitreal RBZ in case of persistent DME with vision impairment. The results at year-3 demonstrated that prompt laser was no better and possibly worse than deferring laser for 24 weeks or more in the study population [17]. At year-3, fewer RBZ injections were given in the prompt laser group causing a difference in BCVA compared to previous published results. Sixty-seven percent of patients completed the 5-year follow-up [18]. The study showed that patients treated with RBZ with immediate or deferred laser achieved significant BCVA and retinal thickness improvements that were sustained over time. At year-5, subjects treated with RBZ for center-involving DME achieved better long-term visual outcomes than patients managed with triamcinolone or laser followed by very deferred RBZ for persistent DME and vision impairment.

The effects of RBZ in the case of persistent macular thickening despite therapy have been investigated through a recent post-hoc, exploratory analysis of the DRCR.net Protocol I trial [19]. Patients randomly assigned to the RBZ arm with DME persisting for 24 weeks after initiating therapy were included in this post-hoc assessment. Forty percent of included patients had chronic persistent DME at 3 years despite therapy. Nevertheless, vision outcomes were only slightly worse compared to the remaining 60% of patients in who DME did not persist. The authors concluded that substantial vision loss (2 or more lines of BCVA drop) was uncommon at 3 years despite chronic persistent DME.

Pooled data from the RBZ + prompt or deferred laser treatment arms of the Protocol I study were analyzed through a post-hoc analysis, to determine whether early visual acuity response to RBZ is associated with long-term outcomes [20]. The authors classified the BCVA improvement in 3 groups: <5-letter, 5- to 9-letter, or ≥10-letter change at 12 weeks compared to baseline. They found that 39.7, 23.2, and 37.1% of eyes, respectively, at 12 weeks, and 34.2, 16.5, and 49.3% of eyes at 156 weeks reached a BCVA improvement of <5-letter, 5- to 9-letter, or ≥10-letters. This post-hoc assessment demonstrated that eyes with suboptimal (<5 letter) early BCVA improvement reached a poorer long-term visual gain than eyes with pronounced (≥10-letter) response.

Another exploratory post-hoc assessment of the DRCR.net Protocol I trial evaluated the effectiveness of RBZ on patients with DME who previously underwent vitrectomy [21]. The analysis did not identify any substantial differences compared to patients without vitrectomy in terms of visual acuity or CRT outcomes.

In the more recent READ-3 trial (RBZ for edema of the mAcula in Diabetes-Protocol 3 with high dose), intravitreal RBZ was tested at different dosages: 2.0 versus 0.5 mg [22]. At month-6 (primary outcome), after 6 monthly injections in both groups, there was no statistically significant difference in the 2 arms in terms of the number of letters gained. Thus, the authors concluded that 2 mg intravitreal RBZ did not provide additional benefits compared to 0.5 mg RBZ. After month-6, enrolled subjects received RBZ injections based on a PRN regimen [23]. At month-24, patients in both groups showed a further improvement in vision and retinal thickness, sustaining the benefits achieved at month-6. The results at 24 months confirmed PRN 2.0 mg intravitreal RBZ did not seem to provide additional benefits over PRN 0.5 mg RBZ after 6 month loading doses. In a retrospective cohort study of month-6 primary outcomes in the READ-3 study, patients with DME and vitreomacular adhesion (VMA) were analyzed [24]. The study showed that intravitreal RBZ has a greater potential for visual improvement in DME patients with VMA.

Nowadays, current investigations are also targeting the treatment schedule to define individualized dosing regimens of RBZ, to reduce the frequency of visits and patients' treatment burden. While in real world, most of the clinicians used a PRN regimen in which patients who came for monthly visits were retreated on the basis of active signs of disease activity; new treatment strategies are presently under assessment. In RELIGHT study, an individualized treatment of DME with RBZ injections followed by bimonthly monitoring has been investigated [25]. Patients underwent 3 monthly injections followed by 3 monthly visits with PRN retreatment and then bimonthly monitoring with PRN injections. The mean BCVA gain was +6.6, +4.8, and + 6.5 letters at 6, 12, and 18 months, respectively. The study demonstrated that the initial BCVA gain obtained at 6 months with monthly follow-up was maintained at 18 months with bimonthly visits.

The authors concluded that a less strict follow-up regimen could be considered as a possible strategy for a mid- and long-term management of DME.

Another treatment approach to individualize DME management currently under investigation is the treat-and-extend (T&E) regimen. This alternative scheme allows incremental augmentation in treatment intervals targeted to identify the longest possible treatment interval, reducing the number of visits. The RETAIN study evaluated the non-inferiority of the T&E regimen with/without laser to RBZ PRN in patients with DME [26] in 24 months of follow-up. Patients were randomized in 3 groups: T&E + laser, T&E, and PRN. They underwent monthly RBZ until BCVA stabilization and then according to the treatment regimen. The study showed that the T&E and T&E + laser groups were non-inferior to PRN. The mean BCVA change from baseline to month-24 was similar across groups: +8.3, +6.5, and +8.1 letters in T&E + laser, T&E and PRN groups, respectively. The mean number of injections was 12.4, 12.8, and 10.7 in the 3 arms, respectively. The 2 T&E regimens revealed 46% reduction in the number of follow-up visits. In conclusion, T&E regimen could be considered a feasible treatment option for patients with DME, requiring less clinical visits, but slightly more number of injections.

In conclusion, the results of these and other randomized clinical trials demonstrated a substantial improvement in vision and anatomic outcomes in patients treated with RBZ for DME. Patient and clinician expectation of increased visual outcome is increasing over time following these promising results. Nevertheless, in the future, developing treatment strategies, including new anti-VEGF therapies or combined treatment, may emerge to improve the visual acuity outcomes and will require additional studies.

Financial Disclosures

I.Z.: none.

F.B.: consultant for Alcon, Allergan, Alimera Science, Bayer, Bausch&Lomb, Boehringer-Ingelheim, Farmila Thea, Genentech, Hofmann La Roche, Novagali Pharma, Novartis, Sanofi Aventis, Santen, Sifi, Sooft, Thrombogenics, Zeiss.

References

1 Funatsu H, Yamashita H, Nakamura S, Mimura T, Eguchi S, Noma H, Hori S: Vitreous levels of pigment epithelium-derived factor and vascular endothelial growth factor are related to diabetic macular edema. Ophthalmology 2006;113:294–301.

2 Roh MI, Kim HS, Song JH, Lim JB, Kwon OW: Effect of intravitreal bevacizumab injection on aqueous humor cytokine levels in clinically significant macular edema. Ophthalmology 2009;116:80–86.

3 Ferrara N, Davis-Smyth T: The biology of vascular endothelial growth factor. Endocr Rev 1997;18:4–25.

4 Nguyen QD, Tatlipinar S, Shah SM, Haller JA, Quinlan E, Sung J, Zimmer-Galler I, Do DV, Campochiaro PA: Vascular endothelial growth factor is a critical stimulus for diabetic macular edema. Am J Ophthalmol 2006;142:961–969.

5 Massin P, Bandello F, Garweg JG, Hansen LL, Harding SP, Larsen M, Mitchell P, Sharp D, Wolf-Schnurrbusch UE, Gekkieva M, Weichselberger A, Wolf S: Safety and efficacy of ranibizumab in diabetic macular edema (RESOLVE study): a 12-month, randomized, controlled, double-masked, multicenter phase II study. Diabetes Care 2010;33:2399–2405.

6 Nguyen QD, Brown DM, Marcus DM, Boyer DS, Patel S, Feiner L, Gibson A, Sy J, Rundle AC, Hopkins JJ, Rubio RG, Ehrlich JS; RISE and RIDE Research Group: Ranibizumab for diabetic macular edema: results from 2 phase III randomized trials: RISE and RIDE. Ophthalmology 2012;119:789–801.

7 Pieramici DJ, Wang PW, Ding B, Gune S: Visual and anatomic outcomes in patients with diabetic macular edema with limited initial anatomic response to ranibizumab in RIDE and RISE. Ophthalmology 2016;123:1345–1350.

8 Wykoff CC, Elman MJ, Regillo CD, Ding B, Lu N, Stoilov I: Predictors of diabetic macular edema treatment frequency with ranibizumab during the open-label extension of the RIDE and RISE trials. Ophthalmology 2016;123:1716–1721.

9 Domalpally A, Ip MS, Ehrlich JS: Effects of intravitreal ranibizumab on retinal hard exudate in diabetic macular edema: findings from the RIDE and RISE phase III clinical trials. Ophthalmology 2015; 122:779–786.
10 Singh RP, Habbu K, Ehlers JP, Lansang MC, Hill L, Stoilov I: The impact of systemic factors on clinical response to ranibizumab for diabetic macular edema. Ophthalmology 2016;123:1581–1587.
11 Nguyen QD, Shah SM, Heier JS, Do DV, Lim J, Boyer D, Abraham P, Campochiaro PA; READ-2 Study Group: Primary end point (six months) results of the Ranibizumab for Edema of the mAcula in Diabetes (READ-2) study. Ophthalmology 2009;116:2175–2181.e1.
12 Nguyen QD, Shah SM, Khwaja AA, Channa R, Hatef E, Do DV, Boyer D, Heier JS, Abraham P, Thach AB, Lit ES, Foster BS, Kruger E, Dugel P, Chang T, Das A, Ciulla TA, Pollack JS, Lim JI, Eliott D, Campochiaro PA; READ-2 Study Group: Two-year outcomes of the Ranibizumab for Edema of the mAcula in Diabetes (READ-2) study. Ophthalmology 2010;117:2146–2151.
13 Do DV, Nguyen QD, Khwaja AA, Channa R, Sepah YJ, Sophie R, Hafiz G, Campochiaro PA; READ-2 Study Group: Ranibizumab for Edema of the Macula in Diabetes study: 3-year outcomes and the need for prolonged frequent treatment. JAMA Ophthalmol 2013;131:139–145.
14 Mitchell P, Bandello F, Schmidt-Erfurth U, Lang GE, Massin P, Schlingemann RO, Sutter F, Simader C, Burian G, Gerstner O, Weichselberger A; RESTORE Study Group: The RESTORE study: ranibizumab monotherapy or combined with laser versus laser monotherapy for diabetic macular edema. Ophthalmology 2011;118:615–625.
15 Diabetic Retinopathy Clinical Research Network, Elman MJ, Aiello LP, Beck RW, Bressler NM, Bressler SB, Edwards AR, Ferris FL 3rd, Friedman SM, Glassman AR, Miller KM, Scott IU, Stockdale CR, Sun JK: Randomized trial evaluating ranibizumab plus prompt or deferred laser or triamcinolone plus prompt laser for diabetic macular edema. Ophthalmology 2010;117:1064–1077.e35.
16 Elman MJ, Bressler NM, Qin H, Beck RW, Ferris FL 3rd, Friedman SM, Glassman AR, Scott IU, Stockdale CR, Sun JK; Diabetic Retinopathy Clinical Research Network: Expanded 2-year follow-up of ranibizumab plus prompt or deferred laser or triamcinolone plus prompt laser for diabetic macular edema. Ophthalmology 2011;118:609–614.
17 Diabetic Retinopathy Clinical Research Network, Elman MJ, Qin H, Aiello LP, Beck RW, Bressler NM, Ferris FL 3rd, Glassman AR, Maturi RK, Melia M: Intravitreal ranibizumab for diabetic macular edema with prompt versus deferred laser treatment: three-year randomized trial results. Ophthalmology 2012;119: 2312–2318.
18 Bressler SB, Glassman AR, Almukhtar T, Bressler NM, Ferris FL, Googe JM Jr, Gupta SK, Jampol LM, Melia M, Wells JA 3rd; Diabetic Retinopathy Clinical Research Network: Five-year outcomes of ranibizumab with prompt or deferred laser versus laser or triamcinolone plus deferred ranibizumab for diabetic macular edema. Am J Ophthalmol 2016;164: 57–68.
19 Bressler SB, Ayala AR, Bressler NM, Melia M, Qin H, Ferris FL 3rd, Flaxel CJ, Friedman SM, Glassman AR, Jampol LM, Rauser ME; Diabetic Retinopathy Clinical Research Network: Persistent macular thickening after ranibizumab treatment for diabetic macular edema with vision impairment. JAMA Ophthalmol 2016;134:278–285.
20 Gonzalez VH, Campbell J, Holekamp NM, Kiss S, Loewenstein A, Augustin AJ, Ma J, Ho AC, Patel V, Whitcup SM, Dugel PU: Early and long-term responses to anti-vascular endothelial growth factor therapy in diabetic macular edema: analysis of protocol I data. Am J Ophthalmol 2016;172:72–79.
21 Bressler SB, Melia M, Glassman AR, Almukhtar T, Jampol LM, Shami M, Berger BB, Bressler NM; Diabetic Retinopathy Clinical Research Network: Ranibizumab plus prompt or deferred laser for diabetic macular edema in eyes with vitrectomy before anti-vascular endothelial growth factor therapy. Retina 2015;35:2516–2528.
22 Do DV, Sepah YJ, Boyer D, Callanan D, Gallemore R, Bennett M, Marcus DM, Halperin L, Sadiq MA, Rajagopalan N, Campochiaro PA, Nguyen QD; READ-3 Study Group: Month-6 primary outcomes of the READ-3 study (Ranibizumab for Edema of the mAcula in Diabetes-Protocol 3 with high dose). Eye (Lond) 2015;29:1538–1544.
23 Sepah YJ, Sadiq MA, Boyer D, Callanan D, Gallemore R, Bennett M, Marcus D, Halperin L, Hassan M, Campochiaro PA, Nguyen QD, Do DV; READ-3 Study Group: Twenty-four-month outcomes of the Ranibizumab for Edema of the Macula in Diabetes – protocol 3 with high dose (READ-3) study. Ophthalmology 2016;123:2581–2587.
24 Sadiq MA, Soliman MK, Sarwar S, Agarwal A, Hanout M, Demirel S, Rentiya ZS, Khan W, Do DV, Nguyen QD, Sepah YJ; READ-3 Study Group: Effect of vitreomacular adhesion on treatment outcomes in the Ranibizumab for Edema of the Macula in Diabetes (READ-3) study. Ophthalmology 2016;123:324–329.
25 Pearce I, Banerjee S, Burton BJ, Chakravarthy U, Downey L, Gale RP, Gibson J, Pagliarini S, Patel J, Sivaprasad S, Andrews C, Brittain C, Warburton J; RELIGHT Study Group: Ranibizumab 0.5 mg for diabetic macular edema with bimonthly monitoring after a phase of initial treatment: 18-month, multicenter, phase IIIB RELIGHT study. Ophthalmology 2015;122:1811–1819.
26 Prünte C, Fajnkuchen F, Mahmood S, Ricci F, Hatz K, Studnička J, Bezlyak V, Parikh S, Stubbings WJ, Wenzel A, Figueira J; RETAIN Study Group: Ranibizumab 0.5 mg treat-and-extend regimen for diabetic macular oedema: the RETAIN study. Br J Ophthalmol 2016; 100:787–795.

Ilaria Zucchiatti, MD
Department of Ophthalmology, Vita-Salute University
Scientific Institute San Raffaele
IT–20132 Milan (Italy)
E-Mail ilaria.zucchiatti@gmail.com

Bandello F, Zarbin MA, Lattanzio R, Zucchiatti I (eds): Management of Diabetic Retinopathy.
Dev Ophthalmol. Basel, Karger, 2017, vol 60, pp 71–77 (DOI: 10.1159/000460220)

Intravitreal Aflibercept in Diabetic Macular Edema: Long-Term Outcomes

Ugo Introini · Giuseppe Casalino

Department of Ophthalmology, University Vita-Salute, San Raffaele Scientific Institute, Milan, Italy

Abstract

For decades, macular laser photocoagulation has been the standard of care in the treatment of diabetic macular edema (DME). With the relatively recent advent of anti-vascular endothelial growth factor (VEGF) agents, DME treatment has entered a new era. VEGF is a well-known pro-angiogenic and pro-permeability factor involved in the pathogenesis of DME. VEGF blockade has proven remarkably effective at reducing DME and improving visual acuity (VA) in eyes with center involved DME causing VA loss in several randomized controlled trials (RCTs). Intravitreal aflibercept, ranibizumab, and bevacizumab (the latter used off-label) are 3 anti-VEGF molecules currently available for DME treatment. Aflibercerpt is a 115-kDA recombinant fusion protein consisting of VEGF binding domains of human VEGF receptors-1 and -2 fused to the Fc domain of human immunoglobulin-G1. The ability to bind placental growth factors 1 and 2 (which is another pro-permeability mediator) and a theoretically long half-life are potential advantages of aflibercept over other anti-VEGF agents. The use of intravitreal aflibercept in DME treatment has been investigated in several RCTs. The aim of this chapter is to briefly report on the current evidence for treating DME with intravitreal aflibercept.

Introduction

Current treatment options for diabetic macular edema (DME) include macular laser photocoagulation, corticosteroids, and anti-vascular endothelial growth factor (VEGF) agents (i.e., intravitreal aflibercept, ranibizumab, and off-label use of bevacizumab). While use of macular laser photocoagulation has been the standard of care for decades, a substantial group of patients are unresponsive and fail to improve after laser photocoagulation [1]. The relatively recent intravitreal use of agents aimed at neutralizing the effects of VEGF, which is a critical factor in promoting angiogenesis and vascular leakage [2], has been regarded as paradigm-shifting in DME treatment [3].

Aflibercept, previously known as VEGF Trap-EYE, is a 115-kDA recombinant fusion protein consisting of VEGF binding domains of human VEGF receptors-1 and -2 fused to the Fc domain of human immunoglobulin-G1 [4]. In some preclinical studies, intravitreal aflibercept has been shown to have advantages over other anti-VEGF

The authors have no proprietary interest in the materials used in this study.

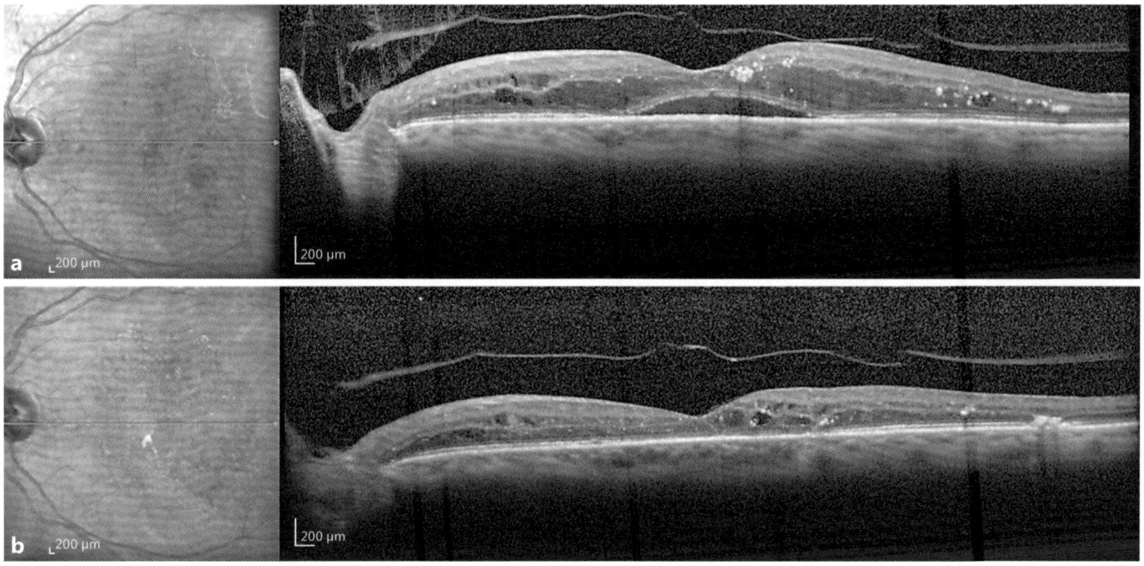

Fig. 1. Imaging of center involved diabetic macular edema (DME) of the left eye of a 62-year-old woman. **a** At the time of presentation, the best corrected visual acuity (BCVA) was 20/125, and the spectral domain optical coherence tomography (SD-OCT) scan showed diffuse center involved DME and subretinal fluid. **b** One month after 3 monthly intravitreal aflibercept injections, BCVA improved to 20/50 and SD-OCT scan showed resolution of subretinal fluid and decreased the thickness of the macula.

agents, such as ranibizumab and bevacizumab. These advantages include: an approximately 100-fold greater binding affinity to VEGF-A [5], although this result was not confirmed in other studies [6, 7]; a longer half-life [8]; and the ability to bind placental growth factors (PlGFs) 1 and 2, which have been shown to contribute to excessive vascular permeability and retinal neovascularization [9–12]. High PlGF-1 levels in the vitreous of patients with diabetic retinopathy [10] and experiments on animal models [11, 12] supported the role of PlGF in the pathogenesis of DME. Evidence that acute injection or sustained induction of PlGF in rat eyes altered the outer retinal barrier and induced vascular and retinal changes similar to those observed in the early stages of diabetic retinopathy represented the rationale of down-regulation of PlGF in DME treatment [11, 12].

Intravitreal aflibercept in patients with DME was first used in a phase 1 study, which showed that a single intravitreal injection of 4.0 mg of this agent had biologic activity by improving the visual acuity (VA) and reducing the excess retinal thickness in 5 eyes with DME [13].

Since then, efficacy and safety of multiple intravitreal aflibercept injections (IAIs) for DME treatment have been evaluated in several randomized controlled trials (RCTs) [14]. In this chapter, we will briefly cover the current evidence for treating DME with intravitreal aflibercept.

The DAVINCI Study

The DAVINCI study was a randomized, double-masked, multicenter phase 2 clinical trial, aimed at comparing different doses and dosing regimens of IAI with laser photocoagulation in eyes with DME [15, 16]. Thirty-nine sites in the United States, Canada, and Austria participated in the trial; 221 patients with center-involved DME (defined as central retinal thickness ≥250 µ in the central subfield based on optical coherence tomography – OCT) were enrolled and assigned randomly to 1 of 5 treatment regimens: (1) 0.5 mg IAI every 4 weeks (0.5q4); (2) 2 mg IAI every 4 weeks (2q4); (3) 2 mg IAI for a loading dose of 3 initial monthly doses and then every 8 weeks (2q8); (4) 2 mg VEGF Trap-Eye for 3 initial monthly doses and then on an as-needed basis (2 PRN); (5) macular laser treatment using the modified ETDRS protocol. Overall, the groups were similar with regard to demographic characteristics. However, the IAI 2q8 group had higher prevalence of type 1 diabetes and history of proliferative diabetic retinopathy compared with other groups. Moreover, the percentage of patients who had previously received grid laser was higher in the 2q8 group (66.7%) than in the other groups (47.7% in the 0.5q4 group, 52.3% in the 2q4 group, and 57.8% in the 2 PRN group). At week 24, the mean improvement in best-corrected VA (BCVA) was significantly greater for the IAI groups compared to the laser group (8.6, 11.4, 8.5, and 10.3 letters for 0.5q4, 2q4, 2q8, and 2 PRN regimens, respectively, versus 2.5 letters for the laser group). These mean improvements were maintained and even improved at week 52 (11.0, 13.1, 9.7, and 12.0 letters for 0.5q4, 2q4, 2q8, and 2 PRN regimens, respectively, versus –1.3 letters for the laser group).

Concomitant anatomical improvement was achieved with mean reduction in central retinal thickness on OCT, which was greater in the IAI groups (–165.4, –227.4, –187.8 and –180.3 microns for 0.5q4, 2q4, 2q8, and 2 PRN regimens, respectively, versus –58.4 for the laser group) at week 52.

While the study was not powered to detect differences between the different aflibercept groups, the VA gains were the highest in the 2q4 and the PRN groups and were the least in the 2q8 and the 0.5q4 groups. Since the low visual gains achieved by the 2q8 group were already evident at 4 weeks, the higher proportion of patients with a history of proliferative diabetic retinopathy, possibly indicating greater ischemia, might have accounted for the observed difference in BCVA outcome for this group. This observation was later supported by a post-hoc analysis of RISE and RIDE studies that showed that the severity of diabetic retinopathy negatively affects the response to ranibizumab injections [17]. The low visual gains achieved by the 0.5q4 group were attributed to the low efficacy of the 0.5 mg dose. With regard to safety, ocular adverse events (AEs) in patients treated with IAI were generally consistent with those seen with other intravitreal anti-VEGF agents and included conjunctival hemorrhage, eye pain, ocular hyperemia, and increased intraocular pressure; uncommon systemic AEs included hypertension, nausea, and congestive heart failure.

VISTA and VIVID

VISTA and VIVID were 2 parallel, double-masked, randomized, phase 3 trials, aimed at comparing the effects of IAI with laser treatment in DME [18]. Encouraged by results of VIEW trials, which showed bimonthly IAI after a loading dose of 3 monthly IAI having equivalent efficacy to monthly ranibizumab in the treatment of neovascular age-related macular degeneration [19], monthly and bimonthly dosing for IAI was also compared in VISTA and VIVID studies.

The VISTA study was conducted across 54 sites in the United States, and the VIVID study was conducted at 73 sites across Europe, Japan, and Australia. Overall, 872 eyes (466 in VISTA and 406 in VIVID) from 872 patients with center involved DME (defined as retinal thickening involving 1-mm central area as measured by OCT) were randomized in 3 treatment groups in a 1:1:1 ratio to receive: (1) 2 mg IAI every 4 weeks (2q4); (2) 2 mg IAI every 8 weeks after 5 initial monthly doses (from baseline to week 16) with sham injections on non-treatment visits (2q8); (3) macular laser photocoagulation at baseline and sham injections at every visit (laser control group). Study eyes in all treatment groups could also receive additional (rescue) laser treatment from week 24 onward if they lost 10 letters on 2 consecutive visits or 15 letters at any visit from the best previous measurement with BCVA worse than baseline. When criteria for additional treatment were met, study eyes in the 2q4 and 2q8 groups received active laser (rather than sham) from week 24 onward, whereas those in the laser group received 5 doses of 2 mg IAI every 4 weeks followed by dosing every 8 weeks.

While demographics and baseline characteristics of patients were similar across all treatment groups in both studies, VISTA included a greater proportion of Black or African-American patients and VIVID had a greater proportion of Asian patients. Also, more eyes in VISTA had prior anti-VEGF therapy for DME compared with VIVID (42.9 vs. 8.9%, respectively).

The mean BCVA gains from baseline to week 52 were significantly greater in the IAI 2q4 and 2q8 groups (12.5 and 10.7, respectively, vs. 0.2 letters for the laser group in VISTA, and 10.5 and 10.7, respectively, vs. 1.2 letters for the laser group in VIVID). At 100 weeks of follow-up, the visual gains in the IAI 2q4 and 2q8 groups were maintained (11.5 and 11.1, respectively, versus 0.9 letters for the laser group in VISTA, and 11.4 and 9.4, respectively, versus 0.7 letters for the laser group in VIVID) [20].

The improvements observed at 100 weeks [20] were maintained over 148 weeks of treatment [21]. The mean BCVA gains from baseline to week 148 with IAI 2q4, IAI 2q8, and laser control were 10.4, 10.5, and 1.4 letters in VISTA and 10.3, 11.7, and 1.6 letters in VIVID, respectively.

Therefore, the difference in BCVA gain between the 2 IAI treatment regimens was small at week 52, and it was absent at 100 weeks and 148 weeks. This indicates that unlike DAVINCI, visual gains were similar for IAI 2q4 and 2q8 groups with advantages of less frequent injections in terms of reduced treatment burden for 2q8 group compared to 2q4.

Also, the proportion of patients with improvements on the ETDRS Diabetic Retinopathy Severity Scale score at weeks 52, 100, and 148 was also significantly greater with IAI than with laser control, suggesting beneficial effects of intravitreal aflibercept on the severity of underlying diabetic retinopathy.

With regard to eyes that needed rescue therapy, at 52 weeks 31 and 24% of eyes in the laser group in VISTA and VIVID, respectively, needed IAI as a rescue treatment. These eyes had a gain of 4.2 and 3.5 letters compared with 0.2 and 1.2 in the group that received laser alone in VISTA and VIVID, respectively. At 100 weeks, these gains increased up to 6.3 and 5.5 letters in the rescue IAI group compared with 0.9 and 0.7 letters in the laser only group in VISTA and VIVID, respectively. Only a small percentage of patients in the IAI groups ended up receiving laser treatment as rescue treatment; 5.8% in the 2q4 group and 2.9% in the 2q8 group in VIVID and VISTA, collectively. These latter data indicate that only very few patients in the IAI group lost vision.

From week 100, patients in the laser control group who had not received IAI rescue treatment during weeks 24–96 received IAI as needed [21].

Considering IAI treatment given 'as needed' from week 100 to week 148, 87.0% of laser control eyes in VISTA and 82.0% of laser control eyes in VIVID received IAI treatment (rescue or as needed) from weeks 24 to 148.

By including VA values after all IAI treatments (rescue or "as needed"), the between-group differences narrowed but the laser control group gained significantly inferior visual outcome compared to patients who were injected from the baseline (IAI 2q4 and IAI 2q8 groups). However, no between-group differences in terms of central subfield thickness (CST) were present by week 148. This latter finding may indicate that, despite retinal thickness decrease, in eyes that did not receive IAI from baseline (laser control group), irreversible vision loss occurred because of delayed treatment with IAI.

With regard to safety, in both VISTA and VIVID, the overall incidence of ocular and non-ocular AEs was similar across treatment groups and the AE profile of IAI over the 148 weeks of the study was consistent with the known safety profile of IAI [21].

Sixty patients completing VISTA were elected to enter in a phase IV, multicenter, open-label extension study named ENDURANCE [22]. This study was aimed at evaluating both the ability of an individualized IAI retreatment approach to maintain the benefits achieved with IAIs during the VISTA DME trial and the ability of macular laser to decrease the treatment burden among patients requiring at least 2 IAIs within 24 weeks. Visual gains achieved during the 3-year VISTA DME trial were maintained through month 12 of this study with a reduced treatment frequency. In fact, 30% of patients had no clinically relevant disease activity to warrant DME treatment with IAIs suggesting that while ongoing disease monitoring is needed to identify those requiring treatment, some patients may be able to stop treatment during follow-up.

With regard to the possible role of macular laser in reducing IAI frequency among eyes requiring ongoing IAIs, through month 12, 62% of patients met macular laser criteria and no significant reduction in IAI retreatment frequency was observed after macular laser application. However, given that ENDURANCE represents at least the fourth year of treatment for these DME patients, the benefit of macular laser in reducing the injection burden was not realized because the laser was applied too late in the disease course. This observation is further supported by previous results obtained from Diabetic Retinopathy Clinical Research Network (DRCR.net) Protocol I, a RCT involving intravitreal ranibizumab, which showed that the value of macular laser in reducing treatment burden may be observed with longer clinical follow-up [23]. In fact in this study, while no difference in treatment burden was identified through year 1, by 5 years eyes receiving prompt macular laser at the beginning of the trial required fewer ranibizumab injections compared to those randomized to deferred macular laser to achieve similar visual outcome.

DRCR.net Protocol T

The DRCR.net Protocol T was a RCT aimed at comparing the effect of 3 anti-VEGF drugs, namely aflibercept, bevacizumab, and ranibizumab on the treatment of center involved DME [24, 25]. The study involved 660 adults across 89 clinical sites in the United States. Patients were randomly assigned to receive intravitreal aflibercept (2.0 mg), bevacizumab (1.25 mg) or ranibizumab (0.3 mg). Patients were injected at baseline and then every 4 weeks unless VA was 20/20 or better with dry macula on OCT, and there was no improvement or worsening in response to the past 2 injections. Laser photocoagulation therapy (focal, grid, or both) was initiated at or after the 24-week visit for persistent DME. This protocol was supported by results of a previous study that showed greater efficacy of deferred laser in comparison to prompt laser [26]. The groups were well balanced with minimal differences in baseline characteristics except for cardiovascular risk factors, which were more prevalent in the ranibizumab cohort. However, the majority of patients were white with very few Asian patients enrolled in the study. In addition, patients could only be enrolled if they had not received intravitreal anti-VEGF therapy during the year prior to enrollment.

At 12 months, the mean visual gain was significantly greater with aflibercept (+13.3 letters) than with bevacizumab (+9.7 letters) or ranibizumab (+11.2 letters). However, these differences were deemed not clinically meaningful, since they were driven by the eyes with VA of 20/50 or worse at baseline. In fact, there were no significant differences in patients with a VA score from 78 to 69 letters (equivalent to approximately 20/32–20/40), which accounted for the majority of eyes enrolled (51% of participants). A post-hoc analysis looked at the 1-year VA and OCT CST outcomes within pre-specified subgroups based on both baseline VA and CST thresholds, defined as worse (20/50 or worse) or better (20/32–20/40) VA and thicker (≥400 μm) or thinner (250–399 μm) CST [27]. These post-hoc secondary findings suggest that for eyes with better initial VA and thicker CST, some VA outcomes may be worse in the bevacizumab group than in the aflibercept and ranibizumab groups. At 2 years, all 3 anti-VEGF groups showed VA improvement in year 2 with an average of almost half the number of injections and decreased amounts of focal/grid laser photocoagulation. The overall differences in mean VA gain decreased with the mean gain of +12.8 letters for aflibercept, +12.3 letters for ranibizumab, and +10.0 letters for bevacizumab.

Among eyes with better VA at baseline, no difference was observed in vision outcomes through the 2-year visit. Among eyes with worse baseline VA, aflibercept had superior mean gain in vision at year 2 compared with bevacizumab, although the difference may not be clinically meaningful since the percentage of patients with ≥10 or ≥15 letters visual gain and the percentage of patients with ≥10 or ≥15 letters visual loss were not different among the aflibercept, bevacizumab, and ranibizumab cohorts. Of note, at 2 years the superiority of aflibercept over ranibizumab among patients with entry level ETDRS vision of 20/50 or worse, noted at 1 year, was no longer identified.

The median number of injections was similar between the 3 groups; 9 for aflibercept, 10 for bevacizumab, and 10 for ranibizumab at year 1. In year 2, the median number of injections was 5 for aflibercept and 6 for bevacizumab and ranibizumab, respectively.

The number of patients achieving dryness or a CST of 250 μm was significantly higher in the aflibercept group than in the bevacizumab group, but not in the ranibizumab group. However, a subgroup analysis showed that it was significantly higher than ranibizumab in the 20/50 or worse VA group at year 1, but not in the 20/32–20/40 group. By year 2, this difference remained but was no longer significant in the 20/50 or worse group. These data indicate that aflibercept seems to be better at reducing retinal edema than bevacizumab in all VA groups at years 1 and 2 of the trial, and only slightly better than ranibizumab in the 20/50 or worse group. However, since there were no significant differences in vision at the end of 2 years, it is unclear as to whether this anatomic difference is clinically important.

By 2 years, the number of patients needing at least 1 session of focal/grid laser photocoagulation in the aflibercept group was significantly less than in both the ranibizumab and bevacizumab groups (41, 64, and 52% in the aflibercept, bevacizumab, and ranibizumab groups, respectively). In the second year, the number of patients needing at least 1 session of laser was 20, 31, and 27% in the aflibercept, bevacizumab, and ranibizumab groups, respectively. This difference in the frequency of use of laser treatment may be attributed to differences in anatomical improvement between the 3 drugs.

Conclusion

Intravitreal anti-VEGF therapy has been shown to be safe and effective in treating center involved DME. Current evidence supports the use of intravitreal aflibercept as the first-line treatment of DME, especially for patients who have not received anti-VEGF therapy within the previous year and with ETDRS of VA 20/50 or worse at the initiation of treatment. Future studies are warranted to study long-term results of intravitreal aflibercept in DME treatment. The role of combination therapy including macular laser treatment and/or other anti-VEGF molecules and possibly new agents targeting new pathogenetic pathways should be addressed in the future.

References

1 Lee CM, Olk RJ: Modified grid laser photocoagulation for diffuse diabetic macular edema. Long-term visual results. Ophthalmology 1991;98:1594–1602.

2 Nguyen QD, Tatlipinar S, Shah SM, Haller JA, Quinlan E, Sung J, et al: Vascular endothelial growth factor is a critical stimulus for diabetic macular edema. Am J Ophthalmol 2006;142:961–969.

3 Bandello F, Casalino G, Loewenstein A, Goldstein M, Pelayes D, Battaglia Parodi M: Pharmacological approach to diabetic macular edema. Ophthalmic Res 2014;51:88–95.

4 Holash J, Davis S, Papadopoulos N, Croll SD, Ho L, Russell M, et al: VEGF-Trap: a VEGF blocker with potent antitumor effects. Proc Natl Acad Sci U S A 2002; 99:11393–11398.

5 Papadopoulos N, Martin J, Ruan Q, et al: Binding and neutralization of vascular endothelial growth factor (VEGF) and related ligands by VEGF Trap, ranibizumab and bevacizumab. Angiogenesis 2012;15:171–185.

6 Yang J, Wang X, Fuh G, et al: Comparison of binding characteristics and in vitro activities of three inhibitors of vascular endothelial growth factor A. Mol Pharm 2014;11:3421–3430.

7 Yu L, Liang XH, Ferrara N: Comparing protein VEGF inhibitors: in vitro biological studies. Biochem Biophys Res Commun 2011;408:276–281.

8 Stewart MW, Rosenfeld PJ: Predicted biological activity of intravitreal VEGF Trap. Br J Ophthalmol 2008;92:667–668.

9 Rakic JM, Lambert V, Devy L, et al: Placental growth factor, a member of the VEGF family, contributes to the development of choroidal neovascularization. Invest Ophthalmol Vis Sci 2003;44: 3186–3193.

10 Khaliq A, Foreman D, Ahmed A, Weich H, Gregor Z, McLeod D, Boulton M: Increased expression of placenta growth factor in proliferative diabetic retinopathy. Lab Invest 1998;78:109–116.

11 Miyamoto N, de Kozak Y, Jeanny JC, Glotin A, Mascarelli F, Massin P, BenEzra D, Behar-Cohen F: Placental growth factor-1 and epithelial haemato-retinal barrier breakdown: potential implication in the pathogenesis of diabetic retinopathy. Diabetologia 2007;50:461–470.

12 Kowalczuk L, Touchard E, Omri S, Jonet L, Klein C, Valamanes F, Berdugo M, Bigey P, Massin P, Jeanny JC, Behar-Cohen F: Placental growth factor contributes to micro-vascular abnormalization and blood-retinal barrier breakdown in diabetic retinopathy. PLoS One 2011;6:e17462.

13 Do DV, Nguyen QD, Shah SM, et al: An exploratory study of the safety, tolerability and bioactivity of a single intravitreal injection of vascular endothelial growth factor Trap-Eye in patients with diabetic macular oedema. Br J Ophthalmol 2009; 93:144–149.

14 Ashraf M, Souka A, Adelman R, Forster SH: Aflibercept in diabetic macular edema: evaluating efficacy as a primary and secondary therapeutic option. Eye (Lond) 2016;30:1531–1541.

15 Do DV, Nguyen QD, Boyer D, Schmidt-Erfurth U, Brown DM, Vitti R, et al: One-year outcomes of the da Vinci Study of VEGF Trap-Eye in eyes with diabetic macular edema. Ophthalmology 2012;119:1658–1665.

16 Do DV, Schmidt-Erfurth U, Gonzalez VH, Gordon CM, Tolentino M, Berliner AJ, et al: The DA VINCI Study: phase 2 primary results of VEGF Trap-Eye in patients with diabetic macular edema. Ophthalmology 2011;118:1819–1826.

17 Sophie R, Lu N, Campochiaro PA: Predictors of functional and anatomic outcomes in patients with diabetic macular edema treated with ranibizumab. Ophthalmology 2015;122:1395–1401.

18 Korobelnik JF, Do DV, Schmidt-Erfurth U, Boyer DS, Holz FG, Heier JS, et al: Intravitreal aflibercept for diabetic macular edema. Ophthalmology 2014;121: 2247–2254.

19 Heier JS, Brown DM, Chong V, et al; VIEW 1 and VIEW 2 Study Groups: Intravitreal aflibercept (VEGF Trap-Eye) in wet age-related macular degeneration. Ophthalmology 2012;119:2537–2548.

20 Brown DM, Schmidt-Erfurth U, Do DV, Holz FG, Boyer DS, Midena E, et al: Intravitreal aflibercept for diabetic macular edema: 100-week results from the VISTA and VIVID studies. Ophthalmology 2015;122:2044–2052.

21 Heier JS, Korobelnik JF, Brown DM, Schmidt-Erfurth U, Do DV, Midena E, et al: Intravitreal aflibercept for diabetic macular edema: 148-week results from the VISTA and VIVID studies. Ophthalmology 2016;123:2376–2385.

22 Wykoff CC, Le RT, Khurana RN, Brown DM, Ou WC, Wang R, Clark WL, Boyer DS; Endurance Study Group: Outcomes with as-needed aflibercept and macular laser following the phase III VISTA DME Trial: ENDURANCE 12-month extension study. Am J Ophthalmol 2017;173:56–63.

23 Elman MJ, Ayala A, Bressler NM, et al: Intravitreal ranibizumab for diabetic macular edema with prompt versus deferred laser treatment: 5-year randomized trial results. Ophthalmology 2015; 122:375–381.

24 Wells JA, Glassman AR, Ayala AR, Jampol LM, Aiello LP, Antoszyk AN, et al: Aflibercept, bevacizumab, or ranibizumab for diabetic macular edema. N Engl J Med 2015;372:1193–1203.

25 Wells JA, Glassman AR, Ayala AR, Jampol LM, Bressler NM, Bressler SB, et al: Aflibercept, bevacizumab, or ranibizumab for diabetic macular edema: two-year results from a Comparative Effectiveness Randomized Clinical Trial. Ophthalmology 2016;123:1351–1359.

26 Elman MJ, Ayala A, Bressler NM, Browning D, Flaxel CJ, Glassman AR, et al: Intravitreal Ranibizumab for diabetic macular edema with prompt versus deferred laser treatment: 5-year randomized trial results. Ophthalmology 2015; 122:375–381.

27 Wells JA, Glassman AR, Jampol LM, Aiello LP, Antoszyk AN, et al: Diabetic Retinopathy Clinical Research Network. Association of baseline visual acuity and retinal thickness with 1-year efficacy of aflibercept, bevacizumab, and ranibizumab for diabetic macular edema. JAMA Ophthalmol 2016;134:127–134.

Giuseppe Casalino
Department of Ophthalmology, University Vita-Salute
San Raffaele Scientific Institute
Via Olgettina, 60
IT–20132 Milan (Italy)
E-Mail peppecasalino@gmail.com

Bandello F, Zarbin MA, Lattanzio R, Zucchiatti I (eds): Management of Diabetic Retinopathy.
Dev Ophthalmol. Basel, Karger, 2017, vol 60, pp 78–90 (DOI: 10.1159/000459691)

Intravitreal Steroids in Diabetic Macular Edema

Rosangela Lattanzio · Maria Vittoria Cicinelli · Francesco Bandello
Department of Ophthalmology, Scientific Institute San Raffaele, Vita-Salute University, Milan, Italy

Abstract

Over the past decade, great strides have been made in the management of diabetic macular edema (DME). Therapeutic alternatives now include focal/grid laser photocoagulation, vitreo-retinal surgery, and intraocular injection of anti-angiogenic and steroid molecules. Intravitreal administration of steroids represents a fundamental alternative for recalcitrant and naive eyes with DME, especially in those cases when anti-vascular endothelial growth factor (VEGF) agents are contraindicated or a treatment regimen with fewer intravitreal injections is required. Currently, 3 intravitreal corticosteroid options for DME treatment are available: the dexamethasone delivery system, the fluocinolone acetonide insert, and off-label intravitreal triamcinolone acetonide. All 3 agents are associated with risk of cataract progression and intraocular pressure elevation, but they maintain a good safety profile. In patients who remain unresponsive to anti-VEGF therapy, are pseudophakic, at low risk for glaucoma, or who have significant cardiovascular risk, treatment with long-lasting intraocular steroids is suggested. There still remain many unanswered questions about intravitreal drugs, regarding dose, frequency, the correct regimen of each treatment, and the potential long-term side effects.

Diabetic macular edema (DME) is a multifactorial disease in which hyperglycemia initiates pro-inflammatory and pro-angiogenic cascades that lead to vascular abnormalities, breakdown of the blood-retinal barrier, and finally to intraretinal or subretinal edema. A variety of biochemical processes have been implicated in its pathogenesis, including the expression of inflammatory mediators such as intercellular adhesion molecule-1, tumor necrosis factor-α, interleukin-6, and vascular endothelial growth factor (VEGF); the recruitment and adhesion of leukocytes to the retinal vascular endothelium; and the loss of endothelial tight junction proteins [1, 2].

Over the past decade, great strides have been made in DME management. In fact, the recent advances in understanding DME pathophysiology have led to significant improvements in the therapeutic alternatives that now include focal/grid laser photocoagulation, vitreo-retinal surgery, and intraocular injections of anti-VEGF and steroid molecules [3].

Although laser photocoagulation has been considered the standard of care for DME treatment for decades, only 3% of eyes achieve a vision improvement (≥3 lines), and a substantial proportion of treated eyes remain unresponsive [4]; on the contrary, pars plana vitrectomy has generally limited indications and efficacy, being hampered by important side effects and limited visual gain [5].

Anti-VEGF injections have become the first-line medical treatment for DME [6]; randomized, multicenter clinical studies have demonstrated that VEGF inhibitors (specifically, bevacizumab, ranibizumab, and aflibercept) result in a significant gain of visual acuity in eyes with DME and improve DR severity as measured by the ETDRS retinopathy severity scale [7–11]. However, intravitreal anti-VEGF molecules, compared to laser treatment, have shorter duration of action and a higher rate of DME recurrence. This feature leads to more frequent treatment, with increased risk of adverse events related to the intraocular surgical procedure (endophthalmitis, retinal tears and holes, and vitreous hemorrhage) and drug exposure. Moreover, due to the side effects associated with anti-VEGF agents (e.g., risk of stroke, myocardial infarction), treating physicians and patients may wish to avoid anti-VEGF agents if patients have a recent history of myocardial infarction or cerebrovascular accident or are at high risk of such complications.

Due to anti-VEGF limitations, corticosteroids have been gaining great interest in DME management [12]. These molecules have demonstrated the capacity to inhibit leukostasis, adhesion, and transmigration of leukocytes and to downregulate the expression of prostaglandins, cytokines, and growth factors, especially VEGF, in both in vitro and in vivo settings [13]. In a prospective study of eyes with DME, aqueous permeability factors measured before and after dexamethasone injections, showed a significant decrease in aqueous angiopoietin-2, hepatocyte growth factor, and endocrine gland-VEGF concentrations. In addition to their anti-inflammatory function, corticosteroids alter the composition of endothelial basal membrane by changing the local ratio of laminin isoforms, suppressing basement membrane dissolution, and strengthening tight junctions to limit permeability and leakage [14]. Finally, long-term steroid usage may have a neuroprotective effect on the retina [15].

Relevant side effects of steroids are related to intraocular pressure (IOP) increase and cataract progression [16, 17]. The exact mechanism of corticosteroid-induced secondary IOP rise is not known; however, one established contributory factor is increased outflow resistance within the trabecular meshwork.

Three fluorinated synthetic corticosteroids lacking mineralocorticoid activity – triamcinolone acetonide (TA), dexamethasone phosphate, and fluocinolone acetonide (FA) – have been used for DME treatment. They differ according to their glucocorticoid-receptor binding affinities (dexamethasone > triamcinolone > fluocinolone), duration of action (from nearly 1 month to 3 years), and their lipophilicity (triamcinolone > fluocinolone > dexamethasone), characteristics that may partially explain their relative potencies (triamcinolone = 5, dexamethasone = 25, fluocinolone = 25, compared to cortisol = 1). In general, these medications are cleared relatively rapidly after intravitreal injection: all have been reported to have an elimination half-life in the vitreous of 2–3 h in animal models. To increase the duration of action, the medication may be dissolved slowly from a crystal structure (e.g., triamcinolone acetonide) or through specific slow-release drug delivery systems (e.g., dexamethasone, FA) [18]. Currently, only the 2 intravitreal implants of dexamethasone and FA have received FDA approval for the management of DME.

Triamcinolone Acetonide

The first proof of efficacy of intravitreal TA on recalcitrant diabetic maculopathy was published in 2001 [18]; since then intravitreal TA has been used for DME treatment in several clinical trials

[19, 20]. TA remains clinically active for 3 months following a single intravitreal injection and is cleared more rapidly from eyes that have undergone vitrectomy. A single-dose preparation of preservative-free TA (Triesence®; Alcon Laboratories, Inc., Fort Worth, TX, USA) has been approved by the FDA to enhance the visualization of the vitreous during pars plana vitrectomy and to treat some posterior segment inflammatory diseases, but not DME [21].

The Diabetic Retinopathy Clinical Research Network (DRCR.net), in a randomized controlled trial (Protocol B) investigated the efficacy and safety of 1- and 4-mg doses of TA in comparison with focal or grid laser photocoagulation. At the 2-year primary end point, the mean BCVA was significantly better in patients treated with photocoagulation; the year-3 results showed that photocoagulation was more effective over time with fewer side effects [22, 23].

The DRCR.net Protocol I RCT compared ranibizumab plus prompt or deferred photocoagulation vs. TA 4 mg plus prompt photocoagulation vs. sham injection plus prompt photocoagulation. Ranibizumab groups (either prompt or deferred photocoagulation) produced significantly greater mean improvements in BCVA (+9 letters for each group) than did sham injection plus prompt photocoagulation (+3 letters) and TA plus prompt photocoagulation (+4 letters). Among patients who were pseudophakic at baseline, however, TA plus prompt photocoagulation produced a similar improvement in mean BCVA (+8 letters) as ranibizumab plus prompt (+8 letters) or deferred (+7 letters) photocoagulation. At year-5 in Protocol I, the ranibizumab groups continued to feature better visual outcomes than the TA group [24].

Suboptimal improvement in morphological and functional outcomes among the triamcinolone cohort was probably due to the high incidence of cataract and IOP increase in the study population. For these reasons, new sustained release implants of lower-dose corticosteroid have been developed to minimize the treatment complications.

Dexamethasone

Dexamethasone is 5 times more potent than TA and shows less retinal toxicity; its effectiveness in in vitro suppression of inflammation, inhibition of edema, fibrin deposits, capillary leakage, and phagocytic migration is well documented. Dexamethasone can be delivered to the back of the eye via a sustained-release intravitreal implant (DEX implant 0.7 mg; Ozurdex; Allergan, Inc., Irvine, CA, USA) through a 20-gauge transscleral incision that slowly releases the drug for up to 6 months. Sustained delivery of the drug allows for higher doses reaching the retina and lower doses absorbed by the systemic circulation, minimizing the adverse effects associated with systemic exposure to glucocorticoids. Moreover, pharmacokinetic studies have demonstrated DEX to be more long-lasting in vitrectomized eyes vs. anti-VEGF agents [25].

The first evidence of the efficacy of dexamethasone in treating DME was published in 2007 with a phase II trial involving 315 subjects with persistent macular edema arising from various

Fig. 1. A 78-year-old woman with long-lasting type 2 diabetes, poor glycemic control (HbA1c 8.9%), hypertension, hypercholesterolemia, femoral artery stenosis, previous IMA presented with non-proliferative diabetic retinopathy with chronic DME refractory to anti-VEGF (6 IV bevacizumab) and laser photocoagulation. BCVA was 20/125 and IOP was normal. Baseline imaging was collected (**a–e**). Three months after the first Ozurdex injection, optical coherence tomography (**f, g**) showed reduction of macular thickness, BCVA improved to 20/63, and no increase in IOP. After 5 months, DME recurrence occurred and BCVA decreased (20/200), even with no signs of progression of DR on FA (**h–k**). After 4 years, 5 well-tolerated DEX-implants and further macular grid laser, final BCVA was 20/50, DME regressed and hard exudates disappeared (**l–o**). (*For figure see next pages.*)

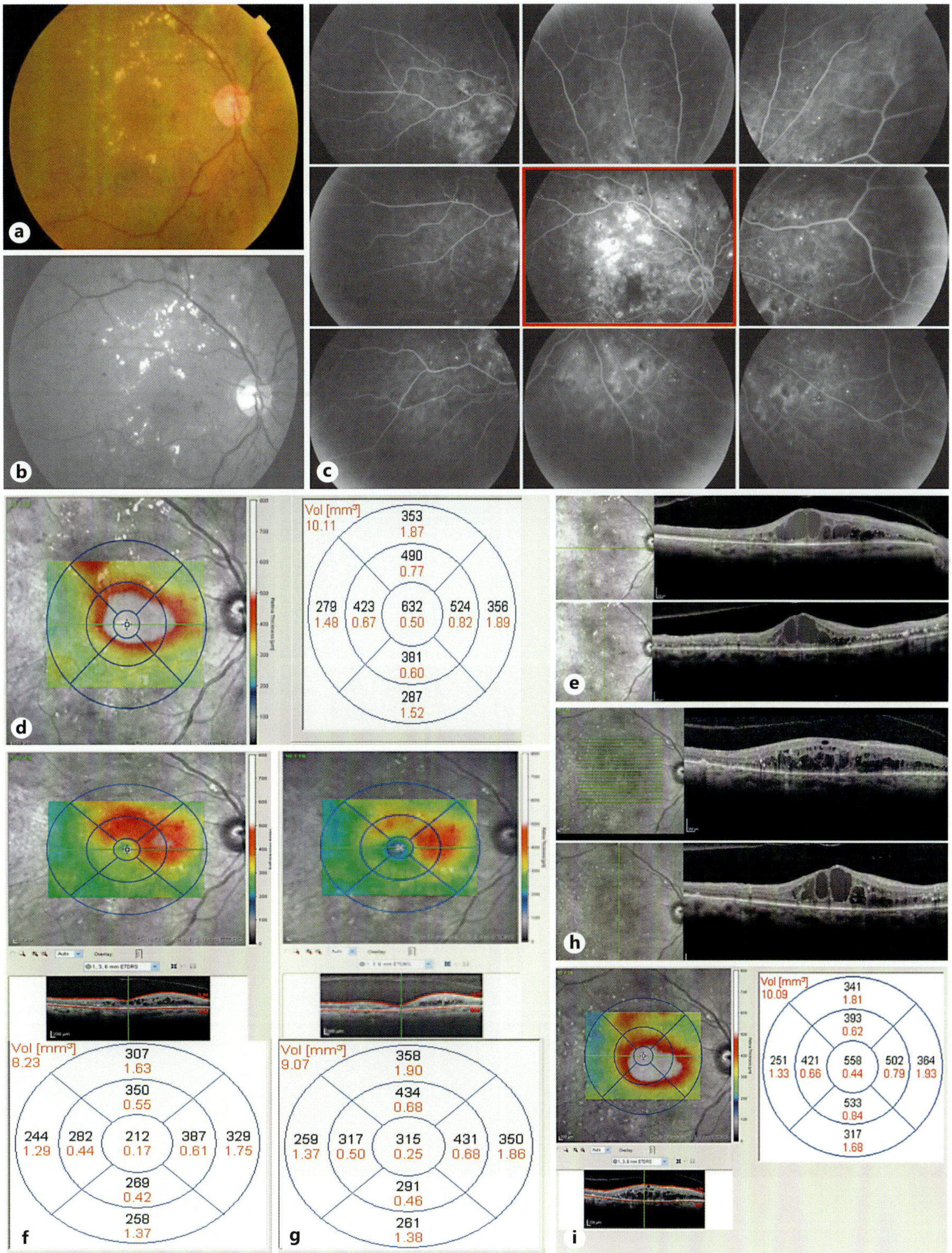
a
b
c
Vol [mm³]
10.11
353
1.87
490
0.77
279
1.48
423
0.67
632
0.50
524
0.82
356
1.89
381
0.60
287
1.52
d
e
h
Vol [mm³]
10.09
341
1.81
393
0.62
251
1.33
421
0.66
558
0.44
502
0.79
364
1.93
533
0.84
317
1.68
Vol [mm³]
8.23
307
1.63
350
0.55
244
1.29
282
0.44
212
0.17
387
0.61
329
1.75
269
0.42
258
1.37
f
Vol [mm³]
9.07
358
1.90
434
0.68
259
1.37
317
0.50
315
0.25
431
0.68
350
1.86
291
0.46
261
1.38
g
i

1

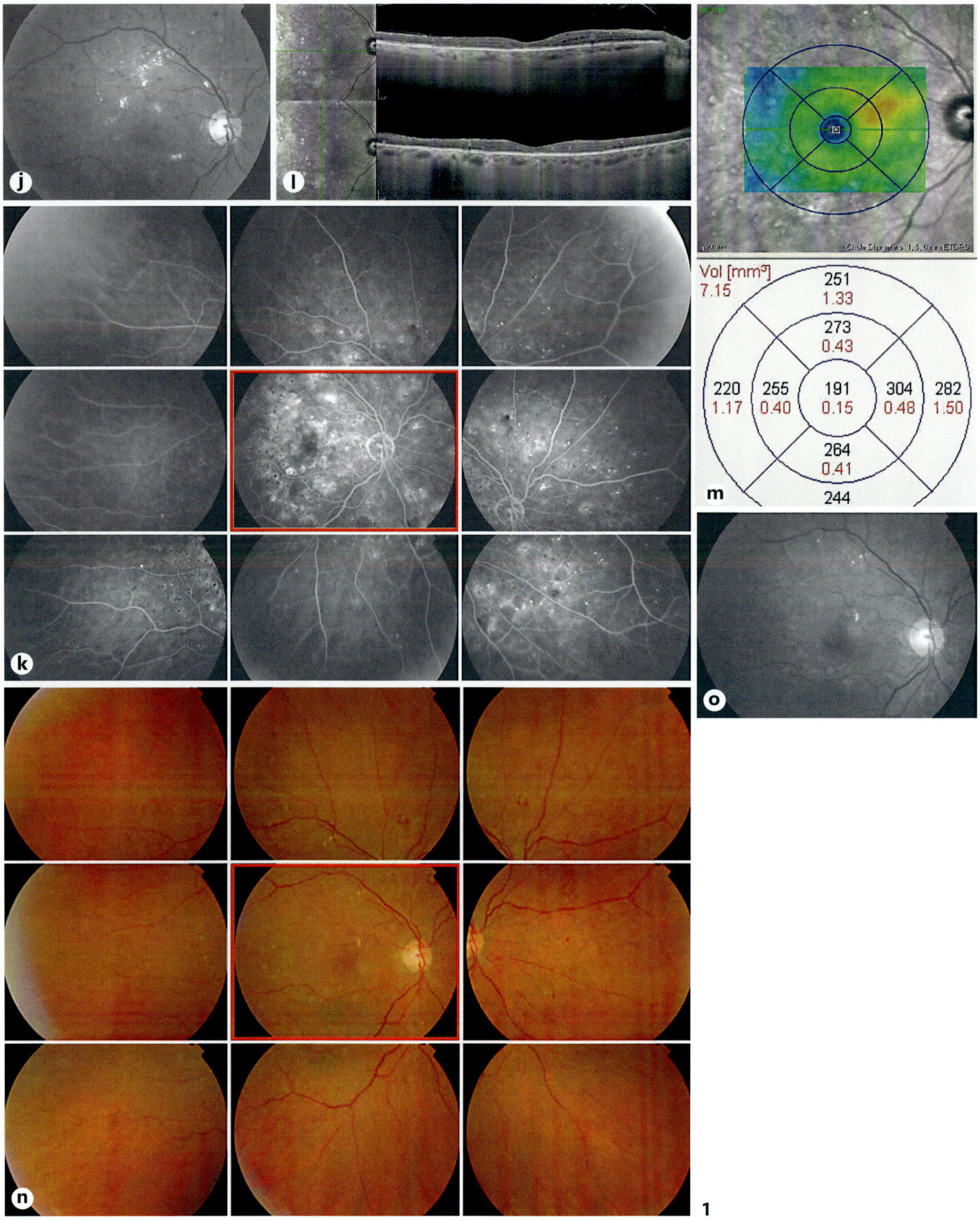
j
l
Vol [mm³]
7.15
251
1.33
273
0.43
220
1.17
255
0.40
191
0.15
304
0.48
282
1.50
264
0.41
244
m
k
o
n

1

causes, including diabetes, central retinal vein occlusion, uveitis, and post-cataract surgery [26]. Haller et al. [27, 28] compared 2 doses of DEX (350 and 700 μg) with no treatment in a trial involving 171 eyes. At 90 days, only the 700-μg group showed a statistically significant higher proportion of patients with ≥10 letter gain compared to sham (33 vs. 12%). Significant improvements in macular thickness and retinal capillary leakage were noted at 6 months in the dexamethasone implant-treated patients compared with controls; visual acuity and anatomic responses tended to be more pronounced with 0.7 mg than with the 0.35 mg dose. In a subsequent analysis of data from this study, the Ozurdex implant was found to display similar efficacy in focal, cystoid, and diffuse DME. The treatment effect appeared to peak at 3 months (Fig. 1–3).

Recent clinical trials, PLACID and MEAD, reported the efficacy of Ozurdex with or without laser photocoagulation in DME management [29, 30]. The PLACID study randomized patients with diffuse DME to 0.7 mg Ozurdex implant followed by laser photocoagulation at 1 month (n = 126) or to sham injection followed by laser photocoagulation at 1 month (n = 127). Subjects were eligible for an additional Ozurdex implant or sham injection 6 months after the first injection. Macular laser could be applied to both groups as needed every 3 months. The percentage of patients who gained 10 letters or more in BCVA at month 12 did not differ between treatment groups. However, there was a significantly greater improvement in BCVA from baseline to various time points up to 9 months in the group receiving the Ozurdex implant. Additionally, area under the curve analysis for BCVA over the 12 months showed a significant benefit for patients treated with the Ozurdex implant in combination with macular laser compared with macular laser alone [29].

Ozurdex intravitreal implants can be considered as the second-line treatment for DME in eyes unresponsive to anti-VEGF therapy [31–33]. However, data from the MEAD and BEVORDEX clinical trials and results from the CHAMPLAIN study suggest that Ozurdex can be considered as a first-line treatment option, especially in pseudophakic and vitrectomized eyes [30, 34, 35].

The MEAD study examined the safety and efficacy of the dexamethasone intravitreal implant in DME over 3 years, by means of 2 parallel randomized, multi-center, masked phase III clinical trials. A total of 1,048 patients with DME were recruited. The patients were randomized 1:1:1 to dexamethasone implant 0.7 mg, dexamethasone implant 0.35 mg, or sham, and they were followed for 3 years. Patients could be retreated no more often than every 6 months. More participants, who received steroid treatment, achieved a ≥15 letter gain: 22.2% in the 0.7 mg group and 18.4% in the 0.35 mg group, compared with only 12.0% in the sham group (p = 0.018). The secondary outcome, mean reduction in central macular thickness (CMT) from baseline, was greater in the groups receiving 0.7 mg (–111.6 μm) and 0.35 mg (–107.9 μm) dexamethasone implants rather than sham (–41.9 μm; p < 0.001). Approximately one-third of patients in each DEX implant group had a clinically significant increase in IOP requiring treatment during the study, but only 2 patients underwent glaucoma incisional surgery. The timing of IOP rises was predictable (IOP peaked at

Fig. 2. A 59-year-old male with type 2 diabetes, chronic kidney failure, ischemic heart disease presented with BCVA of 20/63 and positive Amsler test for metamorphopsia in RE. The patient had undergone pan-retinal photocoagulation, cataract surgery, and vitrectomy for proliferative DR. Baseline imaging showed posterior pole ischemia, DME, but no pre-retinal neovascularization (**a–e**). DME was treated with long-lasting DEX drug delivery system injection. BCVA improved to 20/40, and Amsler test was negative. Photoreceptor damage and macular ischemia (detected by enlarged foveal avascular zone on fluorescein angiography) prevented the patient from full visual acuity recovery after intravitreal medical therapy (**f, g**). After 5 months, macular edema reoccurred (**h, i**), and a second DEX-implant was scheduled. *(For figure see next page.)*

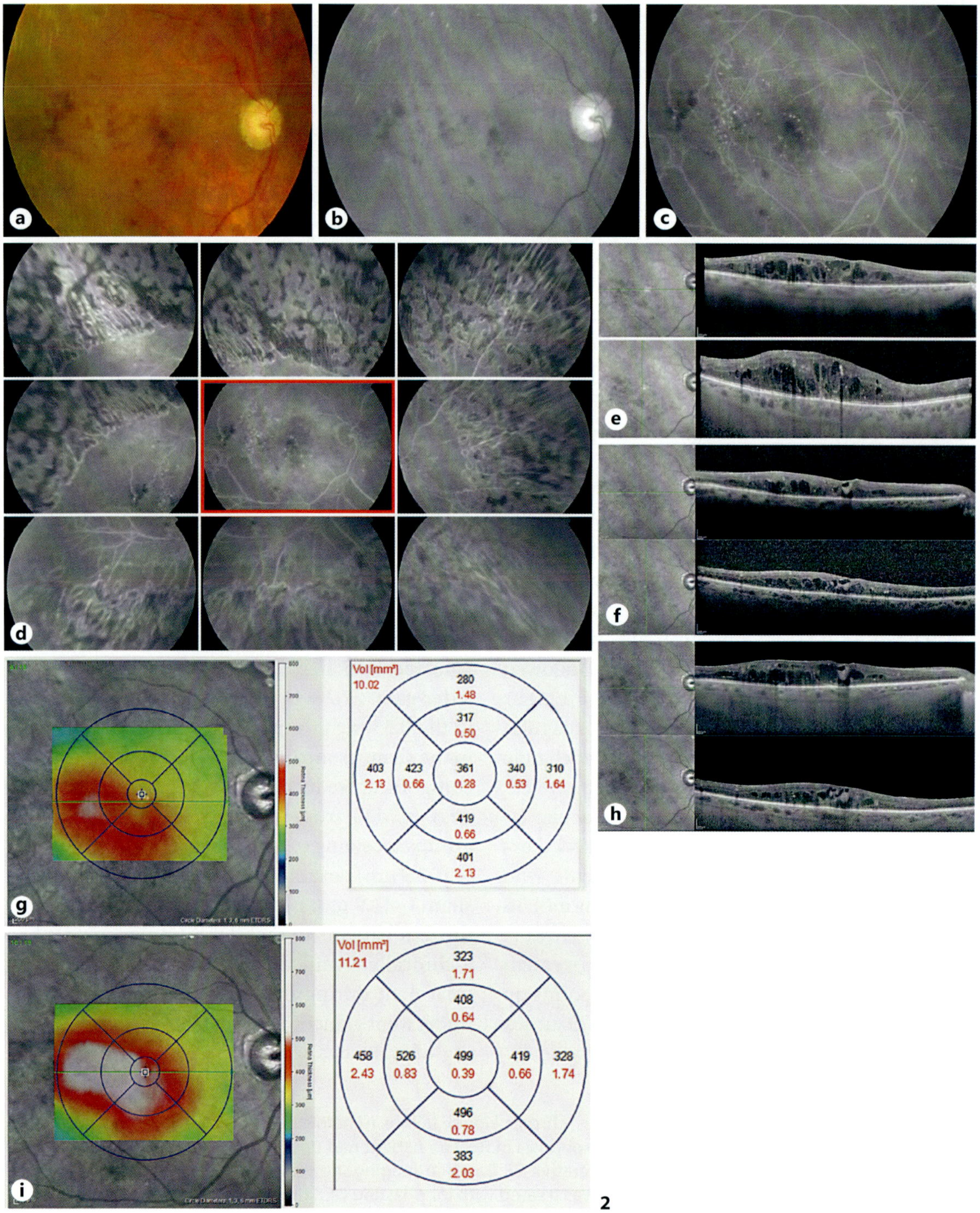
a
b
c
d
e
f
h
Vol [mm³]
10.02
280
1.48
317
0.50
403
2.13
423
0.66
361
0.28
340
0.53
310
1.64
419
0.66
401
2.13
g
Vol [mm³]
11.21
323
1.71
408
0.64
458
2.43
526
0.83
499
0.39
419
0.66
328
1.74
496
0.78
383
2.03
i

2

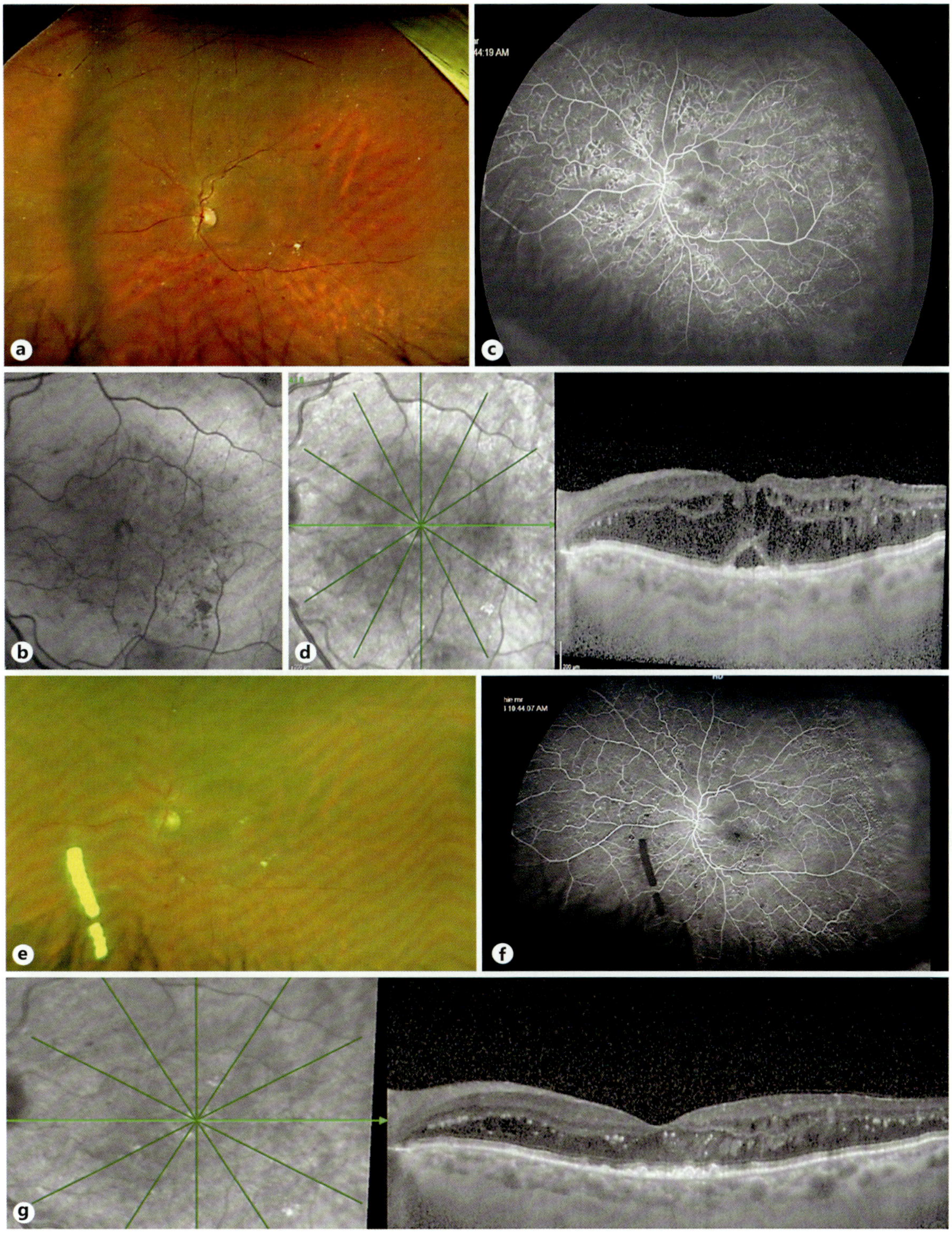

3

(*For figure 3h, i and legend see next page.*)

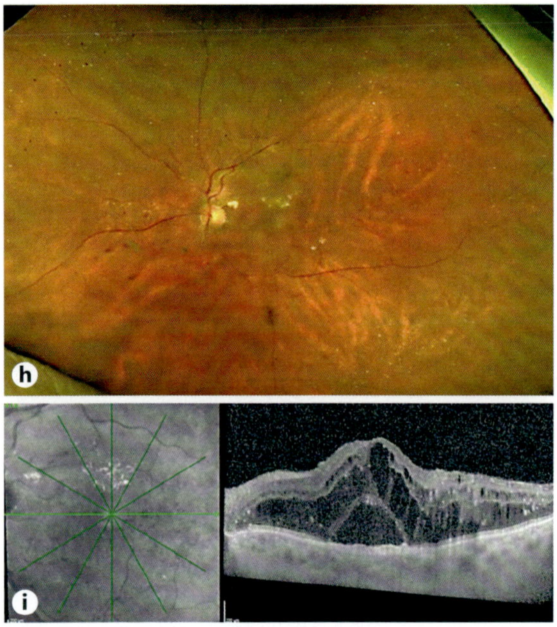

Fig. 3. A 67-year-old man suffering from NIDDM (HbA1c 10.8%), high cholesterol, and high blood pressure, presented with non-proliferative DR and DME; ultra-wide field FA showed non-perfused areas in mid-periphery. OCT scan disclosed neuroepithelium detachment and intraretinal hyperreflective foci, considered as a marker of DME chronicity and high inflammatory response, respectively (**a–d**). Three months after intravitreal DEX implant, BCVA improved to 20/50 (from 20/100). FA showed a reduction of peripheral ischemia, and DME regressed. IOP increased to 32 mm Hg, and topic anti-glaucoma drops were prescribed (**e–g**). DME relapsed after 7 months and required a second DEX-implant (**h**, **i**).

similar intervals and returned to baseline by 6 months after each injection), and the incidence and magnitude of IOP elevations did not increase upon repeated injection or from year to year in the study. These results indicate that there was no cumulative effect of DEX implant on IOP [30].

The BEVORDEX study reported the 12 month results of a randomized head-to-head clinical trial that compared bevacizumab (Avastin, Genentech) with the Ozurdex 0.7 mg implant. There were 88 eyes of 61 patients enrolled; 42 eyes receiving bevacizumab up to every 4 weeks and 46 eyes receiving Ozurdex up to every 16 weeks, both on an as necessary basis (PRN). The proportion of eyes with improvement in BCVA by at least 10 logMAR letters did not differ between the 2 groups, but bevacizumab-treated eyes received a mean of 8.6 injections over 12 months, compared to 2.7 injections for the Ozurdex group [34].

Absolute contraindications for the insertion of Ozurdex implants include advanced or uncontrolled glaucoma, local infection, or communication with the anterior chamber. Patients considered to be at risk for syphilis, tuberculosis, or other potentially infective chorioretinopathies should have these conditions excluded prior to considering intravitreal steroid therapy.

In conclusion, Ozurdex implant represents a fundamental alternative for recalcitrant and naive eyes with DME, with a good safety profile, especially in those cases when anti-VEGF agents are contraindicated, or a regimen with fewer intravitreal injections is required (Fig. 4, 5).

Fluocinolone Acetonide

A non-biodegradable FA sustained-delivery device has been developed (Iluvien®-Alimera Sciences, Alpharetta, GA, USA); the implant can be inserted in the vitreous cavity through a 25-gauge needle and lasts up to 36 months [36]. Unlike the DEX implant, it is not bioerodable. On September 26, 2014, the US Food and Drug Administration approved Iluvien® 190 µg for the treatment of chronic DME resistant to previous treatments (laser and anti-VEGF); subsequently, the drug has received marketing authorization approvals in several European countries. The history of high IOP and signs of intraocular or periocular inflammation are the main contraindications to FA implant injection.

The FAME Study Group aimed to assess the long-term efficacy and safety of intravitreal inserts releasing 0.2 µg/day (low dose) or 0.5 µg/day (high dose) FA versus a sham injection. At both

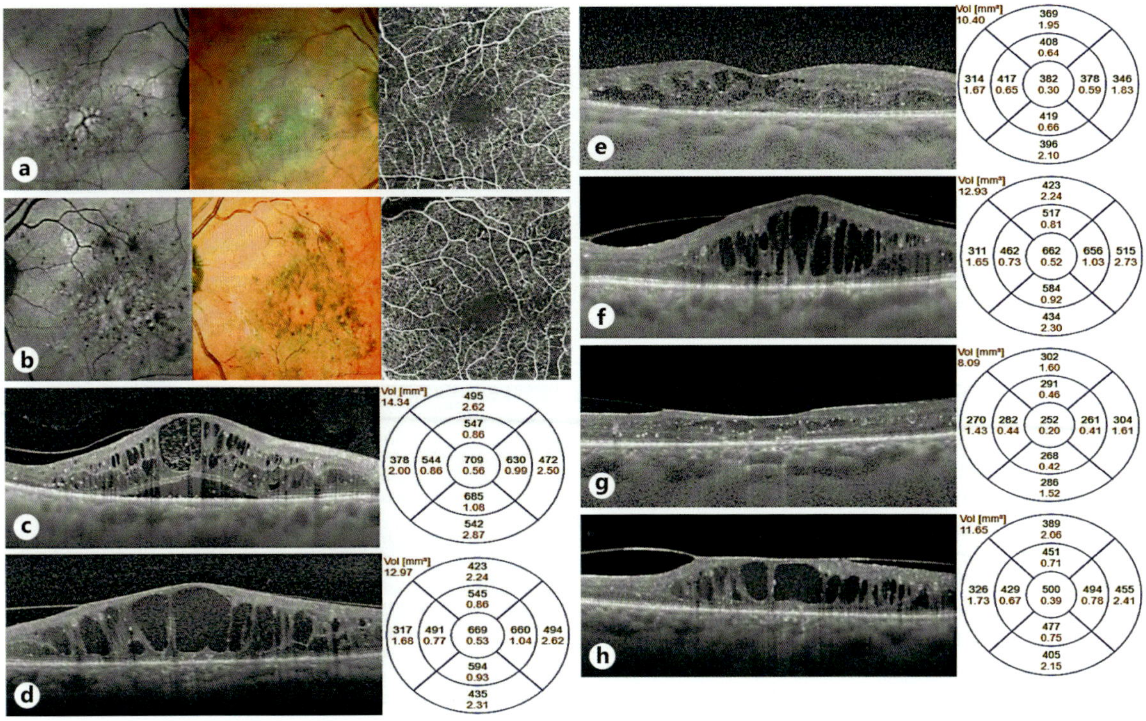

Fig. 4. A 62-year-old patient suffering from type 1 diabetes mellitus for 30 years presented with DME in both eyes. Visual acuity was 20/70 in the RE and 20/100 in the LE. Short-wavelength fundus autofluorescence, multicolor, infrared image, optical coherence tomography (OCT), and OCT angiography confirmed the diagnosis (**a–d**). The RE received a intravitreal dexamethasone implant injection, and after 2 months, CMT was 382 and foveal depression was partially restored (**e**). Visual acuity increased to 20/40. The LE was treated with 3 injections of anti-VEGF, with poor anatomical response (**f**), and then with a dexamethasone implant, with excellent tomographic and functional improvement after 1 month (**g**). After 5 months from steroid injections, DME recurred, vitreo-macular traction increased, and visual acuity decreased to 20/100 (**h**).

24 and 36 months follow-up, the 2 doses of FA showed a statistically significant improvement in the mean BCVA compared to sham; at 2 years, 15-letter improvement in BCVA was achieved in 28.7% of patients treated with the 0.2 μg/day insert (which was then FDA approved), 28.6% with the 0.5 μg/day insert, and 16.2% with sham injection. There was a greater need for surgical glaucoma intervention at the 36 months endpoint in patients receiving the FA injection; 2.5% of the high-dose group, 1.3% of the low-dose group, and 0% of the sham group required laser trabeculoplasty. Incisional glaucoma surgery was needed in 8.1% of the high-dose group, 4.8% of the low-dose group, and 0.5% of the sham injection group [36, 37].

Recently, Cunha-Vaz et al. [38] demonstrated that the percentage of patients treated with FA 0.2 mg/day who gained ≥15 letters after 36 months was significantly greater in chronic DME (34.0 vs. 13.4%; $p < 0.001$), compared with non-chronic DME cases (22.3 vs. 27.8%; $p = 0.275$). The greater response in patients with chronic DME was not associated with baseline ocular characteristics, changes in anatomic features, or differences in retreatment or ancillary therapies, while the ocular adverse event profile for FA was similar regardless of DME duration.

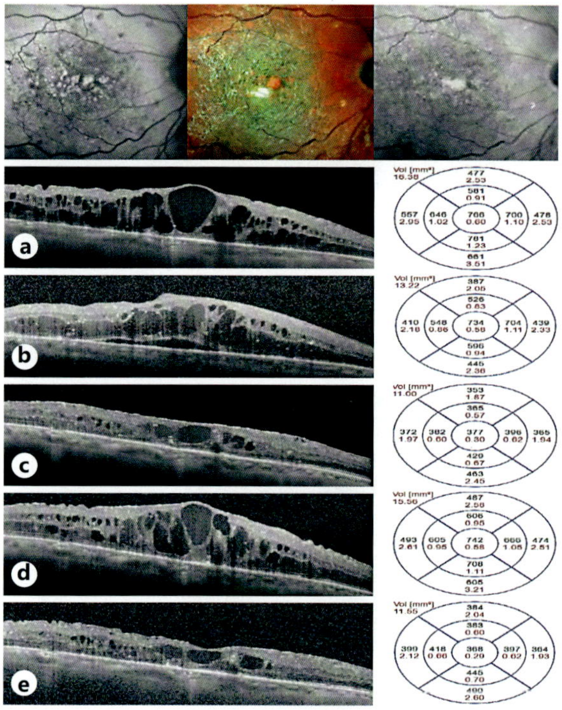

Fig. 5. A 59-year-old patient suffering from type 2 diabetes mellitus with poor glycemic control showed diffuse DME, with CMT of 766 μm and visual acuity of 20/70 (**a**). The patient was treated with 6 monthly injections of anti-VEGF, but both intraretinal and subretinal fluid worsened (**b**). The patient underwent dexamethasone implant injection with excellent optical coherence tomography (OCT) and functional improvement after 2 months (**c**). OCT after 4 months disclosed recurrence of DME and thickening of the internal limiting membrane (ILM). Visual acuity decreased to 20/100 (**d**). The patient was treated with a second injection of dexamethasone implant, with retinal thinning and partial foveal anatomy reestablishment after 2 months (**e**). IOP was within normal limits.

Real-life experience has demonstrated FA effectiveness and safety in the management of recalcitrant DME, in both unilateral and bilateral settings, also in vitrectomized eyes [39–42].

Conclusions

In conclusion, intravitreal administration of intravitreal steroids is able to improve and maintain vision acuity showing a good safety profile and tolerable economic burden, both for patients and the healthcare system. Currently, ophthalmologists have 3 intravitreal corticosteroid options for DME treatment: the dexamethasone delivery system, the FA insert, and off-label intravitreal TA. All 3 agents are associated with risks of cataract progression and IOP elevation. In patients who remain unresponsive to anti-VEGF therapy, are pseudophakic and at low risk for glaucoma or who have significant cardiovascular risk, treatment with long-lasting intraocular steroids is suggested, especially if they require an initial treatment with fewer intravitreal injections. However, there are still many unanswered questions about intravitreal drugs, regarding the doses, the frequency, the correct regimen of each treatment, and the potential side effects, especially at longer follow-up.

References

1 Das A, McGuire PG, Rangasamy S: Diabetic macular edema: pathophysiology and novel therapeutic targets. Ophthalmology 2015;122:1375–1394.

2 Ferrara N, Adamis AP: Ten years of anti-vascular endothelial growth factor therapy. Nat Rev Drug Discov 2016;15:385–403.

3 Bandello F, Cunha-Vaz J, Chong NV, et al: New approaches for the treatment of diabetic macular oedema: recommendations by an expert panel. Eye (Lond) 2012;26:485–493.

4 Photocoagulation for diabetic macular edema. Early Treatment Diabetic Retinopathy Study Report Number 1. Early Treatment Diabetic Retinopathy Study Research Group. Arch Ophthalmol 1985; 103:1796–1806.
5 Modarres M: Vitrectomy for diabetic macular edema; where are we? J Curr Ophthalmol 2016;28:161–162.
6 Bandello F, Casalino G, Loewenstein A, et al: Pharmacological approach to diabetic macular edema. Ophthalmic Res 2014;51:88–95.
7 Massin P, Bandello F, Garweg JG, et al: Safety and efficacy of ranibizumab in diabetic macular edema (RESOLVE study): a 12-month, randomized, controlled, double-masked, multicenter phase II study. Diabetes Care 2010;33: 2399–2405.
8 Schmidt-Erfurth U, Lang GE, Holz FG, et al; RESTORE Extension Study Group: Three-year outcomes of individualized ranibizumab treatment in patients with diabetic macular edema: the RESTORE extension study. Ophthalmology 2014; 121:1045–1053.
9 Wykoff CC, Elman MJ, Regillo CD, Ding B, Lu N, Stoilov I: Predictors of diabetic macular edema treatment frequency with ranibizumab during the open-label extension of the RIDE and RISE trials. Ophthalmology 2016;123:1716–1721.
10 Brown DM, Schmidt-Erfurth U, Do DV, et al: Intravitreal aflibercept for diabetic macular edema: 100-week results from the VISTA and VIVID studies. Ophthalmology 2015;122:2044–2052.
11 Wells JA, Glassman AR, Ayala AR, et al; Diabetic Retinopathy Clinical Research Network: Aflibercept, bevacizumab, or ranibizumab for diabetic macular edema: two-year results from a comparative effectiveness randomized clinical trial. Ophthalmology 2016;123:1351–1359.
12 Bandello F, Battaglia Parodi M, Tremolada G, et al: Steroids as part of combination treatment: the future for the management of macular edema? Ophthalmologica 2010;224(suppl 1):41–45.
13 Antonetti DA, Wolpert EB, DeMaio L, et al: Hydrocortisone decreases retinal endothelial cell water and solute flux coincident with increased content and decreased phosphorylation of occludin. J Neurochem 2002;80:667–677.
14 Silva PS, Sun JK, Aiello LP: Role of steroids in the management of diabetic macular edema and proliferative diabetic retinopathy. Semin Ophthalmol 2009; 24:93–99.
15 Bhisitkul RB, Winn BJ, Lee OT, et al: Neuroprotective effect of intravitreal triamcinolone acetonide against photoreceptor apoptosis in a rabbit model of subretinal hemorrhage. Invest Ophthalmol Vis Sci 2008;49:4071–4077.
16 Edelman JL: Differentiating intraocular glucocorticoids. Ophthalmologica 2010; 224(suppl 1):25–30.
17 Campochiaro PA, Brown DM, Pearson A, et al: Long-term benefit of sustained-delivery fluocinolone acetonide vitreous inserts for diabetic macular edema. Ophthalmology 2011;118:626–635.e2.
18 Jonas JB, Sofker A: Intraocular injection of crystalline cortisone as adjunctive treatment of diabetic macular edema. Am J Ophthalmol 2001;132:425–427.
19 Gillies MC, Sutter FK, Simpson JM, et al: Intravitreal triamcinolone for refractory diabetic macular edema: two-year results of a double-masked, placebo-controlled, randomized clinical trial. Ophthalmology 2006;113:1533–1538.
20 Jeon S, Lee WK: Effect of intravitreal triamcinolone in diabetic macular edema unresponsive to intravitreal bevacizumab. Retina 2014;34:1606–1611.
21 Dyer D, Callanan D, Bochow T, et al: Clinical evaluation of the safety and efficacy of preservative-free triamcinolone (triesence [triamcinolone acetonide injectable suspension] 40 mg/ml) for visualization during pars plana vitrectomy. Retina 2009;29:38–45.
22 Elman MJ, Aiello LP, Beck RW, et al; Diabetic Retinopathy Clinical Research Network: Randomized trial evaluating ranibizumab plus prompt or deferred laser or triamcinolone plus prompt laser for diabetic macular edema. Ophthalmology 2010;117:1064–1077.e35.
23 Elman MJ, Bressler NM, Qin H, et al; Diabetic Retinopathy Clinical Research Network: Expanded 2-year follow-up of ranibizumab plus prompt or deferred laser or triamcinolone plus prompt laser for diabetic macular edema. Ophthalmology 2011;118:609–614.
24 Bressler SB, Glassman AR, Almukhtar T, et al; Diabetic Retinopathy Clinical Research Network: Five-year outcomes of ranibizumab with prompt or deferred laser versus laser or triamcinolone plus deferred ranibizumab for diabetic macular edema. Am J Ophthalmol 2016;164: 57–68.
25 Chang-Lin JE, Attar M, Acheampong AA, et al: Pharmacokinetics and pharmacodynamics of a sustained-release dexamethasone intravitreal implant. Invest Ophthalmol Vis Sci 2011;52:80–86.
26 Kuppermann BD, Blumenkranz MS, Haller JA, et al; Dexamethasone DDS Phase II Study Group: Randomized controlled study of an intravitreous dexamethasone drug delivery system in patients with persistent macular edema. Arch Ophthalmol 2007;125:309–317.
27 Haller JA, Dugel P, Weinberg DV, et al: Evaluation of the safety and performance of an applicator for a novel intravitreal dexamethasone drug delivery system for the treatment of macular edema. Retina 2009;29:46–51.
28 Haller JA, Kuppermann BD, Blumenkranz MS, et al; Dexamethasone DDS Phase II Study Group: Randomized controlled trial of an intravitreous dexamethasone drug delivery system in patients with diabetic macular edema. Arch Ophthalmol 2010;128:289–296.
29 Callanan DG, Gupta S, Boyer DS, et al; Ozurdex PLACID Study Group: Dexamethasone intravitreal implant in combination with laser photocoagulation for the treatment of diffuse diabetic macular edema. Ophthalmology 2013;120: 1843–1851.
30 Boyer DS, Yoon YH, Belfort R Jr, et al; Ozurdex MEAD Study Group: Three-year, randomized, sham-controlled trial of dexamethasone intravitreal implant in patients with diabetic macular edema. Ophthalmology 2014;121:1904–1914.
31 Zucchiatti I, Lattanzio R, Querques G, et al: Intravitreal dexamethasone implant in patients with persistent diabetic macular edema. Ophthalmologica 2012;228: 117–122.
32 Pacella E, Vestri AR, Muscella R, et al: Preliminary results of an intravitreal dexamethasone implant (Ozurdex®) in patients with persistent diabetic macular edema. Clin Ophthalmol 2013;7: 1423–1428.

33 Campochiaro PA, Hafiz G, Mir TA, et al: Pro-permeability factors in diabetic macular edema; the diabetic macular edema treated with ozurdex trial. Am J Ophthalmol 2016;168:13–23.
34 Gillies MC, Lim LL, Campain A, et al: A randomized clinical trial of intravitreal bevacizumab versus intravitreal dexamethasone for diabetic macular edema: the BEVORDEX study. Ophthalmology 2014;121:2473–2481.
35 Boyer DS, Faber D, Gupta S, et al; Ozurdex CHAMPLAIN Study Group: Dexamethasone intravitreal implant for treatment of diabetic macular edema in vitrectomized patients. Retina 2011;31: 915–923.
36 Campochiaro PA, Brown DM, Pearson A, et al: Sustained delivery fluocinolone acetonide vitreous inserts provide benefit for at least 3 years in patients with diabetic macular edema. Ophthalmology 2012;119:2125–2132.
37 Campochiaro PA, Brown DM, Pearson A, et al; FAME Study Group: Long-term benefit of sustained-delivery fluocinolone acetonide vitreous inserts for diabetic macular edema. Ophthalmology 2011;118:626–635.e2.
38 Cunha-Vaz J, Ashton P, Iezzi R, et al: Sustained delivery fluocinolone acetonide vitreous implants: long-term benefit in patients with chronic diabetic macular edema. Ophthalmology 2014;121: 1892–1903.
39 Elaraoud I, Attawan A, Quhill F: Case series investigating the efficacy and safety of bilateral fluocinolone acetonide (ILUVIEN(®)) in patients with diabetic macular edema. Ophthalmol Ther 2016; 5:95–104.
40 Elaraoud I, Andreatta W, Kidess A, et al: Use of flucinolone acetonide for patients with diabetic macular oedema: patient selection criteria and early outcomes in real world setting. BMC Ophthalmol 2016;16:3.
41 Kumar A, Alfahad Q, Mitra A, et al: Intravitreal fluocinolone acetonide (Iluvien) for treatment of refractory diabetic macular oedema in vitrectomised eyes. Eye (Lond) 2016;30:763–764.
42 Massin P, Erginay A, Dupas B, Couturier A, Tadayoni R: Efficacy and safety of sustained-delivery fluocinolone acetonide intravitreal implant in patients with chronic diabetic macular edema insufficiently responsive to available therapies: a real-life study. Clin Ophthalmol 2016;10:1257–1264.

Rosangela Lattanzio, MD
Department of Ophthalmology
Scientific Institute San Raffaele, Vita-Salute University
Via Olgettina, 60, IT–20132 Milan (Italy)
E-Mail lattanzio.rosangela@hsr.it

Bandello F, Zarbin MA, Lattanzio R, Zucchiatti I (eds): Management of Diabetic Retinopathy.
Dev Ophthalmol. Basel, Karger, 2017, vol 60, pp 91–108 (DOI: 10.1159/000459692)

Practical Lessons from Protocol I for the Management of Diabetic Macular Edema

Lekha Mukkamala · Neelakshi Bhagat · Marco A. Zarbin

Institute of Ophthalmology and Visual Science, Rutgers-New Jersey Medical School, Rutgers University, Newark, NJ, USA

Abstract

Protocol I, a multicenter randomized clinical trial, compared the visual outcomes of patients treated with 0.5 mg intravitreal ranibizumab with either prompt or deferred (by 24 weeks laser), 4 mg intravitreal triamcinolone with prompt laser, or sham injection with prompt laser for the treatment of center-involving diabetic macular edema (DME). A total of 854 adult patients with type I or II diabetes and any level of non-proliferative diabetic retinopathy or proliferative retinopathy with adequate panretinal photocoagulation, with best-corrected visual acuity (BCVA) of 78 to 24 ETDRS letters (Snellen equivalent of 20/32 to 20/320) and visual loss attributed to macular edema, or retinal thickening with central subfield thickness of at least 250 μm by OCT were enrolled. The main outcomes relevant for practicing clinicians are as follows. (1) Intravitreal ranibizumab treatment provides superior visual outcomes compared to conventional laser treatment. (2) Adjunctive laser treatment does not appear to provide substantial visual benefit compared to ranibizumab treatment alone, but may reduce the number of injections required to resolve DME. Deferral of laser is likely beneficial in patients with worse initial visual acuity. (3) Intravitreal triamcinolone provides similar visual outcomes compared to intravitreal ranibizumab in pseudophakic patients but is associated with a clinically important increased risk of increased intraocular pressure (IOP), need for glaucoma medications, and need for glaucoma surgery. (4) Delayed initiation of intravitreal ranibizumab therapy provides improved visual outcome among patients initially treated with conventional laser photocoagulation or triamcinolone, but the magnitude of the benefit is not as great as is observed when ranibizumab treatment is initiated promptly. (5) The number of ranibizumab injections required to achieve the desired visual outcome decreases substantially after the first year, with the majority of patients not requiring further treatment after 3 years. (6) Patients who do not have a rapid response to ranibizumab still display long-term benefit to continued therapy, although perhaps less than those with immediate improvement. (7) Intravitreal ranibizumab is not only effective in reducing retinal edema and improving BCVA among patients with DME, it is also a disease modifying therapy and induces improvement of the diabetic retinopathy severity score by 2 or more steps in approximately one third of patients. Triamcinolone injection also induces improvement in diabetic retinopathy severity in DME patients, but perhaps to a lesser degree.

(8) No increased risk of systemic adverse events was observed among patients treated with intravitreal ranibizumab compared to sham-injected controls or triamcinolone-treated patients, but the low frequency of adverse events, restrictive enrollment criteria, and specific posology employed in this study limit the generalization of this conclusion to patients routinely encountered in clinical practice. (9) There was no clinically important increased risk of major ocular complications among patients treated with intravitreal ranibizumab (including the risk of glaucoma), although endophthalmitis is a potentially devastating outcome should it occur. In addition to the risk of endophthalmitis, intravitreal triamcinolone injection was associated with clinically important increased risk of cataract progression and increased IOP.

Protocol I Findings

Introduction

Diabetic macular edema (DME) is a common retinal manifestation of diabetic retinopathy and is the most common cause of visual loss among patients with diabetic retinopathy. Anti-vascular endothelial growth factor (VEGF) therapy results in substantially better visual outcomes for DME compared to traditional laser (focal or macular grid). Identification of the optimal treatment regimen is ongoing, yet a number of studies have provided important information that guides the current practice patterns for anti-VEGF therapy for DME. Protocol I, conducted by the Diabetic Retinopathy Clinical Research (DRCR) Network, or DRCR.net, investigated the visual outcomes of patients treated with one of 4 regimens: 0.5 mg intravitreal ranibizumab with deferred laser (by at least 24 weeks), 0.5 mg intravitreal ranibizumab with prompt laser (within 3–10 days after ranibizumab injection), sham injection with prompt laser (within 3–10 days of sham injection), and 4 mg intravitreal triamcinolone with prompt laser (within 3–10 days after injection). The initial protocol was designed to follow patients for 3 years after study initiation [1], and was later extended to 5 years follow-up [2]. In the subsequent sections, we review the results of this pivotal study emphasizing issues that are critical to the practicing physician: inclusion criteria, main outcome measures, treatment regimens, visual acuity (VA) and anatomic outcomes, and impact on diabetic retinopathy progression.

Inclusion Criteria

Patients 18 years or older with type I or II diabetes with best corrected ETDRS VA (BCVA) of 78 to 24 ETDRS letters (i.e., 20/32 to 20/320) and visual loss attributed to macular edema or retinal thickening with central subfield thickness (CST) of at least 250 μm by OCT were enrolled. Patients with any level of non-proliferative diabetic retinopathy or proliferative diabetic retinopathy with adequate panretinal photocoagulation (PRP) were enrolled [1, 3]. Patients were required to have a 4-month "washout" period prior to enrollment during which they received no intravitreal anti-VEGF or steroid treatment and no PRP, with no anticipated need for PRP in the coming 6 months. Patients who had undergone ocular surgery within the previous 4 months, with a history of glaucoma or steroid-induced intraocular pressure (IOP) elevation requiring treatment, or with IOP >25 mm Hg were also excluded. Systemic conditions excluding participation included: significant renal disease, uncontrolled hypertension (systolic blood pressure >180 mm Hg or diastolic >110 mm Hg); history of myocardial infarction, cerebrovascular accident, or transient ischemic attack, or acute congestive heart failure in the previous 4 months. Patients with bilateral involvement were required to have one eye assigned to the sham + prompt laser group [1]. The number of patients in each cohort is shown in Table 1.

Main Outcome Measures

Protocol I investigated several outcomes, the most important of which was BCVA and anatomic success measured as CST. The number of

Table 1. Definitions of various outcomes of each study visit

Term	Definition
Success	BCVA score ≥84 ETDRS letters (20/20 equivalent) CST <250 µm since last non-sham injection or since baseline visit
Improvement	BCVA ETDRS letter score improvement of at least 5 letters Decrease in CST by at least 10% since last non-sham injection or since baseline visit
Failure	BCVA 10 or more ETDRS letters worse than baseline CST >250 µm DME judged to be the cause of VA loss At least 13 weeks since "complete laser" with "no improvement" after
Futility	After 52-week visit: OCT CST ≥250 µm DME judged to be the cause of VA loss At least 29 weeks since "complete laser" with "no improvement" after
No improvement	Definition of success or failure/futility not met BCVA change ± <5 ETDRS letters CST ± <10% since last non-sham injection or since baseline visit
Complete laser	Treatment of all microaneurysms within areas of macular edema Grid laser treatment to other areas of macular edema
Center-involving edema	CST ≥250 µm
Center-threatening edema	Edema on clinical examination within 500 µm of foveal center Edema associated with lipid within 500 µm of foveal center 1 disc area of edema within 1 disc area of the foveal center

Adapted from the work of DRCR Network [1].

injections, time of injection, IOP, and need for intraocular surgery including cataract and vitrectomy, were among the outcome measures recorded [1].

At year-3, patients were asked to participate for an additional 2 years. The majority of patients (77% of the initial cohort) consented and maintained participation through 5 years of follow-up. There were no significant differences in baseline characteristics between patients who completed and did not complete the 5-year follow-up [2]. Initial results regarding the primary outcomes listed above raised additional questions that were explored in subsequent analyses of the Protocol I cohorts. The results of these post-hoc analyses are also reported in this chapter.

Treatment Regimens

The protocol-defined treatment regimen was somewhat complex and is detailed in this section. Patients were followed monthly for the first year at which time the primary outcome measure was evaluated. The patients in each of the laser cohorts were masked until the 1-year time point. Patients were required to receive a baseline injection followed by a study drug or sham injection every 4 weeks for the first 12 weeks. From week-16 visit onward, a retreatment algorithm was followed that required retreatment unless the patient demonstrated "success" or "no improvement" (Table 1 for definitions), at which time the treatment was at the investigator's discretion. If the retreatment

Table 2. Visual acuity outcomes at 1-year follow-up in Protocol I

	Ranibizumab + prompt laser	Ranibizumab + deferred laser	Triamcinolone + prompt laser	Sham injection + prompt laser
Number of eyes, *n*	187	188	186	293
Mean change in BCVA ETDRS letters from BL	+9±11	+9±12	+4±13	+3±13
Difference in mean change compared to sham + prompt laser (*p* value)	+5.8 (<0.001)	+6.0 (<0.001)	+1.1 (0.31)	–
Proportion of eyes with ≥10 ETDRS letters of improvement, %	50	47	33	28
Proportion of eyes with ≥15 ETDRS letters of improvement, %	30	28	21	15
Proportion of eyes with >10 ETDRS letters of worsening, %	4	3	14	13
Proportion of eyes with ≥15 ETDRS letters of worsening, %	2	2	8	8

Adapted from the work of DRCR.net [1]. BL, baseline.

protocol was followed, ranibizumab could be given as often as every 4 weeks and triamcinolone as often as every 16 weeks (with sham injections in between as frequently as every 4 weeks). After the 24-week follow-up, the retreatment decision was left to the investigator if the study visit showed "no improvement." If criteria for "failure" were met, any alternative treatment (ranibizumab, corticosteroids, or laser) could be pursued.

After the first year of monthly follow-up examinations, extension of time interval between visits was permitted to once every 2 months, and then doubled again to once every 4 months if no injection was given for the previous 2 visits and there was no worsening in edema, or if there was no improvement despite repeated injections. Subsequent visit frequency was tailored to the patient's VA and CST, and was determined based on a live computerized feedback system [3].

The retreatment algorithm for patients in the sham + prompt laser group required additional laser applications if there was center-involving or center-threatening edema or the laser was not yet complete (Table 1), with the last treatment at least 13 weeks prior. In patients in the ranibizumab + deferred laser group, laser was initiated after 24 weeks only if "no improvement" was noted after 2 consecutive injections [1].

A Practical, Clinically Applicable Follow-Up Method for Patients with DME

The study protocol followed in the DRCR.net study Protocol I may be difficult to reproduce in clinical practice. Therefore, general guidelines for more practical follow-up have been recommended as follows [3]:

- Monthly ranibizumab injections until an eye reaches success or displays low likelihood for further benefit given that no further improvement has been noted despite repeated injections, or if no response to treatment is noted.
- Ranibizumab should be restarted if edema worsens.
- If treatment is withheld and edema is stable, the follow-up interval can be doubled.

Short-Term VA Outcomes

Year one results revealed significantly better VA than baseline in patients receiving ranibizumab, either with prompt or deferred laser, compared to the sham injection + prompt laser ($p < 0.001$; Table 2). There was no statistically significant difference in the mean change from baseline in the triamcinolone + prompt laser cohort compared to the sham injection + prompt laser cohort ($p = 0.31$; Table 2). A greater proportion of patients had an improvement of >10 or 15 letters, with a lesser proportion of patients displaying a worsening of ≥10 or 15 letters in the 2 ranibizum-

Table 3. Change in central subfield thickness at 1-year follow-up in Protocol I

	Ranibizumab + prompt laser	Ranibizumab + deferred laser	Triamcinolone + prompt laser	Sham injection + prompt laser
Number of eyes, *n*	171	175	173	271
Overall mean change in thickness from BL	−131±129	−137±136	−127±140	−102±151
Difference in mean change from sham + prompt laser	−55 ($p < 0.001$)	−49 ($p < 0.001$)	−52 ($p < 0.001$)	–
Mean change in thickness from BL of <400 μm	−65±78	−64±73	−53±85	−21±88
Mean change in thickness from BL of >400 μm	−225±128	−226±142	−239±134	−174±158

Adapted from the work of DRCR.net [1]. BL, baseline.

ab cohorts compared to the sham injection + prompt laser group (Table 2) [1]. Similar outcomes were found at year-2 follow-up [4].

Based on the retreatment protocol, after the 16-week visit, additional ranibizumab injections were not required in patients who met the criteria for success unless there was a worsening of VA or increase in CST at a subsequent visit. More than 2/3 of these eyes received at least 1 more injection, and at least 1/3 of eyes in the ranibizumab + deferred laser required laser treatment between week-24 and year-1 visits. Therefore, although success may have been achieved early in patients receiving ranibizumab, ongoing treatment with additional injections and/or laser was required to maintain this benefit at least to the year-2 time point [4].

Short-Term Anatomic Outcomes

At 1 year, the decrease in CST revealed a similar trend to that of the VA results, with greatest reduction in thickness being in patients receiving ranibizumab (Table 3). However, less discrepancy in thickness was found between patients in the ranibizumab versus triamcinolone cohorts compared to the difference in VA. Of note, a much greater response was found in patients who had a baseline CST >400 μm compared to those with CST <400 μm [1], suggesting that patients with profound edema can achieve an excellent anatomical response to therapy. The analysis of 2 year results showed similar findings [4].

VA Outcomes Are Sustained Over Time

After the primary endpoint of the study was reached, clinicians were given the option to initiate the ranibizumab treatment protocol for patients in the sham injection + prompt laser and triamcinolone + prompt laser cohorts at years 1.5 or 3. These cohorts were termed "very deferred" ranibizumab cohorts [2].

At year-5 follow-up, patients in the ranibizumab plus deferred laser group continued to demonstrate the greatest improvement in VA with a mean improvement from baseline of 10 ± 13 ETDRS letters. This was a gain of 4.4 letters more than the sham injection + prompt laser/very deferred ranibizumab ($p < 0.01$). Patients in the ranibizumab + prompt laser cohort demonstrated 8 ± 13 letters ($p = 0.186$ compared to ranibizumab + deferred laser) improvement. Over 60% of patients in both the cohorts had a gain of at least 10 letters, with approximately 1/3 achieving at least 15 letters of improvement (Table 4; Fig. 1). Patients in the ranibizumab + prompt laser group demonstrated an improvement later in the follow-up compared to patients in the ranibizumab + deferred laser group, but this outcome may be related to delayed initiation of anti-VEGF therapy as detailed below [2].

Over half the patients in the sham injection + prompt laser and triamcinolone + prompt laser cohorts received ranibizumab as a "very deferred treatment" (58 and 62%, respectively). The tim-

Table 4. Visual acuity outcomes, central subfield thickness, and number of injections at year-5 follow-up in Protocol I

	Ranibizumab + deferred laser	Ranibizumab + prompt laser	Sham injection + prompt laser/ very deferred ranibizumab	Triamcinolone + prompt laser/very deferred ranibizumab
Number of eyes, *n*	111	124	198	125
Mean BCVA ETDRS letter score at 5 years	74	71	68	70
Mean gain in BCVA ETDRS letters from BL at 5 years	10±13	8±13	5±14	7±14
Difference in BCVA ETDRS letters vs. ranibizumab + deferred laser		2.0 ($p = 0.186$)	4.4 ($p = 0.01$)	2.8 ($p = 0.67$)
Gain of 5–14 ETDRS letters, *n* (%)	40 (36)	48 (38)	72 (36)	38 (31)
Gain of ≥15 ETDRS letters, *n* (%)	42 (38)	34 (27)	48 (24)	41 (33)
Loss of 5–14 ETDRS letters, *n* (%)	10 (9)	7 (5)	18 (9)	9 (7)
Loss of ≥15 ETDRS letters, *n* (%)	6 (5)	7 (6)	20 (10)	11 (9)
Median number of ranibizumab injections during years 1–3 (% of patients)	15 (100)	12 (100)	5 (40)	6 (37); 4 triamcinolone injections
Median number of ranibizumab injections during 5 years, *n* (%)	17 (100)	13 (100)	8 (58)	9 (62); 4 triamcinolone injections

Adapted from the work of Bressler et al. [2].

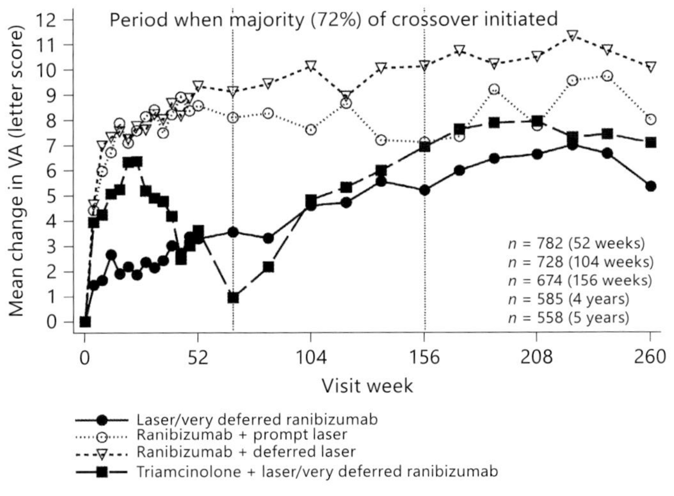

Fig. 1. Mean change in VA letter score over 5-year follow-up in Protocol I [2].

ing and number of injections as well as visual and structural response 6 months after initiation are shown in Table 4. These patients demonstrated an improvement of 5 ± 14 and 7 ±14 letters from baseline, respectively. Much of this gain in BCVA, however, was noted within 24 weeks of the initiation of ranibizumab injections (Table 5; Fig. 2). Only 1/3 of patients received laser during the 24 weeks after the initial injection [2].

Table 5. Visual and anatomic outcomes and number of injections in cohorts receiving very deferred ranibizumab in Protocol I

	Sham + prompt laser/very deferred ranibizumab	Triamcinolone + prompt laser/very deferred ranibizumab
Number of eyes in which ranibizumab was initiated, *n* (%)	130 (57)	89 (62)
Timing of initiation, between years	2 and 3	2 and 3
Median # of injections at 24 weeks after initiation	5 injections	5 injections
Improvement in BCVA ETDRS letters at 24 weeks after initiation	3	4
CST at time of initiation, μm	357	361
Mean decrease in thickness, μm	57	78

Adapted from the work of Bressler et al. [2]. CST, central subfield thickness.

Long-Term Anatomic Outcomes

Among all cohorts, 2/3 of patients had a CST <250 μm at 5 years. Patients in the laser + very deferred ranibizumab had the greatest absolute decrease from baseline, which was 32 μm greater than the ranibizumab plus deferred laser group ($p = 0.009$; Table 6; Fig. 3). Patients enrolled in the laser + very deferred ranibizumab group demonstrated a decrease in CST after ranibizumab injection, during which period very few had laser treatment as well. Study investigators noted that it is not clear whether the thinning of retinal tissue was a result of the ranibizumab injection or a delayed outcome of laser. As noted earlier, the groups receiving ranibizumab had the greatest improvement in BCVA; therefore, better anatomic outcomes may not always mean better VA outcomes. Less than or equal to 6% of patients in all groups had worsening of approximately 20% from baseline [2].

An immediate effect of ranibizumab on CST was evident in the cohorts that received very deferred injections. The average CST at the time of the ranibizumab in the sham injection + prompt laser and triamcinolone + prompt laser was 357 and 361 μm, respectively, and these cohorts achieved a 57 and 78 μm decrease in CST, respectively, most of which was observed after the first ranibizumab injection (Table 5; Fig. 2) [2].

Average Number of Injections Needed during the First 5 Years of Therapy

During 5 years follow-up, patients in the ranibizumab + deferred laser cohort received a median of 17 injections, compared to the ranibizumab + prompt laser cohort, who received 13 injections. In both cohorts, the majority of injections was given during the first 3 years (Table 4). A median of 0–1 injections were given among all patients in either cohort during year-4 and -5. Only half or less of patients in the ranibizumab + prompt or deferred laser cohorts received injections during year-4 and -5 (Fig. 4), and those that did received 3–4 injections per year (Fig. 5) [2].

Fewer triamcinolone injections were given in the triamcinolone + prompt laser/very deferred ranibizumab cohort, with a median of 4 injections during 5 years follow-up. However, ranibizumab treatment was initiated in 62% of patients (see above) between years-2 and -3 follow-up, who then received a median of 9 injections. A similar number of ranibizumab injections was administered in the sham injection + prompt laser cohort, with a median of 8 injections in 58% of patients [2].

Median Number of Laser Treatments Needed during 5 Years of Therapy

Patients in the prompt laser cohort received laser within 3–10 days of injection (ranibizumab,

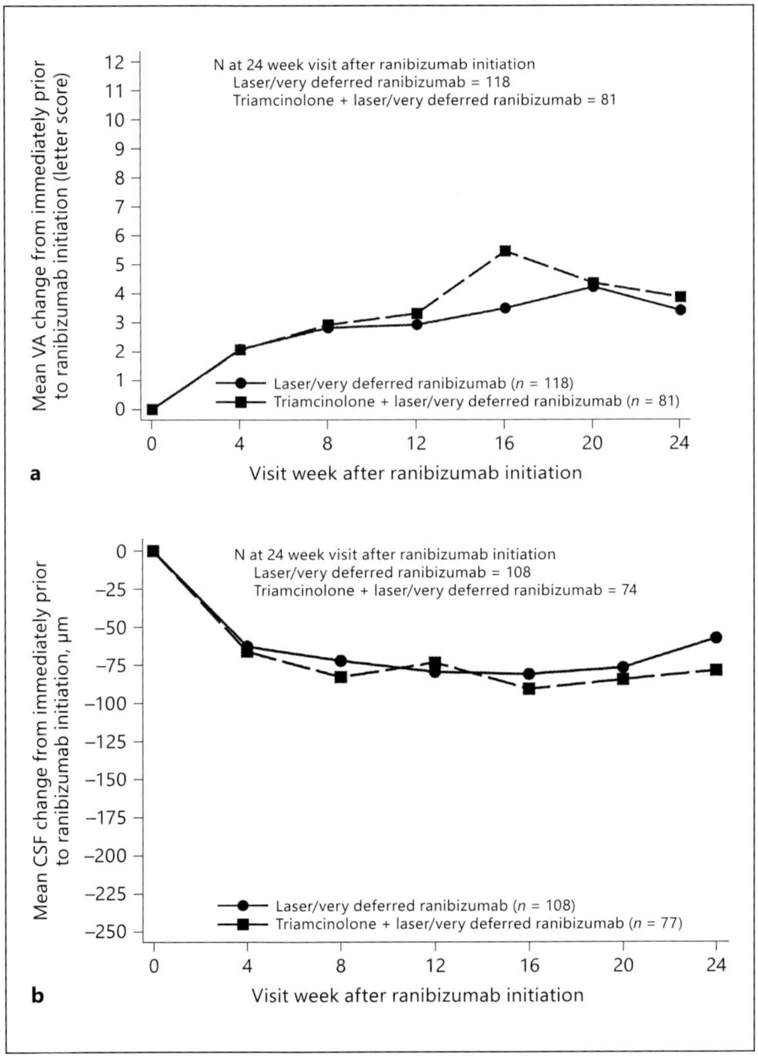

Fig. 2. Mean change in VA (**a**) and central subfield thickness (**b**) 24 weeks after initiation of very deferred ranibizumab in eyes originally in sham injection + laser or triamcinolone + laser cohorts [2].

triamcinolone, or sham). A median of 3 laser treatments were performed in patients in the triamcinolone + prompt laser and ranibizumab + prompt laser cohorts, and a median of 4 was done in the sham injection + prompt laser cohort. Laser was initiated in the ranibizumab + deferred laser group if edema persisted despite injections every 4 weeks on 2 consecutive injections. Less than half (46%) of the patients in this cohort met these criteria and received laser treatment during the first 3 years of the study, resulting in a median of 0 laser treatments. Substantially fewer laser treatments were applied during year-4 and -5 among all cohorts, with the most being 13% in the triamcinolone + prompt laser cohort (Table 7) [2].

Does Combining Laser Photocoagulation with Ranibizumab Improve Visual Outcome in DME

In most patients enrolled in Protocol I, adding laser treatment to ranibizumab therapy did not seem to confer a clinically important benefit.

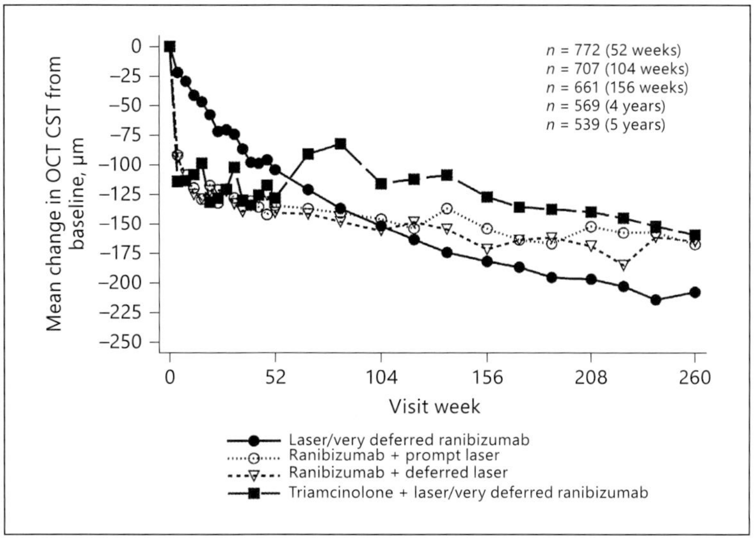

Fig. 3. Mean change in CST from baseline over 5-year follow-up [2].

Table 6. Anatomic outcomes measured by central subfield thickness (CST) at year-5 follow-up in Protocol I [2]

	Ranibizumab + deferred laser	Ranibizumab + prompt laser	Sham + prompt laser/ very deferred ranibizumab	Triamcinolone + prompt laser/very deferred ranibizumab
Number of eyes, *n*	111	124	198	125
CST at 5 years, mean ± SD	256±110	239±90	233±98	245±99
Change from BL, mean ± SD	−165±165	−167±168	−208±164	−159±154
Difference in mean change vs. ranibizumab + deferred laser	–	17 ($p = 0.20$)	32 ($p = 0.009$)	7 ($p = 0.61$)

BL, baseline.

Patients in the deferred laser cohort were eligible for laser photocoagulation after week-24 if center-involving edema persisted without improvement despite monthly ranibizumab injections. Laser treatment was applied in only 44% of patients in the deferred laser group during the entire 5-year follow-up. However, this cohort underwent more injections compared to patients receiving prompt laser (median of 17 vs. 13, respectively). At year-5, the improvement in VA after adjusting for baseline acuity was somewhat greater in the deferred laser group, 9.8 versus 7.2 ETDRS letters, respectively (p = 0.09). However, after adjustment for confounding variables (lens status, severity of retinopathy, CST, prior PRP, and age), there was no substantial difference (p = 0.15). The percentage of patients with ≥15 letters of improvement was 38 versus 27% (p = 0.03) in the ranibizumab + deferred versus + prompt laser cohorts. The percentage of patients with vision loss was similar in the 2 cohorts [5].

The advantage of deferring laser photocoagulation among patients receiving intravitreal ranibizumab versus combining ranibizumab with prompt laser was clear, however, it was unclear

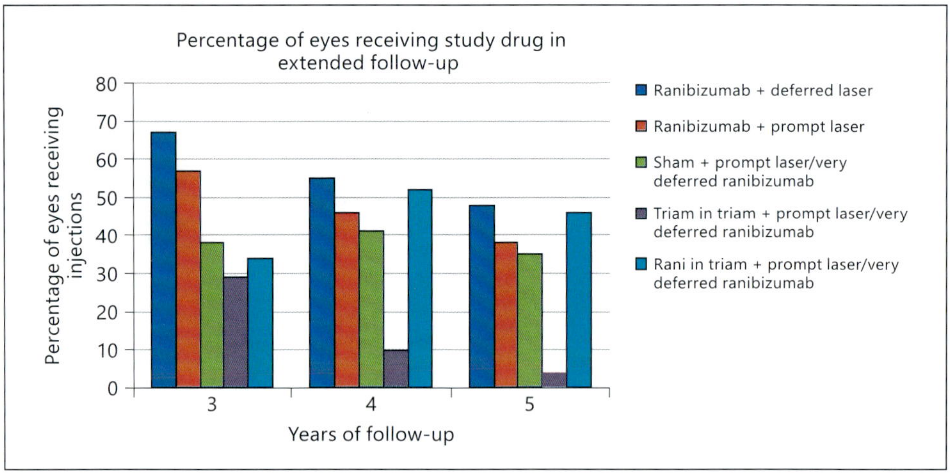

Fig. 4. Percentage of total patients in each cohort receiving study drug during 5-year follow-up in Protocol I. Rani, ranibizumab; triam, triamcinolone. Adapted from the work of Bressler et al. [2].

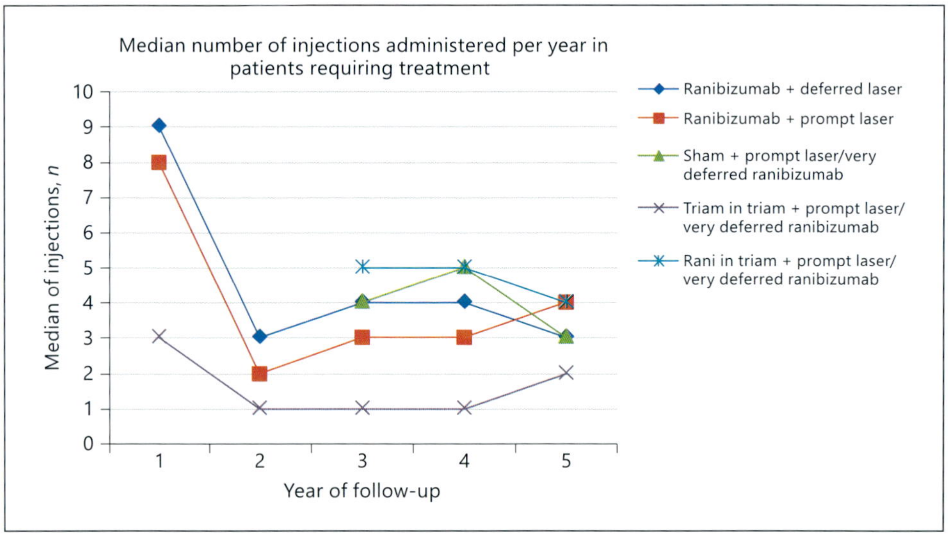

Fig. 5. Median number of injections administered in patients receiving treatment during years 3–5 follow-up in Protocol I. rani, ranibizumab; triam, triamcinolone. Adapted from the work of Bressler et al. [2].

among patients with baseline BCVA of 20/50 or worse. Differences in VA at 5 years were noted to be greater in patients that had worse baseline VA of 20/50 or worse ($p < 0.001$; Fig. 6). The CST, however, did not exhibit the same differences. The percentage of patients with CST >250 µm was 35% in both groups ($p = 0.91$). Although the deferred laser group underwent more injections, no higher rate of endophthalmitis or other complications was noted [5].

Table 7. Number of eyes requiring laser treatment and median number of laser treatments during 5-year follow-up in Protocol I

	Ranibizumab + deferred laser	Ranibizumab + prompt laser	Sham + prompt laser/very deferred ranibizumab	Triamcinolone + prompt laser/very deferred ranibizumab
Percentage of eyes with laser treatment years 1–3 (*n*)	46 (68)	100 (127)	99 (232)	100 (150)
Percentage of eyes with laser treatment years 4–5 (*n*)	3 (3)	10 (12)	11 (21)	13 (16)
Percentage of eyes with laser treatments all years (*n*)	44 (49)	100 (124)	100 (198)	100 (125)
Median number of laser treatments years 1–3 (*n*)	0	3	4	3
Median number of total laser treatments (*n*)	0	3	4	3

Adapted from the work of Bressler et al. [2].

Green Laser versus Yellow Laser

Protocol I data do not demonstrate a clinically important difference in visual outcome for patients with DME when treated with green versus yellow wavelength laser photocoagulation. A subanalysis of specific cohorts of patients in 2 studies assessed the primary outcome measures of VA and OCT thickness between patients treated with green and yellow lasers. Patients who received sham injection or ranibizumab + prompt laser in the Intravitreal Ranibizumab or Triamcinolone Acetonide in combination with Laser Photocoagulation for Diabetic Macular Edema trial (LRT-DME), and patients who received prompt laser only in the randomized trial comparing Intravitreal Triamcinolone Acetonide and Laser Photocoagulation for Diabetic Macular Edema (IVT), were compared. In patients concurrently treated with ranibizumab, no difference was noted between patients who received green versus yellow laser. In patients treated with sham + prompt laser in the LRT-DME, there was a mean improvement of 2.4 ETDRS letters for green and 5.1 ETDRS letters for yellow at 1 year ($p = 0.06$), and 2.4 versus 6.0 letters at 2 years ($p = 0.13$); however, OCT thickness was not different among patients receiving green versus yellow laser treatment. No meaningful differences were noted between patients who received yellow or green laser in patients in the ranibizumab + prompt laser or the prompt laser only groups. Therefore, although a trend of improved VA was observed in one subcohort treated with yellow laser, anatomic results were not congruent, and were not established in patients in the other 2 cohorts [6].

Correlation between CST and BCVA

Using the gross measure of CST, there was no strict correlation between retinal thickness on OCT and BCVA in Protocol I. Among the patients receiving ranibizumab, thinner retinas were paralleled by better BCVA. However, in the sham + prompt laser group, 2-year thickness results revealed thinner retinas, but this benefit was not associated with improvement in BCVA. The triamcinolone cohort showed a mild increase in retinal thickness that was accompanied by a slight decrease in BCVA [4]. A similar finding was noted when ranibizumab + prompt or deferred laser cohorts were compared, in which a greater improvement in BCVA was noted in the deferred laser group, but CST was similar among the cohorts [5].

Influence of Anti-VEGF Therapy on Diabetic Retinopathy Progression

The severity of diabetic retinopathy was judged using 7-field or 4-field wide fundus photographs that were evaluated by masked graders at baseline, year-1, and -3 (or one additional time point

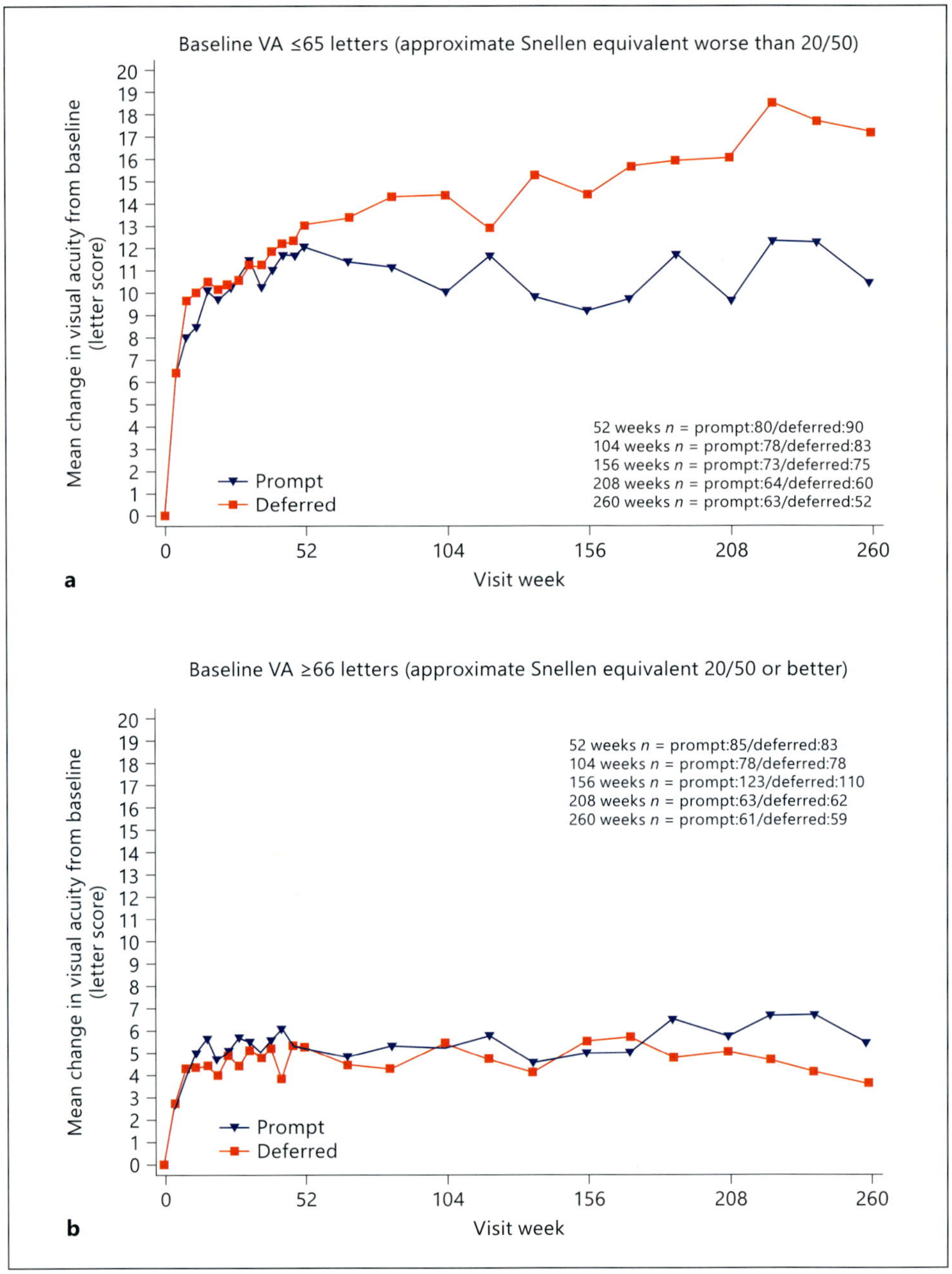

Fig. 6. Mean change in ETDRS letters in patients receiving prompt or deferred laser in patients with baseline vision worse than 20/50 (**a**), or 20/50 or better (**b**) [5].

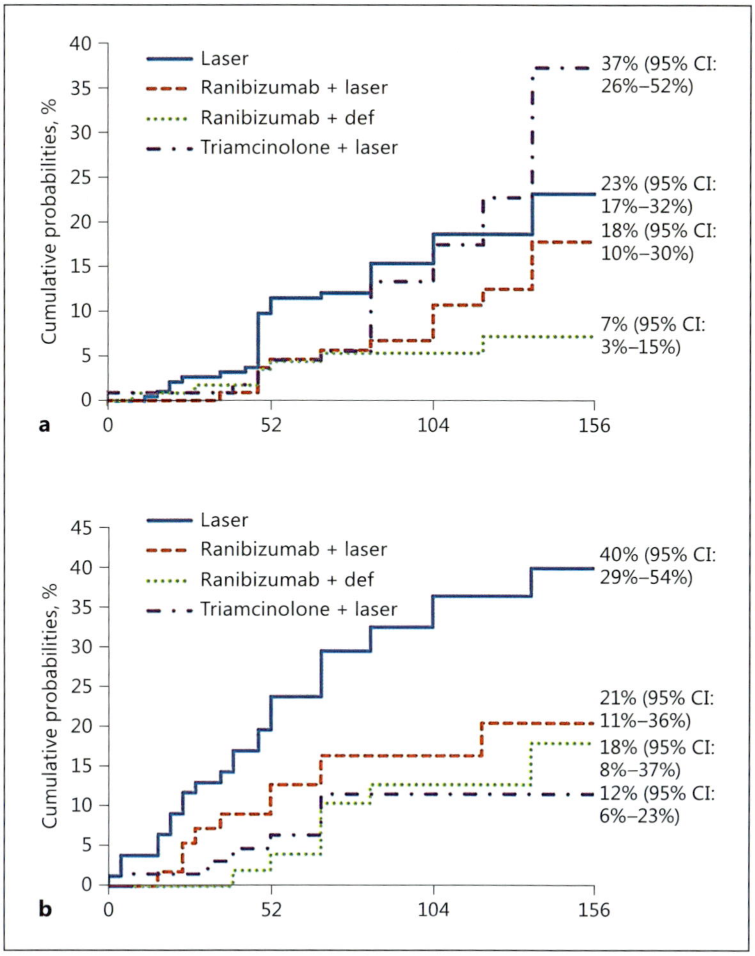

Fig. 7. Cumulative probability of worsening of diabetic retinopathy in eyes without proliferative diabetic retinopathy (PDR) (**a**) and with PDR (**b**) [7].

between years 1 and 3). Diabetic retinopathy progression was defined as: (1) progression from NPDR to PDR; (2) worsening of retinopathy by 2 or more levels; (3) requiring PRP; (4) vitreous hemorrhage; or (5) requiring vitrectomy for PDR. The cohorts were sub-analyzed based on those with PDR ($n = 254$) and without PDR ($n = 538$) at baseline.

In the cohort without PDR at baseline, eyes receiving ranibizumab or triamcinolone showed less risk of progression at 1 year (Fig. 7, $p = 0.04$). This effect was sustained for the ranibizumab + deferred laser group at year-3 ($p = 0.001$) and showed some decreased risk for the ranibizumab + prompt laser (18%, $p = 0.25$) versus the 23% risk of progression in the sham + prompt laser cohort. A greater risk of progression at 3 years was noted in eyes without PDR receiving triamcinolone (37%), but the difference was not statistically significant ($p = 0.10$). In eyes with PDR at baseline, all injection groups had less likelihood of worsening retinopathy throughout the 3 years of follow-up (Fig. 7, $p = 0.05$, $p = 0.02$, and $p < 0.001$ in the ranibizumab + prompt laser, ranibizumab + deferred laser, and triamcinolone + prompt laser groups, respectively).

In an attempt to minimize the influence of systemic control of diabetes on the results of progression of retinopathy, patients with bilateral involvement were analyzed separately. In the subgroup without PDR, the findings were very similar to the entire study group without PDR. Therefore, at 3 years of follow-up, ranibizumab was associated with decreased probability of worsening retinopathy in eyes with and without PDR. The treatment effect was greater in patients in the deferred laser group, possibly because these patients received more injections than those in the prompt laser group. The greater risk of worsening retinopathy at 3 years in patients receiving triamcinolone may have been confounded by the higher chance of these patients requiring cataract surgery. Therefore, it is unknown if the worsening retinopathy was due to inferior treatment by triamcinolone or due the confounding effect of cataract surgery [7].

A limitation in the strength of these conclusions is that the investigators were not masked at the time of assessment of severity, although the results were similar to other studies in which the graders were masked [7]. Additionally, fundus photography was not performed as frequently during the second and third years of follow-up, and therefore worsening may have been missed. Lastly, this cohort of patients represents only those with DME and not retinopathy more broadly [7]. Protocol S has confirmed the disease modifying effect of ranibizumab on diabetic retinopathy progression [8].

Influence of Vitrectomy on DME Management

Vitrectomy enhances the clearance of anti-VEGF antibodies in rat eyes. To determine whether anti-VEGF therapy efficacy differs among patients that have undergone pars plana vitrectomy (PPV) versus non-vitrectomized eyes, patients who received ranibizumab (either with prompt or deferred laser) were grouped according to whether they had undergone PPV ($n = 25$ eyes) or not ($n = 335$ eyes). At baseline, the PPV cohort exhibited severe diabetes and diabetic retinopathy (longer duration of diabetes, worse retinopathy severity, higher prevalence of PDR, greater prevalence of PRP or treatment for DME prior to enrollment), slightly worse BCVA (but same Snellen equivalent), and thinner CST. Both groups received a similar number of injections during 3 years. After correction for differences in baseline characteristics, no meaningful difference between the 2 cohorts was identified at 1, 2, or 3 years follow-up. However, the response of the CST was slower in patients with a history of PPV, which may have been due to differences in drug clearance [9].

Identification of Patients Most Likely to Respond to Ranibizumab Therapy

One subanalysis investigated 37 different baseline demographic, systemic, ocular, OCT, and fundus photo variables to identify associations with change in BCVA or CST between baseline and year-1 follow-up. Factors associated with worsening of vision or edema were not identified, but there were very few such patients at year-1.

Among patients in whom BCVA improved, however, younger age ($p < 0.001$), less severe diabetic retinopathy ($p = 0.003$), and lack of surface wrinkling retinopathy ($p < 0.001$) were associated with greater BCVA improvement after correcting for baseline vision. CST resolution over the first year was also associated with better VA outcomes ($p < 0.001$), and the presence of lipid within 6 mm of the fovea was predictive of more favorable OCT improvement, after correcting for baseline thickness ($p = 0.004$). The presence of lipid may indicate a disrupted blood-retinal barrier and hyperpermeability, which are abnormalities that could be most affected by anti-VEGF therapy [10].

Management of Patients Who Do Not Show Rapid Response to Ranibizumab Therapy

A cohort of patients who demonstrated persistent DME (defined as CST >250 μm) through the 24-week visit were analyzed to assess whether they demonstrated chronic persistent DME (failure to achieve CST <250 μm and at least 10% reduction

Table 8. IOP elevation at 1 and 3 years in patients receiving ranibizumab in Protocol I

	Sham injection + prompt laser	Ranibizumab (+ prompt or deferred laser)
Percentage of eyes that met primary outcome at 1 year (*n*)	2.0 (260)	5.7 (322)
Number of eyes that met primary outcome at 3 years	6	22
3-Year cumulative probability, %	3.4	9.5
Mean IOP, mm Hg	23	28
Mean change in IOP from BL, mm Hg	+7	+9
Number of eyes that had a history of glaucoma (angle closure) or IOP meds	1	2
Need for IOP lowering procedure (surgery or laser)	0	0

Adapted from Bressler et al. [12]. BL, baseline.

from 24-week visit) on at least 2 consecutive study visits. Data revealed that the probability of chronic persistent DME decreased at year-1, -2, and -3 visits from 81 to 55.8%, and 40%, respectively. At year-3, these eyes still had an improvement in VA but with a more modest gain than those patients without chronic persistent DME (mean of 7 ETDRS letters vs. 13 letters, respectively). Of the 40 eyes with chronic persistent DME at year-3, 17 (42.5%) still demonstrated a gain of ≥10 letters from baseline, while only 5 eyes (12.5%) lost ≥10 letters from baseline. Therefore, even with persistent DME at 24-week follow-up, continued ranibizumab injections can improve the macular thickness and VA over the long-term [11].

Risk of IOP Elevation in Patients Receiving Ranibizumab

Triamcinolone acetonide is known to increase the risk of IOP elevation, mandating medical or surgical therapy. The risk of IOP elevation has not been established in patients receiving intravitreal ranibizumab. A post-hoc analysis of a cohort of 582 eyes with DME but without pre-existing open-angle glaucoma, known history of steroid response, neovascular glaucoma, or IOP >25 mm Hg at baseline was undertaken. The primary outcome measure was an elevation in IOP, defined as IOP ≥22 mm Hg, an increase of at least 6 mm Hg from baseline in 2 visits, or initiation or augmentation of ocular hypotensive therapy over the 3-year follow-up. Response of patients in the prompt or deferred laser + ranibizumab cohorts was compared to sham injections (Table 8). The mean baseline IOP was 16 ± 3 mm Hg. The cumulative 3-year probability of meeting the primary outcome measure was 6.1% higher in the ranibizumab cohorts versus sham (99% CI –0.2 to 12.3%, hazard ratio (HR) for ranibizumab/sham = 2.9; 99% CI 1.03–7.9, p = 0.01), with a mean IOP of 28 and 23 mm Hg, respectively. A mean of 7 ± 4 injections were given to the 22 eyes that met the primary outcome measure, compared to 15 ± 8 in the remaining eyes. Therefore, the number of injections was not associated with an increased risk of sustained IOP elevation [12]. No patients required laser or incisional surgery to achieve IOP control.

In an attempt to minimize confounding variables such as genetic predisposition to the development of IOP elevation, a sub-analysis of 96 patients who had 1 eye enrolled in sham and one eye in ranibizumab cohorts was performed. These patients revealed an 8.3 versus 15.0% cumulative probability of the primary outcome measure at 3 years in the ranibizumab and sham cohorts, respectively, thereby resulting in a 6.6% difference (99% CI –8 to 21%; HR ranibizumab/sham = 1.9; 99% CI 0.7–5.1, p = 0.11) [12]. In summary,

Table 9. Response in the mean gain of ETDRS letters in the subgroup of pseudophakic eyes at year-5 follow-up in Protocol I

	Ranibizumab + deferred laser	Ranibizumab + prompt laser	Sham injection + prompt laser/very deferred ranibizumab	Triamcinolone + prompt laser/very deferred ranibizumab
Number of eyes, *n*	28	34	67	36
Mean gain in ETDRS letters (95% CI) from BL at 5 years	10 (4, 16)	10 (6, 14)	6 (3, 9)	6 (1, 11)

Adapted from the work of Bressler et al. [2]. BL, baseline.

Protocol I data demonstrate no definitive link between ranibizumab and increased risk of glaucoma, but a trend of increased IOP was noted, and therefore the investigators suggested IOP monitoring during follow-up visits.

Results in Pseudophakic Eyes

Results at year-1 and -2 in pseudophakic eyes (n = 273) were similar to those of the overall cohort in the case of the sham + prompt laser and both ranibizumab groups. In the triamcinolone cohort, however, pseudophakic patients had better BCVA outcomes than phakic eyes and had outcomes similar to those of the ranibizumab cohorts [1]. Therefore, induction of cataract progression by triamcinolone may have confounded VA results in phakic eyes assigned to receive triamcinolone.

By year-5, patients who were pseudophakic at baseline in the triamcinolone + prompt laser/very deferred ranibizumab had similar outcomes as the full triamcinolone cohort. The mean change in BCVA in each pseudophakic cohort is shown in Table 9 [2]. Perhaps cataract surgery performed during this longer follow-up period minimized the difference between the initially phakic and pseudophakic patients seen in the first 2 years of the study. In addition, precipitation of edema by the patients undergoing cataract surgery may have confounded the results. The mean decrease in retinal thickness over the 5-year follow-up period was similar to that of the full cohort in each treatment group [2].

Adverse Systemic Effects

There was no increased risk of systemic cardiovascular/cerebrovascular events among patients receiving ranibizumab versus sham injections or triamcinolone-treated patients at year-5. The number of patients who experienced severe systemic events is shown in Table 10.

Major Ocular Adverse Events

The incidence of major ocular adverse events was low and similar across all groups, with 4 (0.05%) of 8,051 injections resulting in endophthalmitis. The risk of cataract and increased IOP was significantly higher in the triamcinolone group (p < 0.01) compared to all cohorts [2]. The specific rates of major ocular adverse events are summarized in Table 11.

Take Home Points from Protocol I for the Practicing Clinician

Protocol I provides useful information for the practicing clinician regarding the management of DME. The main results are as follows:

1. Intravitreal ranibizumab treatment provides superior visual outcomes compared to conventional laser treatment.

2. Adjunctive laser treatment does not appear to provide substantial visual benefit compared to ranibizumab treatment alone, but may reduce the injection load. Deferral of laser is likely beneficial in patients with worse initial VA.

Table 10. Incidence of systemic adverse events and death among all patients over 5 years

Systemic adverse event	Ranibizumab + deferred laser	Ranibizumab + prompt laser	Sham + prompt laser/very deferred ranibizumab	Triamcinolone + prompt laser/very deferred ranibizumab
Number of patients, *n*	188	187	130	186
Any death, %	32 (17)	17 (9)	32 (17)	21 (11)
Non-fatal myocardial infarction, %	8 (4)	7 (4)	8 (4)	11 (6)
Non-fatal stroke of any etiology, %	7 (4)	8 (4)	7 (4)	10 (5)
Vascular death of any cause, %	21 (11)	10 (5)	21 (11)	11 (6)
Any APTC event, %	32 (17)	21 (11)	32 (1)	29 (16)

Patients with bilateral involvement were included in the cohort of pharmacologic therapy. Adapted from the work of Bressler et al. [2] online supplemental Table 5 (APTC, antiplatelet trialists collaboration).

Table 11. Rate of major ocular adverse events in each cohort over 5-year follow-up in Protocol I [2]

	Ranibizumab + deferred laser	Ranibizumab + prompt laser	Sham injection + prompt laser/very deferred ranibizumab	Triamcinolone + prompt laser/very deferred ranibizumab
Major ocular adverse event				
Number of eyes, *n*	188	187	293	186
Endophthalmitis, %	2 (1)	2 (1)	2 (1)	1 (<1)
Vitreous hemorrhage, %	20 (11)	18 (10)	20 (11)	22 (12)
Inflammation, %	3 (2)	2 (1)	3 (2)	9 (5)
Retinal detachment, %	1 (<1)	0	1 (<1)	2 (1)
Retinal tears, %	1 (<1)	0	1 (<1)	0
Cataract surgery during study, %	40 (32)	38 (31)	40 (32)	98 (81)
Elevated IOP/glaucoma				
IOP increase ≥10 mm Hg from baseline at any visit, %	15 (8)	26 (14)	15 (8)	83 (45)
IOP ≥30 mm Hg at any visit, %	7 (4)	7 (4)	7 (4)	56 (30)
Initiation of IOP-lowering meds at any visit, %	14 (7)	22 (12)	14 (7)	67 (36)
Number of eyes meeting ≥1 of above criteria, %	25 (13)	38 (20)	25 (13)	102 (55)
Glaucoma surgery, %	0	2 (1)	0	2 (1)

3. Intravitreal triamcinolone provides similar visual outcomes compared to intravitreal ranibizumab in pseudophakic patients, but is associated with a clinically important increased risk of increased IOP, need for glaucoma medications, and need for glaucoma surgery.

4. Delayed initiation of intravitreal ranibizumab therapy provides improved visual outcome among patients initially treated with conventional laser photocoagulation or triamcinolone, but the magnitude of the benefit is not as great as is observed when ranibizumab treatment is initiated promptly.

5. The number of injections required to achieve the desired visual outcome decreases substantially after the first year, with the majority of patients not requiring further treatment after 3 years.

6. Patients who do not respond rapidly to ranibizumab still display long-term benefit to continued therapy, although perhaps less than those with immediate improvement.

7. Intravitreal ranibizumab is not only effective in reducing retinal edema and improving BCVA among patients with DME, it also is a disease modifying therapy and reduces the progression of diabetic retinopathy severity score by 2 or more steps in approximately one third of patients. Triamcinolone injection also reduces the progression of diabetic retinopathy in DME patients, but perhaps to a lesser degree.

8. No increased risk of systemic adverse events was observed among patients treated with intravitreal ranibizumab compared to sham-injected controls or triamcinolone-treated patients, but the low frequency of adverse events, restrictive enrollment criteria, and specific posology employed in this study limit the generalizability of this conclusion to patients routinely encountered in clinical practice.

9. There was no clinically important increased risk of major ocular complications among patients treated with intravitreal ranibizumab (including the risk of glaucoma) although endophthalmitis is a potentially devastating outcome, should it occur. In addition to the risk of endophthalmitis, intravitreal triamcinolone injection was associated with clinically important increased risk of cataract progression and increased IOP.

References

1 Diabetic Retinopathy Clinical Research Network, Elman MJ, Aiello LP, et al: Randomized trial evaluating ranibizumab plus prompt or deferred laser or triamcinolone plus prompt laser for diabetic macular edema. Ophthalmology 2010;117:1064–1077.e35.

2 Bressler SB, Glassman AR, Almukhtar T, et al: Five-year outcomes of ranibizumab with prompt or deferred laser versus laser or triamcinolone plus deferred ranibizumab for diabetic macular edema. Am J Ophthalmol 2016;164:57–68.

3 Diabetic Retinopathy Clinical Research Network, Writing Committee, Aiello LP, et al: Rationale for the diabetic retinopathy clinical research network treatment protocol for center-involved diabetic macular edema. Ophthalmology 2011; 118:e5–e14.

4 Elman MJ, Bressler NM, Qin H, et al: Expanded 2-year follow-up of ranibizumab plus prompt or deferred laser or triamcinolone plus prompt laser for diabetic macular edema. Ophthalmology 2011;118:609–614.

5 Elman MJ, Ayala A, Bressler NM, et al: Intravitreal Ranibizumab for diabetic macular edema with prompt versus deferred laser treatment: 5-year randomized trial results. Ophthalmology 2015; 122:375–381.

6 Bressler SB, Almukhtar T, Aiello LP, et al: Green or yellow laser treatment for diabetic macular edema: exploratory assessment within the Diabetic Retinopathy Clinical Research Network. Retina 2013;33:2080–2088.

7 Bressler SB, Qin H, Melia M, et al: Exploratory analysis of the effect of intravitreal ranibizumab or triamcinolone on worsening of diabetic retinopathy in a randomized clinical trial. JAMA Ophthalmol 2013;131:1033–1040.

8 Writing Committee for the Diabetic Retinopathy Clinical Research Network, Gross JG, Glassman AR, et al: Panretinal photocoagulation vs intravitreous ranibizumab for proliferative diabetic retinopathy: a randomized clinical trial. JAMA 2015;314:2137–2146.

9 Bressler SB, Melia M, Glassman AR, et al: Ranibizumab plus prompt or deferred laser for diabetic macular edema in eyes with vitrectomy before anti-vascular endothelial growth factor therapy. Retina 2015;35:2516–2528.

10 Bressler SB, Qin H, Beck RW, et al: Factors associated with changes in visual acuity and central subfield thickness at 1 year after treatment for diabetic macular edema with ranibizumab. Arch Ophthalmol 2012;130:1153–1161.

11 Bressler SB, Ayala AR, Bressler NM, et al: Persistent macular thickening after ranibizumab treatment for diabetic macular edema with vision impairment. JAMA Ophthalmol 2016;134:278–285.

12 Bressler SB, Almukhtar T, Bhorade A, et al: Repeated intravitreous ranibizumab injections for diabetic macular edema and the risk of sustained elevation of intraocular pressure or the need for ocular hypotensive treatment. JAMA Ophthalmol 2015;133:589–597.

Marco A. Zarbin, MD, PhD, FACS
Institute of Ophthalmology and Visual Science
Rutgers-New Jersey Medical School, Rutgers University, Doctors Office Center
90 Bergen Street
Newark, NJ 07103 (USA)
E-Mail zarbin@earthlink.net

Bandello F, Zarbin MA, Lattanzio R, Zucchiatti I (eds): Management of Diabetic Retinopathy.
Dev Ophthalmol. Basel, Karger, 2017, vol 60, pp 109–124 (DOI: 10.1159/000459694)

Practical Lessons from Protocol T for the Management of Diabetic Macular Edema

Lekha Mukkamala • Neelakshi Bhagat • Marco Zarbin

Institute of Ophthalmology and Visual Science, Rutgers-New Jersey Medical School, Rutgers University, Newark, NJ, USA

Abstract

Purpose: To review the results of Diabetic Retinopathy Clinical Research Network Protocol T, as applied to clinical practice. ***Methods:*** Review of major publications reporting the results of Protocol T, a randomized single-masked (in year-1 only), multicenter clinical trial comparing aflibercept, bevacizumab, and ranibizumab as treatment option for center-involving diabetic macular edema (DME). The main outcome measures were change in visual acuity (VA), central subfield thickness (CST) on optical coherence tomography, cost effectiveness, burden of care, and safety. ***Results:*** A total of 660 participants (mean age 61 ± 10 years, 47% women, 65% Caucasian) were randomized to treatment with aflibercept (n = 224), ranibizumab (n = 218), or bevacizumab (n = 218). The majority of patients (90%) had type II diabetes, with an average duration of 17 ± 11 years. About half the patients had baseline ETDRS VA of 20/32 to 20/40, and half had ETDRS VA of 20/50 to 20/320 in all 3 cohorts. Patients in all 3 cohorts received a similar number of injections during the study period (9–10 in year-1; 5–6 in year-2). The year-1 improvement in ETDRS letters was significantly higher for aflibercept than for ranibizumab and bevacizumab in patients with baseline VA 20/50 or worse ($p = 0.003$ and $p < 0.001$, respectively), but was no different in patients with better baseline VA of 20/32 to 20/40 ($p = 0.69$). By year-2, among patients with poorer baseline VA, there was a difference in mean letters gained between aflibercept and bevacizumab ($p = 0.02$), but no difference between aflibercept and ranibizumab ($p = 0.18$). At year-2, there was no clinically meaningful difference in VA improvement (i.e., gain or loss of ≥10 or ≥15 letters) among any of the agents ($p > 0.74$). Bevacizumab was less effective than the other agents in decreasing CST at years-1 and -2 in the overall cohort of patients ($p < 0.001$). However, bevacizumab is substantially cheaper and much more cost-effective (when comparing expense and quality of life measures) than aflibercept and ranibizumab. The cost of other agents would have to decrease by 80–90% to be cost-effective relative to bevacizumab. Intravitreal administration of anti-VEGF therapy has relatively few ocular and systemic side effects, but caution may be warranted for patients with a recent history or high risk of myocardial infarction or stroke. ***Conclusions:*** Aflibercept, bevacizumab, and ranibizumab are highly effective treatments for DME. Bevacizumab is more cost-effective than aflibercept and ranibizumab. Intravitreal administration of drugs is relatively safe; however, intravitreal administration may be associated with severe systemic side effects in a small percentage of patients, particularly in those with a prior history of or high risk of Anti-Platelet Trialists' Collaboration events.

Introduction

Diabetic macular edema (DME) is a leading cause of vision loss in the United States, affecting about 750,000 people [1], and its prevalence will likely increase as the prevalence of diabetes increases. The advent of intravitreal administration of anti-vascular endothelial growth factor (VEGF) agents has revolutionized the treatment of DME and substantially improved the visual outcome compared with traditional therapy using laser photocoagulation. The 3 main anti-VEGF agents in practice are aflibercept (Eylea, Regeneron Pharmaceuticals), ranibizumab (Lucentis, Genentech), and bevacizumab (Avastin, Genentech); aflibercept and ranibizumab have been approved by the US Food and Drug Administration (FDA) for the treatment of DME, and bevacizumab is used off-label at 1/500th of the dose for cancer therapy [1]. Previous studies have demonstrated the advantages of these anti-VEGF agents compared to other treatments [2]. Protocol T was designed by the Diabetic Retinopathy Clinical Research Network to compare the efficacy and safety of aflibercept, ranibizumab, and bevacizumab. Several post-hoc analyses have also been completed to provide insight into the cost effectiveness of the treatments and other measures of visual acuity (VA) outcomes. The findings of these reports are summarized here.

Description of Study and Protocol

Protocol T was conducted at 89 sites across the United States. Adult patients with either type I or type II diabetes with impaired VA of 20/32 to 20/320 (ETDRS letters of 78–24, respectively), secondary to center-involving macular edema, diagnosed on clinical examination and with optical coherence tomography (OCT) (as measured by central subfield thickness [CST]) were included in the study. Patients were randomized 1:1:1 to 1 of 3 treatment groups for each of the study drugs: 2.0 mg of aflibercept, 0.3 mg of ranibizumab, and 1.25 mg of bevacizumab. If both eyes were involved (approximately 60% of patients in each cohort), the fellow eye was also treated with the same agent but was not included in the study. Patients were required to have a 1-year period without anti-VEGF treatment to be part of the study [1].

Patients were treated at baseline and every 4 weeks unless (1) vision was 20/20 with a CST below the eligibility criteria (250 μm) and (2) the patient had 2 consecutive injections without improvement or worsening. Improvement was defined as an increase in VA letter score of 5 or more (Snellen equivalent of approximately 1 line) or a decrease in CST of 10% or more. Conversely, a decrease in VA letters ≥5 or increase in CST of at least 10% defined worsening. Starting at the 24-week follow-up, injections were withheld if the patient had no change (improvement or worsening) of vision after 2 consecutive injections, regardless of the VA or CST. However, if the vision decreased or CST thickened from the previous injection, treatments were reinitiated [1].

Laser treatment (focal, grid, or both) was given at or after the 24-week visit if there was persistent DME. If criteria for treatment failure were met, anti-VEGF or laser therapy other than the study drug was permitted. Failure was defined as CST ≥250 μm, VA ≥10 letters worse than baseline at 2 consecutive visits, no improvement since either of last 2 injections or last laser treatment, and complete laser treatment performed at least 13 weeks prior [1].

Follow-up during the first year was every 4 weeks [1], which could be extended up to every 16 weeks depending on the treatment rendered [3]. The study was partially masked. The patients and technicians measuring VA and performing OCT analysis were masked to the treatment. The study investigators were aware of the drug, and patients were unmasked after the 1-year follow-up, at which time they could request to alter the treatment. (Only 1 patient asked for treatment

Table 1. Baseline ocular characteristics and treatment during first year of follow-up of each cohort in Protocol T

	Aflibercept	Ranibizumab	Bevacizumab
Number of participants	224	218	218
Median baseline ETDRS VA letter score (Snellen equivalent)	69 (20/40)	68 (20/50)	69 (20/40)
Mean baseline ETDRS VA letter score of patients with VA 20/32 to 20/40 (*n*)	73.5±2.6 (106)	73.4±2.7 (105)	72.8±2.9 (104)
Mean baseline ETDRS VA letter score of patients with VA 20/50 to 20/320 (*n*)	56.2±11.1 (102)	56.5±9.9 (101)	56.6±10.6 (102)
Baseline CST, μm	387	390	376
Median number of injections			
Overall (IQR)	9 (8–11)	10 (8–12)	10 (8–11)
VA 20/32 to 20/40	9	9	9
VA 20/50 to 20/320	10	10	11
Percentage of patients with laser treatment			
Overall	76 of 208 (37)	115 of 206 (56)	95 of 206 (46)
VA 20/32 to 20/40	36	43	47
VA 20/50 to 20/320	37	50	65

VA, visual acuity; CST, central subfield thickness; IQR, interquartile range. Adapted from Wells et al. [1].

reassignment.) Analyses were conducted for the entire study population, and for those with better VA (Snellen of 20/32 to 20/40) and worse VA (20/50 to 20/320) at baseline.

Baseline Characteristics

A total of 660 participants (mean age 61 ± 10 years, 47% women, 65% Caucasian) were randomized to treatment with aflibercept (n = 224), ranibizumab (n = 218), or bevacizumab (n = 218). The majority of patients (90%) had type II diabetes, with an average duration of 17 ± 11 years.

The mean baseline VA for the entire study population was 64.8 ± 11.3 letters (i.e., 20/50 Snellen equivalent), with CST of 412 ± 130 μm. The baseline VA letter score and CST of each cohort are shown in Table 1. Half of the patients in each group had baseline ETDRS VA (i.e., VA measured on an ETDRS chart) of 20/32 to 20/40 (78 to 69 letters), and half had ETDRS VA 20/50 or worse (<69 letters); the baseline VA is shown in Table 1. All 3 cohorts received a similar number of injections during the first year. A lower percentage of patients in the aflibercept cohort received laser treatment compared to the other 2 agents; the percentage was higher in patients who had worse baseline VA among all cohorts (Table 1).

Year-1 Results

Follow-up through 1 year showed a substantial improvement in VA by 4 weeks after the initial injection, accompanied by a decrease in CST on OCT (Table 2). This improvement was maintained for 1 year of follow-up, congruent with the results of prior studies [2]. Aflibercept resulted in greater improvement in ETDRS VA letters compared to ranibizumab and bevacizumab, but this

Table 2. Visual acuity (VA) and central subfield thickness (CST) outcomes at 1 year in Protocol T [1]

	Aflibercept	Ranibizumab	Bevacizumab	Aflib vs. Rani	Aflib vs. Beva	Rani vs. Beva
Improvement in ETDRS letters from baseline						
Overall, mean ± SD	+13.3±11.1	+11.2±9.4	+9.7±10.1	+2.1 ($p = 0.03$)	+3.5 ($p < 0.001$)	+1.4 ($p = 0.12$)
VA 20/32 to 20/40, mean ± SD	+8.0±7.6	+8.3±6.8	+7.5±7.4	−0.4 ($p = 0.69$)	+0.7 ($p = 0.69$)	+1.1 ($p = 0.69$)
VA 20/50 to 20/320, mean ± SD	+18.9±11.5	+14.2±10.6	+11.8±12.0	+4.7 ($p = 0.003$)	+6.5 ($p < 0.001$)	+1.8 ($p = 0.21$)
≥15 letter improvement						
VA 20/32 to 20/40, *n* (%)	19 (18)	16 (15)	17 (16)	+4 ($p = 0.73$)	+2 ($p = 0.73$)	−2 ($p = 0.73$)
VA 20/50 to 20/320, *n* (%)	68 (67)	50 (50)	42 (41)	+18 ($p = 0.008$)	+24 ($p < 0.001$)	+6 ($p = 0.34$)
≥15 letter decline						
VA 20/32 to 20/40, *n* (%)	2 (2)	1 (1)	1 (1)	+1 ($p = 0.99$)	+1 ($p = 0.99$)	0 ($p = 0.99$)
VA 20/50 to 20/320, *n* (%)	1 (1)	2 (2)	2 (2)	−1 ($p = 0.85$)	0 ($p = 0.85$)	1 ($p = 0.85$)
Decrease in CST from baseline, μm						
Overall, mean ± SD	−169±138	−147±134	−101±121	−18.6 ($p = 0.036$)	−69.9 ($p < 0.001$)	−51.2 ($p < 0.001$)
VA 20/32 to 20/40, mean ± SD	−129±110	−119±109	−67±65	−18 ($p = 0.06$)	−56 ($p < 0.001$)	−38 ($p < 0.001$)
VA 20/50 or 20/320, mean ± SD	−210±151	−176±151	−135±152	−19 ($p = 0.22$)	−86 ($p < 0.001$)	−67 ($p < 0.001$)

Aflib, aflibercept; Rani, ranibizumab; Beva, bevacizumab.

difference was largely driven by the subgroup with worse baseline VA. In patients with better VA, no significant difference in VA improvement was found ($p = 0.69$ in all pairwise comparisons, Table 2, Fig. 1). To better identify the clinically significant VA changes, the percentage of patients who had a ≥15 ETDRS letter improvement or loss of vision was also calculated and is shown in Table 2. Among the cohort with worse baseline vision, a significantly higher number of patients had a substantial improvement in VA after injection with aflibercept compared to the other 2 agents ($p = 0.008$ for aflibercept vs. ranibizumab and $p < 0.001$ for aflibercept vs. bevacizumab). In contrast, the vision in patients with better baseline vision was similar at 1-year between all 3 agents ($p = 0.93$, Table 2, Fig. 1). Very few patients experienced a loss of more than 15 letters, and therefore no significant differences were found between the 3 cohorts regarding vision loss (Table 2, Fig. 1) [1].

CST also improved at 1-year. Bevacizumab had less effect on reducing CST than aflibercept and ranibizumab in cohorts with better and worse baseline visions ($p < 0.001$) (Table 2, Fig. 2) [1].

Year-2 Results

Patients were followed for an additional year to determine if the disparities noted between the treatments at year-1 were sustained for 2 years. Only 1 patient switched the treatment drug from the initial study agent at year-1 after unmasking. Most eyes (84%) received at least 1 injection during year-2. All 3 treatment arms received a median of 5 injections in year-2, which was about half of the number needed in year-1 (Table 3). Follow-up intervals during year-2 ranged from every 4 to 16 weeks, depending on the treatment. Correspondingly, the percentage of visits in

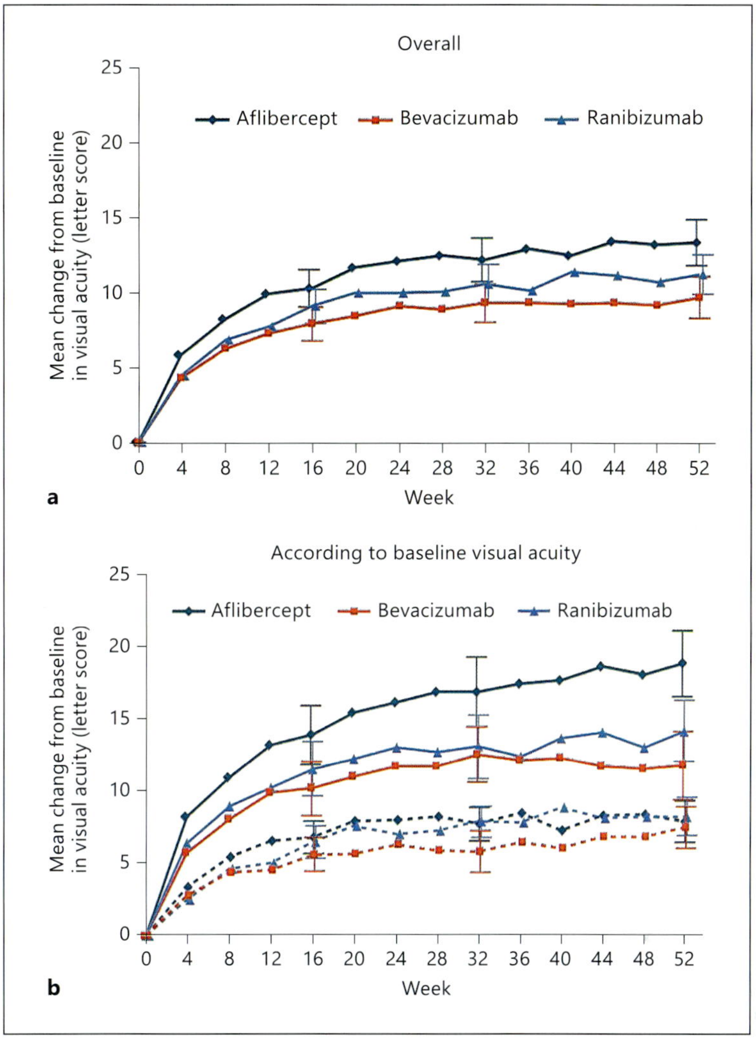

Fig. 1. Mean change from baseline in VA letter score for all patients (**a**) and based on baseline visual acuity (**b**), with dotted lines representing patients with baseline VA of 20/32 to 20/40 [1]. Reproduced with kind permission.

which injections were received was also similar (approximately 70%, Table 3). Therefore, not only was the median number of injections similar, but also the burden of care represented by the median number of visits, was also the same for all 3 treatment arms [3].

Changes in VA at Year-2

VA for the overall cohorts at year-2 maintained the improvement noted at year-1. However, differences noted between agents at year-1 did not persist at year-2. Among patients with worse baseline ETDRS VA, the mean number of letters gained by aflibercept was superior only to bevacizumab at 2 years ($p = 0.18$ for aflibercept vs. ranibizumab, $p = 0.02$ for aflibercept vs. bevacizumab, Table 4). However, when comparing the percentages of patients achieving at least a 15 ETDRS letter gain to characterize a more clinically meaningful outcome, no difference was seen between any of the treatment arms ($p = 0.74$ or 0.75 for aflibercept vs. ranibizumab and bevacizumab, respectively). Consistent with the year-1 follow-up analyses, the cohort of patients with better VA

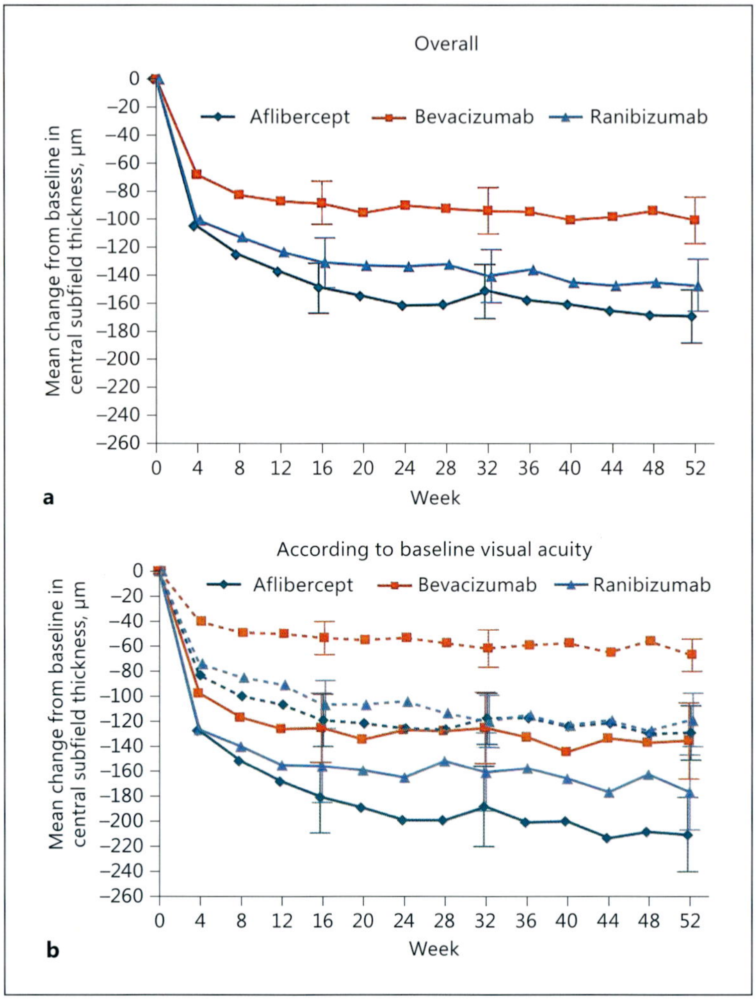

Fig. 2. Mean change central subfield thickness from baseline for all patients (**a**) and stratified based on baseline visual acuity (**b**), with dotted lined representing patients with VA of 20/32 to 20/40 [1]. Reproduced with kind permission.

(20/32 to 20/40) revealed no statistically significant differences between the 3 treatment arms at year-2 ($p = 0.51$ for aflibercept vs. ranibizumab or bevacizumab and $p = 0.31$ for ranibizumab vs. bevacizumab, Table 4), both in terms of the mean number of letters gained and with respect to the percentage of patients with a gain of ≥15 letters ($p = 0.89$ for aflibercept vs. ranibizumab or bevacizumab) [3].

The data mentioned thus far describe the differences in final VA at year-2 follow-up. However, the mean VA improvement sustained throughout the follow-up period provides insight into the changes in vision that patients experienced over the entire study time. This quantity can be represented by the area under the curve (AUC) of the change in VA measured at each follow-up visit, averaged over each follow-up visit, and was investigated in a post-hoc analysis. It was further analyzed based on whether the study eye received laser treatment. The results over the 2 years are shown in Table 5 [4], and demonstrate that patients with worse baseline VA treated with aflibercept resulted in a greater mean improvement in ETDRS VA letters over 2 years compared to the other 2 agents ($p = 0.009$ for aflibercept vs.

Table 3. Characteristics of treatment during year-2 of follow-up

	Aflibercept	Ranibizumab	Bevacizumab
Completion rate (excluding deaths), %	91	91	90
Median number of visits in year 2	10	10	10
Percentage of visits in which injection was given, %	66	70	71
Injections in year 2, median (IQR)[#]	5 (2–7)	6 (2–9)	6 (2–9)
Percentage of patients undergoing at least 1 laser treatment in year 2, %	20	27	31

VA, visual acuity; CST, central subfield thickness; IQR, Interquartile range. Adapted from Wells et al. [3].

Table 4. Visual acuity (VA) and central subfield thickness (CST) outcomes at 2 years

	Aflibercept	Ranibizumab	Bevacizumab	Aflib vs. Rani	Aflib vs. Beva	Rani vs. Beva
Improvement in ETDRS letters from baseline						
Overall, mean ± SD	+12.8±12.4	+12.3±10.5	+10.0±11.8	+2.3 (p = 0.18)	+4.7 (p = 0.02)	+2.4 (p = 0.18)
VA 20/32 to 20/40	+7.8±8.4	+8.6±7.0	+6.8±8.8	–0.7 (p = 0.51)	+1.1 (p = 0.51)	+1.9 (p = 0.31)
VA 20/50 to 20/320	+18.1±13.8	+16.1±12.1	+13.3±13.4	+2.3 (p = 0.18)	+4.7 (p = 0.02)	+2.4 (p = 0.18)
≥15 letter improvement						
VA 20/32 to 20/40, *n* (%)	21 (20)	18 (19)	16 (17)	+2 (p = 0.89)	+1 (p = 0.89)	–1 (p = 0.89)
VA 20/50 to 20/320, *n* (%)	57 (58)	52 (55)	48 (52)	+2 (p = 0.75)	+8 (p = 0.74)	+6 (p = 0.75)
≥15 letter decline						
VA 20/32 to 20/40, *n* (%)	3 (3)	1 (1)	2 (2)	+2 (p = 0.69)	+1 (p = 0.69)	–1 (p = 0.69)
VA 20/50 to 20/320, *n* (%)	2 (2)	2 (2)	4 (4)	0 (p = 0.86)	–2 (p = 0.86)	–2 (p = 0.86)
Decrease in CST from baseline						
Overall, μm	–171±141	–149±141	–126±143	–15.5 (p = 0.08)	–48.5 (p < 0.001)	–33.0 (p < 0.001)
VA 20/32 to 20/40, μm	–13±115	–125±118	–68±98	–11.8 (p = 0.26)	–57.3 (p < 0.001)	–45.4 (p < 0.001)
VA 20/50 to 20/320, μm	–211±155	–174±159	–185±158	–19.3 (p = 0.19)	–42.1 (p = 0.01)	–22.8 (p = 0.19)

Afib, aflibercept; Rani, ranibizumab; Beva, bevacizumab. Adapted from Wells et al. [3].

ranibizumab and $p < 0.001$ for aflibercept vs. bevacizumab). Aflibercept also maintained at least a 15-letter improvement in VA for a greater percentage of the time (58%) compared to both ranibizumab (46%) and bevacizumab (43%) (p = 0.05 for aflibercept vs. ranibizumab and p = 0.02 for aflibercept vs. bevacizumab, Table 5) [4]. However, if one examines the more clinically meaningful outcome of the fraction of patients who experienced a ≥10 or ≥15 letter gain, the results are not consistent (Table 5).

Changes in Retinal Thickness at Year-2

Bevacizumab had been found to decrease the retinal thickness less than both aflibercept and ranibizumab at year-1; however, this difference

Table 5. Area under the curve (AUC) analysis over 2 years with respect to baseline visual acuity (VA)

	Aflibercept	Ranibizumab	Bevacizumab	Aflib vs. Rani	Aflib vs. Beva	Rani vs. Beva
VA worse than 20/50						
Number of eyes	98	92	94			
Mean AUC (SD)	+17.1 (9.7)	+13.6 (8.5)	+12.1 (9.4)	+3.4 ($p = 0.009$)	+4.5 ($p < 0.001$)	+1.1 ($p = 0.35$)
Mean % of time per eye with VA improved by ≥10 letters from BL	73	66	60	+7 ($p = 0.29$)	+11 ($p = 0.04$)	+5 ($p = 0.29$)
Mean % of time per eye with VA improved by ≥15 letters from BL	58	46	43	+11 ($p = 0.05$)	+13 ($p = 0.02$)	+2 ($p = 0.64$)
VA 20/32-20/40						
Number of eyes	103	93	97			
AUC (SD)	+7.5 (5.2)	+7.5 (4.9)	+6.5 (5.5)	+0.0 ($p = 0.96$)	+1.4 ($p = 0.12$)	+1.4 ($p = 0.12$)
Mean % of time per eye with VA improved by ≥10 letters from BL	42	42	36	+1 ($p = 0.79$)	+9 ($p = 0.15$)	+8 ($p = 0.18$)
Mean % of time per eye with VA improved by ≥15 letters from BL	15	13	12	+3 ($p = 0.50$)	+5 ($p = 0.35$)	+2 ($p = 0.50$)

BL, baseline; VA, visual acuity; Aflib, aflibercept; Rani, ranibizumab; Beva, bevacizumab. Adapted from Jampol et al. [4].

reduced at year-2 in the cohort with worse baseline VA and was inferior only to aflibercept (Table 4) [3]. Congruently, bevacizumab decreased the retinal thickness more during year-2 (–42 μm, $p < 0.001$ from year-1 to year-2) than the other 2 drugs, as aflibercept and ranibizumab had much more modest changes after year-1 (–2 μm, $p = 0.82$ and +4, $p = 0.66$, respectively). However, laser treatments were also administered more frequently with bevacizumab than the other 2 agents. Therefore, to discern which eyes had the greatest response of reduced CST thickness from year-1 to -2, a post-hoc analysis was done dividing patients by whether or not laser treatment was administered [4]. It was found that only patients with worse baseline VA in the bevacizumab cohort, who received laser treatment, had a significant decrease in CST (–55 μm, $p < 0.001$) from year-1 to -2. The final CST at year-2 in this group with poorer baseline VA and laser treatment was similar among all treatment arms. However, in those not receiving laser, the reduction in thickness from baseline was greater with aflibercept (–209 μm) compared to bevacizumab (–144 μm) but not ranibizumab (–153 μm). Such findings were not seen in the cohort with better baseline acuity. Among the cohort of eyes with worse baseline vision who received bevacizumab, the change from 1 to 2 years was similar for eyes with and without laser treatment (+0.03 vs. +0.75 letter score, respectively) [4].

There are several potential reasons for the continued thinning of retinal thickness in the bevacizumab group as identified in the post-hoc analysis, which may be prone to selection bias. Some reasons include the effect of laser treatment, persistent administration of anti-VEGF injections, and natural history. In addition, eyes that received aflibercept and ranibizumab may have achieved the maximal amount of thinning by year-1, and therefore, additional improvement was not possible during year-2 [4].

Analysis of Cost Effectiveness and Burden of Care

Background

Although anti-VEGF drugs are highly effective in preventing visual loss from DME and in restoring vision lost due to DME, access to such treatments can be limited by cost. Aflibercept and ranibizumab are substantially more expensive than bevacizumab. A post-hoc analysis was conducted to calculate the clinical costs, benefits, and cost effectiveness of each drug. The overall medical costs and quality-adjusted life-years (QALY) were calculated based on published cost and quality-of-life data, and VA results from the first year of the trial. These costs were also projected and estimated over a 10-year time period. The incremental cost-effectiveness ratio (ICER), defined as the ratio of the incremental cost to a drug's incremental benefit in QALY compared to the next best therapy was also determined. Cost effectiveness was established as USD 100,000 per QALY, based on established standards and US guidelines [5]. These costs were also established for each subgroup: with vision ≤20/40 or ≥20/50.

Determination of Quality of Life

The quality of life was determined based on previously defined conversion tables that linked vision in the better-seeing eye to health-related quality of life. The vision at year-1 was carried forward to represent the vision for the rest of the patient's life, given that previous trials had demonstrated stability of VA between 1 and 5 years after treatment, and with the assumption that the patient would receive anti-VEGF treatments as needed to maintain such vision. The quality of life score for a particular month was decreased if patients experienced an adverse event such as retinal detachment or vitreous hemorrhage. If a patient suffered a myocardial infarction or cerebrovascular accident, the score was reduced for all subsequent visits.

Determination of Drug Cost

Drug cost was calculated based on standardized unit costs of the agent and physician fees for office-based administration. The cost for both the study eye and the non-study fellow eye were included, given that patients with bilateral involvement were required to have treatment with the same agent in both eyes. The cost of adverse events was also incorporated based on prior studies. However, costs that would apply equally to all treatment arms such as indirect medical costs and caregiver burden were not included. Therefore, the costs represent the relative burden of each therapy, but not the overall medical cost of DME treatment [5].

Results: Overall Costs and Cost Effectiveness

In the overall cohort of patients, the mean QALY was higher in the aflibercept group compared to the bevacizumab group. This difference was also noted in the cohort with better baseline vision ($p = 0.03$, 0.02, respectively, Table 6). This finding is likely due to the calculation of the QALYs as a summation of each month versus a comparison at just year-1, and evidence of a non-linear relationship between VA and quality of life.

The mean total cost per patient for anti-VEGF injections (study and non-study eyes), laser photocoagulation, and adverse events are shown in Figure 3 and Table 6. The greatest portion of total costs was the anti-VEGF agent for the study eye, at 68, 63, and 37% of the total cost for aflibercept, ranibizumab, and bevacizumab, respectively. The cost included the cost of the agent and a USD 102.97 professional fee per injection. Aflibercept and ranibizumab were 31× and 20× more expensive than bevacizumab, respectively. There were no differences in the cost of laser or due to adverse events between groups. Patients with worse baseline vision had higher costs than those with better vision. Costs were higher with aflibercept compared to the other 2 agents, and with ranibizumab compared to bevacizumab ($p < 0.001$ for all

Table 6. Various measures of cost and utility for each anti-VEGF agent

	Aflibercept	Ranibizumab	Bevacizumab	*p* value
Cost, USD				
Overall	26,100	18,600	4,100	<0.001 for all differences
VA 20/32 to 20/40	24,100	16,900	3,200	
VA 20/50 to 20/320	28,100	20,400	5,000	
Utility (QALYs)				
Overall	0.869	0.857	0.849	Aflibercept vs. bevacizumab 0.03
VA 20/32 to 20/40	0.901	0.884	0.875	Aflibercept vs. bevacizumab 0.02
VA 20/50 to 20/320	0.835	0.829	0.823	>0.15

VA, visual acuity; QALY, quality-adjusted life-years. Adapted from Ross et al. [5].

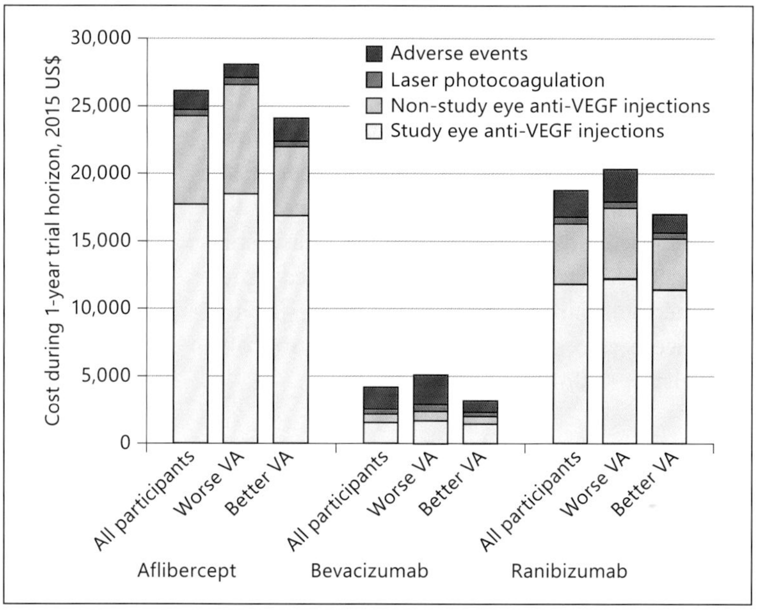

Fig. 3. The overall cost of treatment with each agent, including that of study and non-study eyes, further stratified by baseline visual acuity. From Ross et al. [5].

differences) for the overall study group and each subgroup (Table 6) [5].

The cost effectiveness of treatment with each drug over year-1 and a 10-year projection (expressed as ICER per QALY) compared to that of bevacizumab at USD 100,000 are shown in Table 7. The ICERs were greater in those with worse baseline vision and for patients receiving ranibizumab. Based on these costs, it was calculated that the cost of aflibercept would have to be reduced by 60–90% to be considered as cost-effective as bevacizumab; ranibizumab would require an even greater reduction of 75–95%. To achieve cost effectiveness at 10 years with aflibercept compared to ranibizumab, the cost of aflibercept would have to decrease by 18% among all patients (and by 9% for patients with worse vision, 28% for patients with better vision); raw values are shown in Table 8. Scenarios in which aflibercept would be considered cost-effective compared to other agents were also proposed.

Table 7. Cost effectiveness compared to bevacizumab at 1 year and 10 years

	Aflibercept	Ranibizumab
ICER per QALY (USD) compared to bevacizumab (USD/QALY) at 1 year		
Overall	1,110,000	1,730,000
VA 20/32 to 20/40	798,000	1,500,000
VA 20/50 to 20/320	1,870,000	2,450,000
ICER per QALY (USD) compared to bevacizumab (USD/QALY) at 10 years		
Overall	349,000	603,000
VA 20/32 to 20/40	474,000	506,000
VA 20/50 to 20/320	287,000	817,000

VA, visual acuity; QALY, quality-adjusted life-years; ICER, incremental cost-effectiveness ratio. Adapted from Ross et al. [5].

Table 8. Proposed costs to achieve cost effectiveness of bevacizumab

	Current cost, USD	1 year max. cost per dose for ICER of USD 100,000 per QALY relative to Beva., 2015, USD	Relative reduction from current, %	10 year Max. cost per dose for ICER of USD 100,000 per QALY relative to Beva., 2015 (USD)	Relative reduction from current, %
All patients					
Ranibizumab	1,170	100	91	230	80
Aflibercept	1,850	240	87	570	69
VA of 20/32 to 20/40					
Ranibizumab	1,170	94	92	260	77
Aflibercept	1,850	230	88	410	78
VA of 20/50 to 20/320					
Ranibizumab	1,170	94	92	190	84
Aflibercept	1,850	250	87	700	62

VA, visual acuity; QALY, quality-adjusted life-years; ICER, incremental cost-effectiveness ratio; Beva, Bevacizumab. Adapted from Ross et al. [5].

For example, in order for aflibercept to have an ICER below USD 100,000 per QALY, it would have to result in a 12-letter mean gain in VA during years 2–10, and bevacizumab would have to have a 13-letter loss [5]. These unrealistic situations emphasized that bevacizumab is much more cost-effective than the other agents.

Another method used to compare the treatments was to predict the likelihood that each of the therapies would be considered optimal (i.e., the greatest QALY with ICER below a specific willingness to pay per QALY). At 10 years, it was predicted that bevacizumab would have greater than 90% likelihood of being optimal for all patients (regardless of the baseline vision), as long as the willingness to pay was less than USD 100,000 per QALY. For the cohort of patients with worse baseline vision, aflibercept was more likely to be optimal than the other 2 agents at values of willingness to pay USD 230,000 or more [5].

Burden of Care
Despite slightly higher quality of life measures among patients receiving aflibercept and ranibizumab compared to bevacizumab, the burden of care in terms of the number of visits and number of injections was similar among all 3 cohorts. As stated previously (Table 3), the number of visits in year-2 was 10 in all 3 groups, with a median of 5, 6, and 6 injections being administered to patients in the aflibercept, ranibizumab, and bevacizumab groups. Over the 2-year study period, injections were administered at 66–71% of the visits for each treatment arm [3]. Therefore, one could consider employing a more expensive drug if the number of administrations and visits could also be decreased; however, the more expensive compounds did not afford this opportunity.

DME Treatment in Clinical Practice

Some important differences exist between the study findings and clinical practice. The VA measured by ETDRS and the Snellen equivalent tends to be 1 or 2 lines better than the vision measured directly by Snellen chart. Therefore, the 20/50 equivalent established to separate "better" and "worse" baseline vision in Protocol T is in reality more comparable to 20/60 or 20/70 in clinical practice [1]. Another factor to consider is that patients in the study had not received anti-VEGF treatment for at least 1 year prior to enrollment. Therefore, findings may not be applicable to patients with persistent or recurrent DME who have undergone recent anti-VEGF therapy. In addition, differences in VA letter scores do not always translate into clinically meaningful differences, which is better reflected in the number of patients achieving a gain or loss of at least 10 or 15 letters [1], as described before. Lastly, although the differences in decrease in retinal thickness existed between treatments, this was not always accompanied by a difference in VA. Therefore, as demonstrated in prior studies, thinner retinas are not always equivalent to better VA.

Of necessity, the opportunity to switch medications was not studied in Protocol T. Based on the fact that very few patients lost ≥15 ETDRS letters during 2 years of treatment, regardless of which drug assignment they received, one reasonable option might be to initiate therapy with any particular drug (e.g., based on cost, possible systemic safety, insurance coverage) and to switch to a more expensive/effective option if the patient does not seem to be responding satisfactorily. Decisions about switching medications are fraught with potential confounding (e.g., regression to the mean) [6], and randomized clinical trials would be helpful in providing guidance regarding this approach.

Studies of the actual administration of anti-VEGF injections in patients have shown that the number of injections tend to be fewer in clinical practice than in clinical trials. One study investigated the frequency of anti-VEGF injections over a 3-year period based on the billing of Medicare patients ($n = 770$) and the timing of the last injection compared to the last diagnosis of DME [7]. During the study period (2008–2010), the average number of anti-VEGF injections per patient increased from 3.2 in 2008 to 4.0, and to 5.0 in 2010 ($p < 0.002$). This number is much lower than those reported in clinical trials. For example, in Protocol T, an average of 9 injections were given during the first year of treatment. The total and mean number of injections and the mean number of anti-VEGF claims per patient are shown in Table 9. In addition to anti-VEGF treatment, 19 and 34% of patients received intravitreal steroid injections (triamcinolone acetonide [IVTA]) and focal laser treatment, respectively. The mean number of claims per patient for IVTA and laser were both variable and were not significantly different from year to year (Table 9, $p = 0.39$ for IVTA and $p = 0.37$ for laser) [7]. The overall frequency of

Table 9. Treatments based on year of patient enrollment

	2008	2009	2010
Number of patients enrolled	101	249	422
Total number of injections	319	1,006	2,106
Mean number of injections per patient	3.2	4.0	5.0
Mean number of anti-VEGF injection claims per patient	3.1	3.8	4.6
Mean number of IVTA claims per patient	2.4	2.8	2.2
Mean number of focal claims per patient	2.1	2.7	2.2

IVTA, intravitreal triamcinolone acetonide. Adapted from Dugel et al. [7].

Table 10. Frequency of various treatments for DME based on the number of claims per patient for the entire study period

	Patients, *n*	Claims, *n*	Patients with claims submitted, %	Mean number of claims per patient
Services for DME	772	6,654	100	8.6
Anti-VEGF	772	3,220	100	4.2
IVTA	149	363	19	2.4
Focal	260	611	34	2.4

IVTA, intravitreal triamcinolone acetonide. Adapted from Dugel et al. [7].

various treatment claims for the entire study period is shown in Table 10. The duration of DME was established based on the year in which the diagnosis was made for the final time and was in years 1, 2, or 3 for 46, 18, and 36% of patients, respectively. Therefore, close to half of the patients had a DME resolution after 1 year of treatment. Regarding the pattern of treatment, 65% of patients received their final anti-VEGF treatment for DME within 1 year of diagnosis, whereas 35% continued to be treated throughout the study period, and therefore required more injections. This was demonstrated by the fact that patients who submitted their final claims in years 1, 2, and 3 submitted a mean of 1.9, 4.0, and 7.2 anti-VEGF claims respectively ($p < 0.001$). A similar pattern was noted for focal laser treatment [7]. The authors of this study propose that patients are being undertreated with anti-VEGF therapy compared to the protocols of clinical trials. However, the study was conducted in a period in which the use of anti-VEGF for DME was not FDA-approved (approval for ranibizumab for DME was obtained in 2012). Therefore, treatment decisions and reimbursement patterns were different from later studies and present practice. They also emphasize that DME is a multifactorial disease as many patients required concurrent treatment with IVTA and laser. The majority of patients (65%) had DME that persisted longer than 1 year, and some patients did not receive their final DME diagnosis during the study period. In addition, the authors suggest that patients who respond well to anti-VEGF treatment will do so early. Among those who received their final diagnosis of DME in year-1, over 70% had their final anti-VEGF claim in the first quarter after diagnosis. In addition to the study being partially conducted during a time

Table 11. Ocular adverse events for study eye, occurring at least once

	Aflibercept (n = 224)	Ranibizumab (n = 228)	Bevacizumab (n = 218)	Global p value
Number of injections	2,998	3,066	3,115	
Endophthalmitis	0	0	1 (<1)	0.66
Inflammation	6 (3)	4 (2)	3 (1)	0.69
Retinal detachment (any type)	2 (<1)	1 (<1)	2 (<1)	1.0
Retinal tear	1 (<1)	1 (<1)	1 (<1)	1.0
Vitreous hemorrhage	15 (7)	10 (5)	17 (8)	0.37
Injection-related cataract	3 (1)	0	2 (<1)	0.38
IOP elevation	39 (17)	35 (16)	27 (12)	0.31

IOP, intraocular pressure. Adapted from Wells et al. [3].

when anti-VEGF was not approved for DME, other limitations include the small sample size [7].

Safety

Anti-VEGF agents clearly provide visual benefit to DME patients. However, administration of these medications is known to be associated with risks, both ocular and systemic. Intravitreal administration of medications can cause infectious endophthalmitis, retinal tear or detachment, or increased intraocular pressure. All 3 agents had similar incidence of these complications during the study period (Table 11). Systemic vascular events are of particular concern. Between the 3 cohorts, the unadjusted global p value was 0.047 for Antiplatelet Trialists' Collaboration (APTC) events (Table 12). The pairwise comparisons were $p = 0.34$ for aflibercept versus bevacizumab, $p = 0.047$ for aflibercept versus ranibizumab, and $p = 0.20$ for ranibizumab versus bevacizumab. When adjusted for potential confounders (such as gender, age at baseline, hemoglobin A1c at baseline, diabetes type, diabetes duration at baseline, insulin use, prior coronary artery disease, prior myocardial infarction or stroke, prior transient ischemic attack, prior hypertension, smoking status), there was no statistically significant difference in APTC rates (global p value = 0.09). Besides the APTC events, no other differences were found between the 3 groups at 2 years (Table 12) [3]. Evaluation of data from the RIDE/RISE and VIVID/VISTA trials, focused on patients with the highest exposure to ranibizumab (0.5 mg every 4 weeks) and aflibercept (2 mg every 4 weeks), demonstrates a ~3-fold increased risk of all cause mortality for each cohort compared to randomized controls [8]. Thus, both aflibercept and ranibizumab are likely to be associated with a small but definite increased risk of systemic vascular complications (a known class effect for agents that block VEFG signaling) among high-risk patients (e.g., diabetic patients with DME) and high drug exposure.

Take Away Points from Protocol T for the Practicing Clinician:

Protocol T provides valuable information for the practicing ophthalmologist regarding the management of DME with anti-VEGF agents. The major results are:

- Aflibercept, ranibizumab, and bevacizumab are effective in improving the vision by approximately 2 lines and decreasing the central

Table 12. Systemic adverse events for study eye, occurring at least once

	Aflibercept ($n = 224$)	Ranibizumab ($n = 228$)	Bevacizumab ($n = 218$)	Global p value
Vascular events based on APTC occurring at least once, number of patients, %				
Non-fatal myocardial infarction	7 (3)	6 (3)	3 (1)	NA
Non-fatal stroke	2 (<1)	11 (5)	6 (3)	NA
Vascular death	3 (1)	9 (4)	8 (4)	NA
Any APTC event	12 (5)	26 (12)	17 (8)	0.047
APTC event with no history of MI or CVA	10 (5); $n = 203$	17 (9); $n = 193$	12 (6); $n = 193$	NA
APTC event with history of MI or CVA	2 (10); $n = 21$	9 (36); $n = 25$	5 (20); $n = 25$	NA
Pre-specified systemic events occurring at least once, number of participants, %				
Death (any cause)	5 (2)	11 (5)	13 (6)	0.12
Hospitalization	77 (34)	73 (33)	71 (33)	0.93
Serious adverse event	88 (39)	82 (38)	81 (37)	0.90
Gastrointestinal	67 (30)	60 (28)	64 (29)	0.85
Kidney	50 (22)	35 (16)	46 (21)	0.22
Hypertension	39 (17)	44 (20)	27 (21)	0.08

APTC, antiplatelet trialists' collaboration; MI, myocardial infarction; CVA, cerebrovascular accident; NA, not available. Adapted from Wells et al. [3].

retinal thickness in patients with center-involving DME.

- Despite treatment with anti-VEGF agents, many patients still required additional therapies including focal or grid laser treatment.
- At year-1, patients with worse baseline vision (ETDRS VA 20/50 or worse) had greater improvement in VA letters with aflibercept compared to ranibizumab and bevacizumab. However, this difference did not persist at year-2 when comparing aflibercept and ranibizumab. The difference between aflibercept and bevacizumab at year-2 remained statistically significant with regard to the mean gain in ETDRS vision, but the difference may not have been clinically important (see next point).
- There was no clinically meaningful difference between the 3 agents at year-2 in patients with better or worse baseline acuity as judged by the likelihood of a ≥10 or ≥15 letter gain in ETDRS VA or a ≥10 or ≥15 letter loss in ETDRS VA.
- AUC analysis did not demonstrate a consistent, clinically important benefit of aflibercept over bevacizumab or ranibizumab regarding the likelihood of a ≥10 or ≥15 ETDRS letter gain during the 2-year follow-up. The mean difference in the AUCs plotting visual improvement as a function of time was statistically significant and favored aflibercept.
- There was no difference between any of the agents at years-1 or -2 in patients with better baseline VA (20/32 to 20/40) in terms of the number of ETDRS letters gained, the number of patients with a ≥15 letter gain, or the mean improvement over time.
- Central retinal thickness decreased at years-1 and -2 of follow-up with all agents, but bevacizumab yielded less improvement at year-1 than the other agents. This difference diminished by year-2, particularly in patients with poorer baseline acuity who also received more frequent laser treatment.
- The burden of care regarding the number of office visits and number of injections was the same for all 3 agents.

- Aflibercept and ranibizumab are significantly more expensive than bevacizumab.
- Bevacizumab is much more cost effective (factoring expense and quality of life measures) than both aflibercept and ranibizumab; the costs of aflibercept and ranibizumab would have to decrease by approximately 80–90% to be cost effective compared to bevacizumab.
- Investigations of the early use of anti-VEGF agents in practice show that patients receive fewer injections than what is administered in clinical trials; however, many patients still had a resolution of DME.
- Anti-VEGF agents are generally safe and have few ocular and systemic side effects. Increased caution for DME patients with a recent history of myocardial infarction or stroke may be warranted.

References

1 Diabetic Retinopathy Clinical Research Network, Wells JA, Glassman AR, et al: Aflibercept, bevacizumab, or ranibizumab for diabetic macular edema. N Engl J Med 2015;372:1193–1203.

2 Bressler SB, Glassman AR, Almukhtar T, et al: Five-year outcomes of ranibizumab with prompt or deferred laser versus laser or triamcinolone plus deferred ranibizumab for diabetic macular edema. Am J Ophthalmol 2016;164:57–68.

3 Wells JA, Glassman AR, Ayala AR, et al: Aflibercept, bevacizumab, or ranibizumab for diabetic macular edema: two-year results from a comparative effectiveness randomized clinical trial. Ophthalmology 2016;123:1351–1359.

4 Jampol LM, Glassman AR, Bressler NM, Wells JA, Ayala AR, Diabetic Retinopathy Clinical Research Network: Anti-vascular endothelial growth factor comparative effectiveness trial for diabetic macular edema: additional efficacy post hoc analyses of a randomized clinical trial. JAMA Ophthalmol 2016:134, DOI: 10.1001/jamaophthalmol.2016.3698.

5 Ross EL, Hutton DW, Stein JD, et al: Cost-effectiveness of aflibercept, bevacizumab, and ranibizumab for diabetic macular edema treatment: analysis from the diabetic retinopathy clinical research network comparative effectiveness trial. JAMA Ophthalmol 2016;134:888–896.

6 Ferris FL, Maguire MG, Glassman AR, Ying GS, Martin DF: Evaluating effects of switching anti-vascular endothelial growth factor drugs for age-related macular degeneration and diabetic macular edema. JAMA Ophthalmol 2016, DOI: 10.1001/jamaophthalmol.2016.4820.

7 Dugel PU, Layton A, Varma RB: Diabetic macular edema diagnosis and treatment in the real world: an analysis of Medicare claims data (2008 to 2010). Ophthalmic Surg Lasers Imaging Retina 2016;47:258–267.

8 Avery RL, Gordon GM: Systemic safety of prolonged monthly anti-vascular endothelial growth factor therapy for diabetic macular edema: a systematic review and meta-analysis. JAMA Ophthalmol 2016;134:21–29.

Marco A. Zarbin, MD, PhD, FACS
Institute of Ophthalmology and Visual Science
Rutgers-New Jersey Medical School, Rutgers University, Doctors Office Center
90 Bergen Street, Newark, NJ 07103 (USA)
E-Mail zarbin@earthlink.net

Bandello F, Zarbin MA, Lattanzio R, Zucchiatti I (eds): Management of Diabetic Retinopathy.
Dev Ophthalmol. Basel, Karger, 2017, vol 60, pp 125–130 (DOI: 10.1159/000459696)

Is Laser Still Important in Diabetic Macular Edema as Primary or Deferral Therapy?

Maurizio Battaglia Parodi · Francesco Bandello

Department of Ophthalmology, University Vita-Salute, Ospedale San Raffaele, Milan, Italy

Abstract

Laser treatment was used in the past to reduce the visual loss due to diabetic macular edema. The recent advent of anti-vascular endothelial growth factor (anti-VEGF) has completely revolutionized the management of diabetic retinopathy, with a significant improvement in the overall prognosis. Nevertheless, macular laser can still be applied in selected cases characterized by retinal thickness ≤400 microns, high visual acuity, extrafoveal location, and contraindications to the intravitreal approach with anti-VEGF and steroids. In addition, the combined therapy with anti-VEGF and macular laser can exploit the synergistic effects of both therapies, leading to a simpler and more practical management of patients over the long-term follow-up.

Introduction

Laser treatment has been the most used approach to stop the progression of diabetic retinopathy (DR). Laser photocoagulation was normally applied to two major complications of DR: ocular neovascularization and diabetic macular edema (DME). A recent Cochrane review focused on the effects of anti-vascular endothelial growth factor (anti-VEGF) drugs on the management of DME, demonstrating strong evidence in favor of anti-VEGF therapy, with respect to conventional macular laser photocoagulation [1]. Moreover, Protocol S of Diabetic Retinopathy Clinical Research Network (DRCRnet) proved that repeated anti-VEGF treatments are an effective alternative to laser photocoagulation for the management of proliferative DR in patients prepared to comply with frequent office visits [2]. In spite of the positive results of anti-VEGF approach, however, we have to note that in all the trials a variable number of patients received additional laser photocoagulation to control the DME and ocular neovascularization, indirectly showing that conventional laser photocoagulation still has a role.

Laser for Peripheral Retina

The DR study demonstrated the useful effects of panretinal photocoagulation (PRP) for proliferative DR with active neovascularization. In particular, the incidence of severe vision loss (defined as best-corrected visual acuity [BCVA] less than 5/200 at 2 consecutive visits 4 months apart) at 2 years decreased from 26% of controls to 11% of treated eyes, and this trend increased

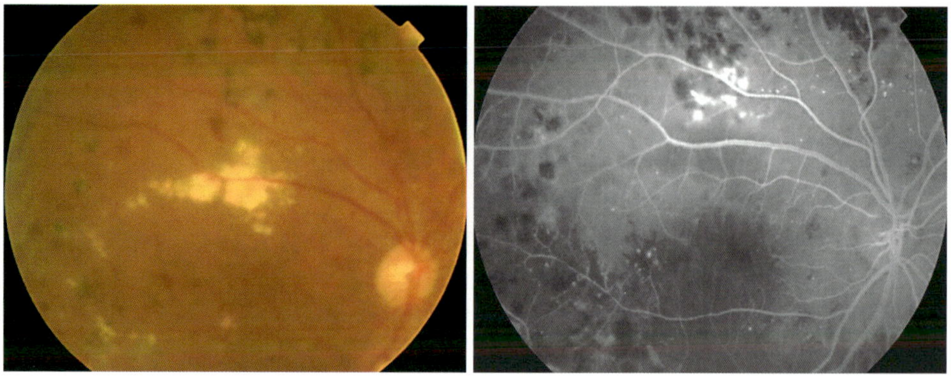

Fig. 1. A case of proliferative diabetic retinopathy with clinically significant macular edema.

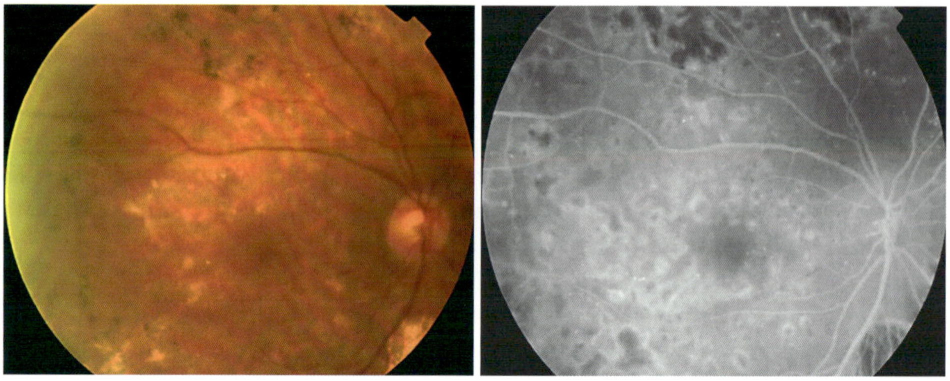

Fig. 2. Same cases 2 years after grid laser photocoagulation, showing resolution of exudative manifestations.

at 4 years with 44% of controls and 20% of treated eyes [3].

Further evidence for the beneficial effects of PRP was provided by the Early Treatment Diabetic Retinopathy Study (ETDRS). The ETDRS found a 5-year rate of severe vision loss of 2.6% in the treatment group and 3.7% in the control group [4].

More recently, the DRCRnet conducted a clinical trial comparing PRP in 1 session versus 4 sessions and found no clinically significant difference [5].

Despite its remarkable effectiveness in the treatment of proliferative DR, PRP can cause side effects, including peripheral visual field defects, night-vision loss, loss of contrast sensitivity, and exacerbation of pre-existing DME with further loss of visual function. Furthermore, 5% of eyes turned out to have severe vision loss despite PRP (BCVA worse than 5/200 at 2 consecutive visits).

Laser for DME

The ETDRS confirmed the beneficial effects of focal/grid laser for DME. Focal photocoagulation consisted of direct focal treatment of microaneurysms more than 500 μm from the foveal center. On the contrary, grid photocoagulation (Fig. 1, 2) was directed to areas of diffuse leakage and capillary non-perfusion on fluorescein angiography [6].

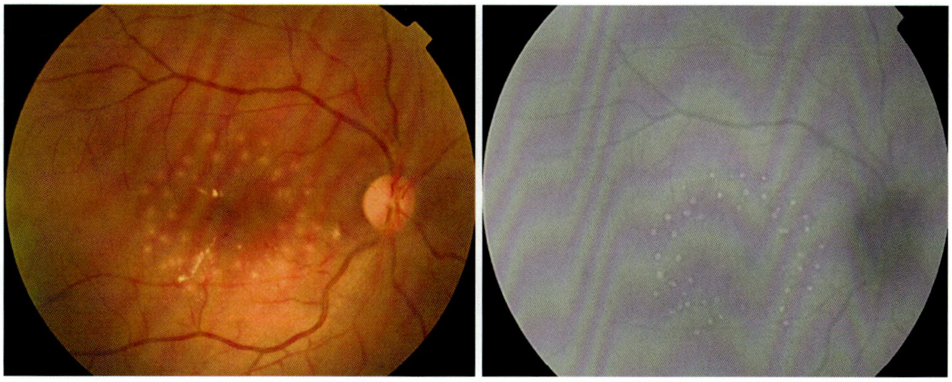

Fig. 3. Color photography and fundus autofluorescence of a case treated with conventional grid laser photocoagulation.

The ETDRS study defined the clinically significant macular edema in 3 different categories: (1) retinal thickening at or within 500 μm of the center of the macula; (2) hard exudates at or within 500 μm of the center of the macula, if associated with adjacent retinal thickening; (3) or a zone or zones of retinal thickening 1 disc area in size, at least part of which is within 1 disc diameter of the center of the macula.

The results at 3 years revealed that the risk of moderate visual loss was 12% in the treated eyes compared to 24% in the untreated eyes, reducing the risk by 50%. The benefits of treatment were present regardless of initial visual acuity, even though the final visual gain increased as baseline visual acuity decreased. In the subgroup of patients with DME involving or threatening the center of the macula, the treatment benefit was greater. Laser scar can be easily identified by means of fundus autofluorescence, to retreat the macula if necessary (Fig. 3).

Current Indications for Macular Laser in DME

Even though intravitreal approach with anti-VEGF agents and steroids is superior to macular laser therapy alone in the management of DME, macular laser treatment can still be considered for some cases.

DME with Central Retinal Thickness <300 μm

A post-hoc subset analysis of the RESTORE trial revealed that macular laser photocoagulation improved BCVA and monthly ranibizumab in eyes affected by DME, which are characterized by baseline central retinal thickness (CRT) less than 300 μm [7]. In addition, taking into consideration eyes with CRT between 300 and 400 μm, the outcomes of macular laser turned out to be comparable with those obtained using intravitreal ranibizumab. This observation led the National Institute for Health Care Excellence in United Kingdom to approve ranibizumab only for eyes with CRT >400 μm. Macular laser can also be performed using new laser applications, including PASCAL or subthreshold treatment, which lessen or completely eliminate the retinal damage (Fig. 4).

DME with High Visual Acuity

DME can be identified in patients with fully preserved or high BCVA (20/20–20/25). To decide on the treatment option, many factors should be considered, including systemic control, age of patients, psychophysical evidence of early retinal impairment (especially by means of

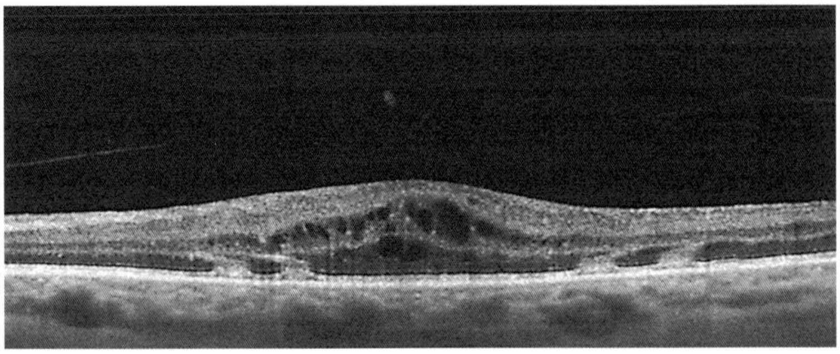

Fig. 4. Grid macular photocoagulation with PASCAL laser in an eye with central retinal thickness of 387 μm. Pascal laser determines a minimal retinal damage at the level of outer retinal layers, due to the reduced choroidal and inner retinal heating secondary to the limited thermal diffusion. The laser spots (white arrows) are confined to the outer retinal layers, with conservation of the inner retina.

microperimetry or mfERG), professional requirements, and psychological profile of the specific patient. Macular laser can be performed, especially using subthreshold laser treatment, which minimizes the retinal damage. Subthreshold laser treatment was employed for DME and other retinal vascular disorders [8–10], especially with the micropulse application, which allows heat dispersion during the treatment avoiding any collateral damage. The mechanism of action of subthreshold laser is still uncertain, but it is thought that laser application initiates the upregulation of several cytoprotective factors (pigment-epithelium-derived factor, thrombospondin-1, heat shock protein) chiefly from the adjacent cells receiving sublethal photothermal damage. Subthreshold laser treatment can be repeated many times in the same macular area of the same patient, if necessary, to control recurrent DME.

DME with Extrafoveal Location

Patients characterized by DME with an extrafoveal location generally have preserved central visual function. Any treatment decision should be made on the basis of the risk of an extension of the DME to the fovea. Macular laser treatment, especially carried out using subthreshold laser application, can be considered to promote edema resolution and to halt the progression in the direction of the fovea.

DME in Patients with Ocular and Systemic Contraindications to Intravitreal Injections

Ocular and systemic conditions can objectively limit the access to intravitreal injections. In particular, patients with a high cardiovascular risk profile may not be ideal candidates to receive anti-VEGF treatment (due to a possible increased risk of stroke and myocardial infarction), and patients affected by glaucoma and chronic infections should not be treated with intravitreal steroids. Under these circumstances, macular laser treatment can be considered and effectively performed.

DME in Patients Unable to Comply with Frequent Office Visits

Older and sick patients, along with patients living far away from the treatment center often have problems complying with the necessity of frequent re-examinations and re-treatment in a chronic disease such as DR. Thus, for practical reasons, macular laser treatment represents the simplest choice under these circumstances.

Combined Therapy of Anti-VEGF and Macular Laser Photocoagulation

Anti-VEGF therapy has been proved to be superior compared to macular laser photocoagulation in improving the vision in center-involving DME, but it is noteworthy that all of the major anti-VEGF trials used laser as a rescue therapy. In particular, a variable figure from 30 to 60% of eyes required supplementary rescue macular laser to control the DME at some time-point over the scheduled follow-up. The DRCRnet with Protocol I assessed the effects of prompt macular laser and deferred macular laser in eyes with DME, showing a visual acuity improvement of 7.2 in the prompt laser subgroup and 9.8 in the deferred laser subgroup at 5 years. Nevertheless, in the deferred laser subgroup, macular laser was required in 44% at some point over the follow-up [11]. Furthermore, the DRCRnet demonstrated in Protocol T that all the 3 anti-VEGF drugs could provide BCVA improvement from baseline to 2 years with a decreased number of injections in year 2. However, macular laser was required in 41% of aflibercept subgroup, 52% of ranibizumab subgroup, and 64% of bevacizumab subgroup over the 24-month follow-up [12]. Thus, it is likely that the combined therapy of anti-VEGF and macular laser is especially beneficial in the long run to control DME, as the laser gradually takes effect, to reduce the number of injections and to achieve the maintenance of early visual acuity gain due initially to the anti-VEGF administration.

Peripheral Retinal Photocoagulation and DME

Large areas of peripheral capillary non-perfusion can sustain the high VEGF intravitreal levels. Peripheral capillary non-perfusion can be visualized with standard fluorescein angiography, but the recent advent of wide-field angiography has enormously implemented the identification of vascular abnormalities in the periphery. Conventional laser photocoagulation could be targeted in those areas in an attempt to stop the up-regulation and release of VEGF. Theoretically, the reduced VEGF concentration could lead to better control of DME [13]. However, clinical results are still controversial and a few randomized clinical trials are ongoing with the specific aim to provide an answer to this question. In this regard, it is interesting that even the recent Protocol S trial of DRCRnet shows that PRP monotherapy has limited effects on the DME course. Indeed, 53% of eyes affected by DME in the subgroup assigned to PRP alone required ranibizumab injections to control DME [11].

Conclusions

Laser treatment still has a place in the management of DME, even in the current era of advanced pharmacotherapy. Further randomized clinical trials are warranted to define the most appropriate approach for each DME subtype. In addition, a more comprehensive treatment algorithm is necessary to improve the management of DME.

References

1 Virgili G, Parravano M, Menchini F, Evans JR: Anti-vascular endothelial growth factor for diabetic macular oedema. Cochrane Database Syst Rev 2014;24:CD007419.

2 Writing Committee for the Diabetic Retinopathy Clinical Research Network, Gross JG, Glassman AR, et al: Panretinal photocoagulation vs. intravitreous ranibizumab for proliferative diabetic retinopathy: A Randomized Clinical Trial. JAMA 2015;314:2137–2146.

3 Indications for photocoagulation treatment of diabetic retinopathy: diabetic retinopathy study report no. 14. The Diabetic Retinopathy Study Research Group. Int Ophthalmol Clin 1987;27: 239–253.

4 Early photocoagulation for diabetic retinopathy. ETDRS report number 9. Early Treatment Diabetic Retinopathy Study Research Group. Ophthalmology 1991; 98(5 suppl):766–785.

5 Diabetic Retinopathy Clinical Research Network, Brucker AJ, Qin H, Antoszyk AN, et al: Observational study of the development of diabetic macular edema following panretinal (scatter) photocoagulation given in 1 or 4 sittings. Arch Ophthalmol 2009;127:132–140.

6 Early Treatment Diabetic retinopathy Study R: Photocoagulation for diabetic macular edema. Early Treatment Diabetic Retinopathy Study report number 1. Early Treatment Diabetic Retinopathy Study research group. Arch Ophthalmol 1985;103:1796–1806.
7 Mitchell P, Bandello F, Schmidt-Erfurth U, Lang GE, Massin P, Schlingemann RO, Sutter F, Simader C, Burian G, Gerstner O, et al: The RESTORE study: ranibizumab monotherapy or combined with laser versus laser monotherapy for diabetic macular edema. Ophthalmology 2011;118:615–625.
8 Figueira J, Khan J, Nunes S, et al: Prospective randomised controlled trial comparing sub-threshold micropulse diode laser photocoagulation and conventional green laser for clinically significant diabetic macular oedema. Br J Ophthalmol 2009;93:1341–1344.
9 Battaglia Parodi M, Spasse S, Iacono P, et al: Subthreshold grid laser treatment of macular edema secondary to branch retinal vein occlusion with micropulse infrared (810 nanometer) diode laser. Ophthalmology 2006;113:2237–2242.
10 Battaglia Parodi M, Iacono P, Pierro L, Papayannis A, Kontadakis S, Bandello FM: Subthreshold laser treatment versus threshold laser treatment for symptomatic retinal arterial macroaneurysm. Invest Ophthalmol Vis Sci 2012;53:1783–1786.
11 Elman MJ, Ayala A, Bressler NM, Browning D, Flaxel CJ, Glassman AR, Jampol LM, Stone TW; Diabetic Retinopathy Clinical Research Network: Intravitreal Ranibizumab for diabetic macular edema with prompt versus deferred laser treatment: 5-year randomized trial results. Ophthalmology 2015;122:375–381.
12 Wells JA, Glassman AR, Ayala AR, Jampol LM, Bressler NM, Bressler SB, Brucker AJ, Ferris FL, Hampton GR, Jhaveri C, Melia M, Beck RW; Diabetic Retinopathy Clinical Research Network: Aflibercept, bevacizumab, or ranibizumab for diabetic maculare: two-year results from a Comparative Effectiveness Randomized Clinical Trial. Ophthalmology 2016;123:1351–1359.
13 Patel RD, Messner LV, Teitelbaum B, Michel KA, Hariprasad SM: Characterization of ischemic index using ultrawidefield fluorescein angiography in patients with focal and diffuse recalcitrant diabetic macular edema. Am J Ophthalmol 2013;155:1038–1044.

Dr. Maurizio Battaglia Parodi
Department of Ophthalmology, University Vita-Salute
Ospedale San Raffaele, Via Olgettina, 60
IT–20132 Milan (Italy)
E-Mail battagliaparodi.maurizio@hsr.it

Bandello F, Zarbin MA, Lattanzio R, Zucchiatti I (eds): Management of Diabetic Retinopathy.
Dev Ophthalmol. Basel, Karger, 2017, vol 60, pp 131–142 (DOI: 10.1159/000459699)

Anti-Vascular Endothelial Growth Factor Injections: The New Standard of Care in Proliferative Diabetic Retinopathy?

Xintong Li • Marco A. Zarbin • Neelakshi Bhagat

Institute of Ophthalmology and Visual Science, Rutgers New Jersey Medical School, Newark, NJ, USA

Abstract

For decades, panretinal photocoagulation (PRP) has been the standard of care for the treatment of proliferative diabetic retinopathy (PDR). The relatively recent advent of anti-vascular endothelial growth factor (VEGF) formulations for intravitreal injection has provided a fresh perspective on PDR treatment, especially in eyes with concurrent diabetic macular edema (DME). The anti-VEGF agent ranibizumab has demonstrated a potentially protective effect on eyes with DME in terms of progression to PDR in the RIDE/RISE trials, as has aflibercept in the VIVID/VISTA trials. In 2015, these 2 agents were approved by the Food and Drug Administration for the treatment of PDR with DME, though PRP still remains the standard of care for eyes without baseline DME. Published results from Protocol S illustrate the non-inferiority of ranibizumab versus PRP in the treatment of PDR, the first prospective study to do so in eyes with and without baseline DME. These results also reveal that treatment with ranibizumab, when compared to standard treatment with PRP, may also lead to less peripheral visual field loss, reduced need for vitrectomy, and reduced chance for developing DME. Both PRP and intravitreal ranibizumab have very low rates of adverse events. However, treatment with anti-VEGF agents generally is associated with higher costs, increased need for follow-up, and the risk of potentially catastrophic ocular complications (e.g., endophthalmitis) and systemic side effects. Anti-VEGF agents should be considered in cases of media opacity preventing completion of PRP in compliant patients without recent cerebrovascular accident or myocardial infarction, though the long-term efficacy of these agents remains to be studied, especially after the discontinuation of injections.

Introduction

Panretinal photocoagulation (PRP) has been the standard of treatment for proliferative diabetic retinopathy (PDR) for the last 40 years. The diabetic retinopathy (DR) study in the late 1970s showed a 50% decrease in the rate of severe vision loss in eyes (i.e., vision worse than 5/200) among patients with PDR treated with PRP compared to untreated eyes [1, 2]. PRP, however, may cause peripheral visual field loss, nyctalopia, and reduced retinal sensitivity [3, 4]. Other adverse effects include worsening of macular edema, uveal effusion, choroidal neovascularization, and pain

[5–9]. Media opacities such as cataract, corneal edema, and vitreous hemorrhage can hinder the application of PRP.

Increased intravitreal levels of vascular endothelial growth factor (VEGF) are present in patients with severe DR [1, 10]. Intravitreal therapy with anti-VEGF agents has shown promise as a potential alternative in treating PDR [11–15]. At 2 years follow-up, a higher proportion of eyes treated with ranibizumab exhibited a 3-step or more improvement of DR compared to sham [16]. The diabetic macular edema (DME) RIDE/RISE and VIVID/VISTA trials showed a lower likelihood of progression to PDR in eyes that received ranibizumab or aflibercept, respectively [14, 15]. Both of these anti-VEGF agents were approved by the Food and Drug Administration for treatment of eyes with PDR and DME in 2015; the approval was, however, based on the effect seen on DR eyes with DME [15, 16].

In 2015, the Diabetic Retinopathy Clinical Research Study group published the findings of Protocol S, a multicenter, randomized, controlled study [13] of 394 eyes with PDR treated with intravitreal ranibizumab 0.5 mg. They noted that initiating treatment in cases of PDR using ranibizumab resulted in final visual acuity (VA) at 2-year follow-up that was no worse than the treatment with PRP (non-inferiority limit was 5 ETDRS letters). Since then, these results have been extrapolated to the use of other anti-VEGF agents (bevacizumab, aflibercept) for PDR with or without DME.

Management of PDR is undergoing a paradigm shift. In this chapter, we review the results of Protocol S in detail and how it impacts the treatment and management of PDR.

Protocol S

Protocol S was designed to determine if visual acuity outcomes at 2 years with intravitreal ranibizumab 0.5 mg were non-inferior to prompt PRP in eyes with PDR. The secondary objectives were to compare the effects of anti-VEGF therapy and PRP on visual function, peripheral vision, DME, and incidence of vitrectomy in these eyes.

Design and Inclusion Criteria (http://drcrnet.jaeb.org/Studies.aspx?RecID = 201)

This prospective, multicenter, randomized study included patients over 18 years of age with either type 1 or 2 diabetes mellitus with PDR without previous PRP treatment, with a best-corrected ETDRS VA of 20/320 or better (letter score of 24 or better) and with media clarity sufficient to perform PRP. Eyes with or without DME could be enrolled.

The study eyes were randomized (1:1) into 2 arms: prompt PRP or intravitreal ranibizumab (0.5 mg) with deferred PRP. If both eyes were recruited in the study, each had to be in a different arm of the study. Exclusion criteria included history of previous PRP, tractional retinal detachment of the macula, neovascularization of the angle, macular edema due to non-diabetic causes, significant cataract causing a VA decline to 20/40, history of anti-VEGF treatment in the previous 2 months, history of intravitreal or peribulbar corticosteroids in the previous 4 months, history of any ocular surgery in the previous 4 months, or aphakia. Intravitreal ranibizumab was given on an as-needed basis for DME. Primary outcome was scheduled at year 2 with a 5-year final follow-up.

Follow-up schedule for the first year in the ranibizumab group included every 4-week follow-up visits. Once the PRP was completed in the laser group within an 8-week time interval, follow-up visits were scheduled every 16 weeks in the first year for eyes in the prompt PRP group. For years 2 and 3, the follow-up visits depended on disease progression and could be every 4–16 weeks. Follow-up after that was as per standard of care but with study visits at years 4 and 5. More frequent visits could be arranged for DME management.

Visual acuity and optical coherence tomography (OCT) was performed at every study visit.

Main Efficacy Measures

The primary outcome measure was mean change in VA in the 2 groups from baseline to year 2. Secondary outcomes were area under the curve analysis for mean VA over 2 years, proportion of eyes with gain or loss of 10 and 15 letters, need for additional PRP after completion or deferred PRP, need for vitrectomy, mean change in retinal thickness on OCT (central subfield thickness [CST] and other subfields), progression of DME in the central subfield in eyes with CST less than 250 microns at baseline, proportion of eyes with vitreous hemorrhage, proportion of eyes with complete regression of neovascularization on fundus photography, associated treatment costs, and proportion of eyes not requiring PRP in the deferred PRP group.

Treatment Regimens

Study eyes were randomized to 2 groups: prompt PRP and ranibizumab with deferred PRP. All eyes in the ranibizumab arm received injections at baseline irrespective of ME status. In both groups, all eyes with center involving (CI)-DME (CST ≥250 microns) and VA 20/32 or worse received intravitreal ranibizumab at baseline. If both eyes of a participant were study eyes and needed intravitreal injections, one eye was done on the day of randomization, and the other eye within 1 week of the first injection.

Prompt PRP

Prompt PRP was delivered in 1–3 sessions within 8 weeks of randomization. Eyes assigned to the PRP group underwent laser the day of randomization unless the eyes also had DME, in which case intravitreal ranibizumab was given immediately after the PRP laser the same day or PRP was performed 0–14 days after baseline injection.

PRP was performed with 500-micron burns for a total of 1,200–1,600 burns, each 1 burn width apart at 0.1 s exposure (acceptable range of 0.05–0.2 s). A wavelength in the green to yellow spectrum was used except in the presence of vitreous hemorrhage, in which case a red wavelength was employed. Burns were distributed from the arcades to at least the equator, with no more than 1–3 sessions, in the temporal arcade >3,000 microns from the fovea, and the nasal limit being >500 microns from the disk. Re-treatment could be performed if increased neovascularization was seen at follow-up.

Ranibizumab Plus Deferred PRP Group

Treatment consisted of a baseline ranibizumab 0.5 mg intravitreal injection followed by 3 monthly injections at the month-1, -2, and -3 follow-up visits, irrespective of the status of neovascularization. At the month-4 and -5 visits, if no neovascularization was seen, the injection was withheld. The injections were continued until neovascularization resolved or was deemed stable clinically for 3 consecutive study follow-up visits.

Re-injection criteria at or after 6 months of follow-up (Table 1) were:

(a) Neovascularization improvement (1 re-injection) or stabilization (2 more monthly injections).

(b) Neovascularization unable to be visualized secondary to vitreous or preretinal hemorrhage (1 re-injection).

In refractory cases, such as eyes with increasing angle neovascularization at any time or elsewhere after the fourth injection, or persisting or recurring neovascularization after 5 or more injections, re-injection or PRP could be considered.

The monthly injections were continued until stabilization or resolution was achieved. If DME or PDR worsened after the injections were deferred, injections were restarted.

Table 1 describes the retreatment criteria in detail.

Diabetic Macular Edema

There were approximately 20% of PDR eyes with DME in the 2 arms that received ranibizumab 0.5 mg at baseline. These eyes were treated with the same algorithm as was used in Protocol I [12].

Table 1. Evaluation for retreatment with ranibizumab

Category	Definition	Re-inject?	PRP?
Resolved	No neovascularization*	No	No
Improvement	Decreased size or density*	Yes	No
Stable	Unchanged neovascularization	Yes (2 more**)	No
Not fully treated	Recurrent or worsening neovascularization of retina, disc, or iris in eye with <4 injections, OR Vitreous/preretinal hemorrhage preventing adequate visualization	Yes	No
Failure	New/worsening neovascularization of retina, disc, or iris to greater than baseline with 4+ study injections, OR New/worsening neovascularization of angle, OR Worsening neovascularization or fibrous proliferation of retina, disc, or iris 1+ day after last injection with strong likelihood of substantial vision loss without PRP	No	Yes
Futility	Persistent/recurrent neovascularization at 1.5 years or more, not improved from baseline, with 5+ study injections	No	Yes

* With adequate visualization of retina, disc, iris, and angle; ** at 4-week intervals.

If DME developed at any point, 4 consecutive monthly injections of ranibizumab 0.5 mg were given, or focal or grid photocoagulation performed. If DME was still present but showed improvement (macular thickness decreased by 10% from onset or 1 Snellen line improvement in VA), re-injection of ranibizumab was given. If DME resolved and vision improved, no more injections were indicated. If only one of the criteria were met or in refractory cases, the clinician would decide whether to continue with re-injection or switch to focal laser.

In case of inability to tolerate ranibizumab or intravitreal injections, or if 6 months had passed since the initial injection without improvement, focal or grid photocoagulation was indicated for DME in eyes with PDR. The same wavelength could be used at a spot size of 50 microns and burn duration of 0.05–0.1 s, with burns 500–3,000 microns from the center of the macula (maximum 3,500 microns permissible temporally for grid photocoagulation). Focal burns were targeted directly at the microaneurysm. Prior to grid photocoagulation, fluorescein angiography was performed; burns were targeted at areas with DME and non-perfusion on angiography with or without microaneurysms.

Results

The 2 groups were balanced in terms of age, gender, duration of diabetes, mean hemoglobin A1C level, and no prior PRP. The mean baseline vision was 75 letters (20/32) in both groups, and the mean OCT CST was 262 microns in the ranibizumab group and 249 in the PRP group (Table 2).

Regression of PDR

Forty percent of eyes had high-risk PDR at baseline in both groups. Around 40% of eyes in both groups had complete regression of neovascularization on fundus photography at 2 years, with no significant difference between groups.

Ninety-eight percent of the PRP group eyes completed initial full PRP. Forty-five percent of eyes in the PRP group, however, needed additional PRP after completion of initial treatment at a

Table 2. Baseline characteristics and study outcomes at 2 years for eyes in each group. Snellen visual acuities provided using the formula 85 + 50*log (Snellen fraction) [17]

	PRP group	Ranibizumab group
Mean visual acuity		
Baseline	75 letters (20/32)	75 letters (20/32)
2 years	76 letters (20/28)	79 letters (20/26)
Mean OCT central subfield thickness		
Baseline	249 microns	262 microns
2 years	243 microns	210 microns

The patients in the anti-VEGF deferred PRP group had 22 median visits over 2 years compared to 16 for the PRP group.

Table 3. Number of intravitreal ranibizumab injections at 1 and 2 years of follow-up

Mean number of injections (median)	Overall	Eyes with baseline DME	Eyes without baseline DME
Prior to 52-week visit	7.3 (7)	8.9 (9)	6.9 (7)
Between 52- and 104-week visits	3.6 (3)	4.6 (5)	3.3 (3)

median time of 7 months. Only 6% of eyes in the ranibizumab group received PRP as well, due to inability to either tolerate ranibizumab or failure or futility (worsening of neovascularization or bleeding despite multiple injections). Two-thirds of the eyes that received PRP did so during vitrectomy.

Ranibizumab injection was added in eyes that failed PRP or those that had DME at baseline or later developed it; 53% of eyes (n = 103) in the PRP group received a ranibizumab injection at some point during the study period. Only 35% of eyes (n = 72) received it at the beginning of the study for concurrent DME.

In the ranibizumab group, eyes with DME received a median of 9 injections in the first year followed by 5 in the second year. In those without DME, a median of 7 injections were given in the first year (6 in the first 6 months) and 3 in the second year. The number of injections given in the second year was fewer than half the number given in the first year irrespective of the status of DME (Table 3).

Approximately half of the eyes in the ranibizumab arm had improvement in DR severity by 2 steps at 2-year follow-up.

Visual Acuity

The mean visual acuity in both groups at baseline was 20/32, which did not change significantly after 2 years of treatment (Table 2). At year-2, the mean visual acuity in the anti-VEGF group was not inferior to that in the PRP group; in fact, it was better in the injection group at 2 years. The mean change in VA was +2.8 letters for eyes treated with ranibizumab versus +0.2 letters in the PRP group (Fig. 1; difference +2.2; 95% CI –0.5 to +5.0; non-inferiority $p < 0.001$).

The mean 2-year change in VA produced by ranibizumab injection was at most 0.5-letter worsening to improvement in 5.0 letters over the PRP therapy [17].

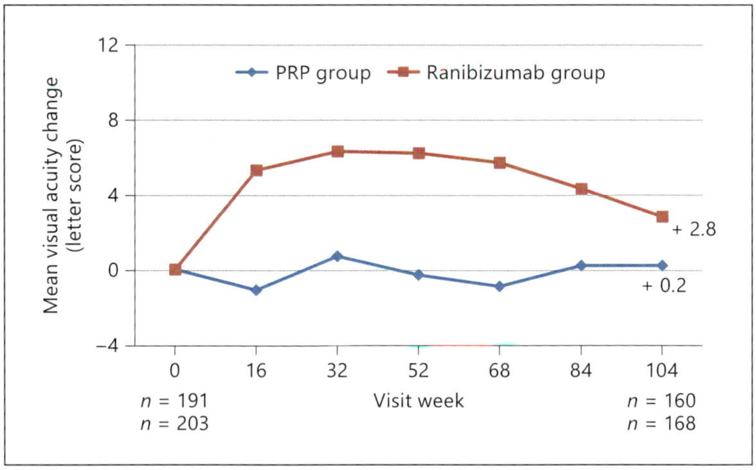

Fig. 1. Mean visual acuity change from baseline over time as measured by letter score, with approximately 5 letters representing 1 line on the Snellen chart. Adapted from Gross et al. [13].

The area-under-the-curve analysis of visual acuity in the anti-VEGF group showed an overall cumulative visual benefit over the 2-year study period, which was significantly greater with ranibizumab injections compared to the PRP group, though this improvement was still less than one line on the Snellen chart. The visual acuity in the PRP group was stable over 2 years; it improved in the injection group initially, peaked between the 32- and 52-week visits, but then regressed somewhat toward baseline. There was still a residual positive mean increase of 4.5 letters over 2 years; the mean treatment group difference in area under the curve analysis was +4.2 letters (95% CI +3.0 to +5.4; $p < 0.001$; Fig. 1) [13].

The greatest visual gains were noted in the eyes with CI-DME, irrespective of being in either arm of the study (Fig. 2) [13].

In eyes with minimal to moderate vision impairment, investigators determined that a change in 10 or 15 letters reflected a clinically significant change. This would equate to 2 or 3 lines on the Snellen chart [18]. Loss of 10 or 15 letters at year-2 was around 10% for each group, with no significant differences between the cohorts; 40% in each group improved by 10 or more letters with no significant difference between the cohorts.

Diabetic Macular Edema

In eyes with no DME (defined as a CST on OCT of 250 microns or more and with a visual acuity of 20/32 or worse) at baseline, DME developed with loss of VA in 28% in the PRP group and only 9% in the anti-VEGF group; the difference (19%) was highly significant (95% CI 10–28; $p < 0.001$). The group treated initially with ranibizumab had a significantly lower cumulative probability of developing DME by year-2.

CST on OCT was significantly different between the groups at year-2, with eyes in the ranibizumab group at a mean of 210 microns and the PRP group at 243 microns. It decreased by a mean of 45 microns in the injection group and 3 microns in the PRP group ($p < 0.001$).

In eyes with DME at baseline, eyes that underwent injections with anti-VEGF had a higher mean change in visual acuity letter score from baseline, measured by area under the curve, versus those that received PRP (+8.0 vs. +3.6, p = 0.08). The same was true in eyes without baseline DME, by +4.9 (around 1 line on the Snellen chart; +3.5 vs. −1.5; $p < 0.001$).

Approximately half of the patients in the PRP cohort needed ranibizumab, because of DME at baseline or development of DME during the course of the study, but only 6% of eyes in the

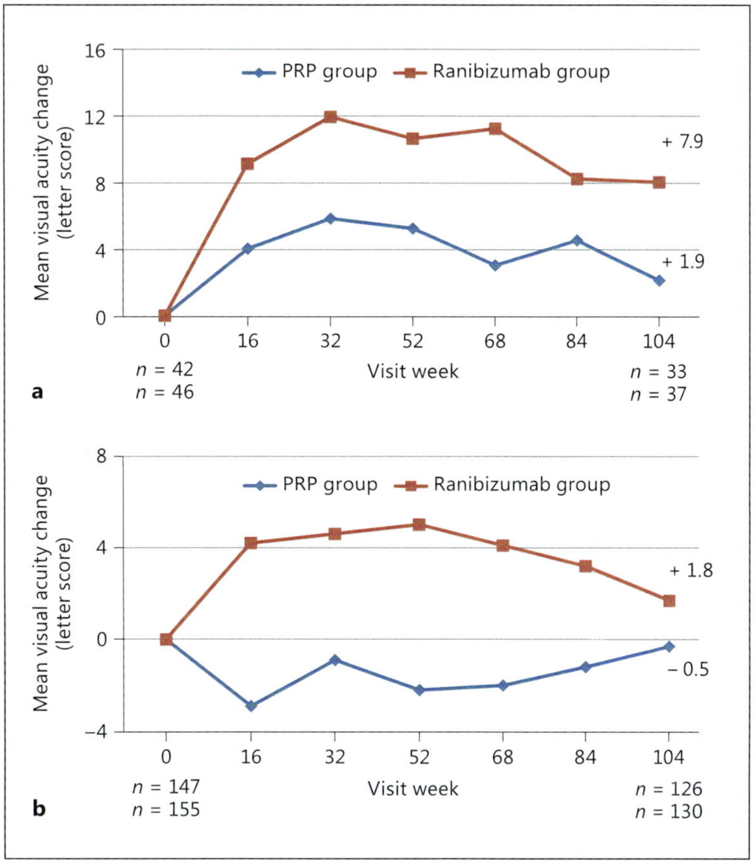

Fig. 2. The mean visual acuity change from baseline over time as measured by letter score, with approximately 5 letters representing 1 line on the Snellen chart, stratified by eyes with (**a**) or without (**b**) baseline DME. Adapted from Gross et al. [13].

ranibizumab group needed PRP. The median number of injections in PDR eyes without DME at baseline was 10 compared to 14 in eyes with DME at baseline at 2 years.

Peripheral Visual Field Outcomes

One of the goals of the study was to also evaluate the potential benefits of intravitreal injection of ranibizumab in preserving the peripheral visual field compared to PRP. Automated peripheral VF testing revealed a significant cumulative worsening in the PRP group. The mean deviation change from baseline was only –0.8 dB in the ranibizumab-treated eyes versus 2.50 dB ($p < 0.001$) in the PRP eyes. The mean peripheral visual field sensitivity loss, as measured by combined 30-2 and 60-4 total point scores, was significantly lower in the ranibizumab group; the mean decibel difference was 372 (95% CI 213–531; $p < 0.001$) [4].

Need for Vitrectomy

The percentage of eyes requiring vitrectomy, as deemed necessary by the treating retina specialist such as for visually significant vitreous hemorrhage, was lower in the ranibizumab group than in the PRP group (4 vs. 15%; difference 9%; 95% CI 4–15). Similar results were found when the eyes were separated into those without baseline DME (2 vs. 14%) versus those with baseline DME (12 vs. 17%). Vitrectomy was performed at a median of 511 days in the anti-VEGF cohort and 465 days in the PRP cohort.

Table 4. Percentage of patients or eyes with adverse events occurring during study period

% Eyes with:	Participants with 2 study eyes, 1 per group ($n = 89$)	Ranibizumab group ($n = 102$)	PRP group ($n = 114$)
Systemic adverse events			
Vascular event	8	9	6
Death (any cause)	4	6	4
Hospitalization	42	47	35
Serious adverse event	43	48	37
Hypertension	16	25	18
Ocular adverse events			
Endophthalmitis	–	0.5	0
Inflammation	–	1	4*
Cataract surgery	–	2	6
IOP elevation	–	9	13

* Indicates statistically significant difference.

Retinal Detachment

The eyes with retinal detachment of the macula were excluded from the study. The frequency of developing a retinal detachment was not significantly different between the laser and injection groups (10 vs. 6%, $p = 0.08$). Traction retinal detachment occurred slightly more in the PRP group (8%) versus the ranibizumab group (5%), while each group had 1 case of rhegmatogenous retinal detachment. The timing of retinal detachment for the ranibizumab group was much shorter at a median of 199 versus 379 days for the PRP group.

Safety

As with any intravitreal injection, injection of ranibizumab carries inherent risks. Protocol S results noted only 1 case of injection-related endophthalmitis out of 299 total cases that received ranibizumab injections. No specific serious adverse reactions were noted in either group (Table 4). Ocular inflammation, excluding endophthalmitis, was significantly higher in the PRP group at 4 versus 1% in the ranibizumab group. No difference in systemic effects was seen between the 2 groups. However, there is strong evidence from randomized prospective clinical trials that DME patients with the highest exposure to intravitreal ranibizumab (0.5 mg monthly) or aflibercept (2 mg monthly) have a 3-fold increased risk of all-cause mortality [19].

Visual field constriction, decreased contrast sensitivity, poor night vision, and worsening of DME are well-documented side effects of PRP. Severe vision loss due to VH may still occur with PRP, which would then require pars plana vitrectomy.

Other Anti-VEGFs

Exploratory analyses in many large DME studies with other anti-VEGF drugs, such as aflibercept, have demonstrated improvement in the DR severity score during the course of DME treatment with intravitreal injections. In the VIVID-DME and VISTA-DME trials, a larger proportion of DME eyes that received aflibercept achieved a 2-step or greater improvement on the ETDRS-DR severity scale (Table 5). In the VIVID-DME trial, one-third of the eyes in the aflibercept group (given monthly or every 2 months) had at least a 2-step improvement in DR, compared to 8% of eyes in the laser group ($p < 0.001$). In the VISTA-DME, 40% of eyes in the aflibercept group had at least a 2-step improvement,

Table 5. Percentage of eyes with 2-step improvement in visual acuity in the VIVID-DME and VISTA-DME trials on aflibercept intravitreal injections in eyes with diabetic macular edema

	VIVID-DME: % with 2-step improvement	VISTA-DME: % with 2-step improvement
Aflibercept injection monthly	29	40
5 initial monthly aflibercept injections then every 2 months	33	40
Laser control	8	17
p value	<0.001	<0.0001

compared to 17% of eyes in the laser group ($p < 0.0001$) [15].

Published data describing the effect of bevacizumab on the progression of DR are limited. Future exploratory analyses using Protocol T [20] may be able to evaluate the efficacy of bevacizumab compared to ranibizumab or aflibercept.

Overview of Results

The primary outcome of the study clearly showed ranibizumab to be at least as effective as PRP in treating PDR in terms of the visual outcome and regression of PDR at 2 years follow-up. Active neovascularization was seen in approximately half of the eyes in each group at the year-2 follow-up. Ranibizumab was superior to PRP in terms of significantly fewer destructive side effects, for example, peripheral visual field loss, contrast sensitivity loss. PDR eyes with baseline DME that underwent injections showed superior year-2 visual acuity gains in the ranibizumab group compared to PRP. There was lesser likelihood by year-2 of developing DME and less likelihood to require vitrectomy in the ranibizumab cohort.

Cost Analyses

There are major differences in the cost burden with the 2 treatments for PDR; PRP is less expensive than ranibizumab injections. The cost of PRP as the initial treatment for PDR is lower by almost 60% than intravitreal ranibizumab 0.5 mg used over the first 2 years. Lin et al. [21] reported the quality-adjusted life year (QALY) value in a non-facility setting for PRP and ranibizumab to be USD 6,297 and 16,238, respectively (accepted QALY value of USD 50,000–100,000 by health policymaker). This value decreases to USD 10,636 for intravitreal ranibizumab 0.3 mg or to USD 2,952 for intravitreal bevacizumab over 2 years. The cost of a specific anti-VEGF drug varies by region; the approximate cost on an average is USD 70 for 1.25 mg of bevacizumab, USD 1,200 for 0.3 mg of ranibizumab, and USD 2,000 for 2.0 mg of aflibercept. The adverse effects of PRP-induced peripheral VF loss, a higher rate of needing vitrectomies with PRP, and regression of retinopathy grade were not included in this analysis, which otherwise would further decrease the cost differential.

Discussion

The visual outcome after 2 years of intravitreal ranibizumab treatment of PDR eyes is at least similar to if not better than what was achieved with PRP, in the presence or absence of DME. The ranibizumab-treated eyes had reduced OCT thickness and a lesser chance of needing a vitrectomy. Furthermore, the secondary outcomes show better preservation of peripheral visual function with ranibizumab injection than with PRP. It is important to know if these differences remain significant at the longer 5-year follow-up and in the course of routine clinical care.

Advantages of PRP treatment are significant; it can be completed in 1–3 sessions, and the effects are long-lasting with fewer follow-up visits. Laser costs less than multiple anti-VEGF injections, and there is no risk of endophthalmitis and no exposure to systemic side effects of VEGF blockade induced by intravitreal injection. PRP has a great record in terms of long-term regression of PDR, with no need of additional treatment [8].

The advantages of ranibizumab injections were superior mean VA compared to PRP over 2 years, with extremely low adverse event rates with minimal peripheral visual field constriction, reduced chance of developing CI-DME, and reduced need for vitrectomy. PRP was rarely given for failure or futility of ranibizumab. The PDR eyes without CI-DME treated with ranibizumab have a significant lower cumulative probability of developing DME by year-2.

Many eyes with PDR have CI-DME or a propensity to develop DME. Eyes with PDR and CI-DME at baseline that received ranibizumab had far better visual outcome than those who received PRP for PDR. This result suggests that PDR eyes with CI-DME should be treated with ranibizumab rather than PRP, at least initially. Ranibizumab treatment for CI-DME eyes with concurrent PDR is considered an effective treatment for both edema and proliferative changes. However, we cannot determine the long-term efficacy of this treatment paradigm when ranibizumab injections are discontinued. Once the CI-DME resolves, the eyes may need to be re-assessed for PDR treatment.

The large prospective DME RISE/RIDE trials did not show recurrence of neovascularization in 60% of eyes, and 25% of patients did not require further treatment after discontinuation of ranibizumab injections at 36 months [22, 23]. We have been treating exudative age-related macular degeneration and CI-DME eyes with monthly anti-VEGF injections for over 5 years and are certainly amenable and comfortable with the idea of monthly anti-VEGF treatment for new cases of PDR, if this were found to be superior to the gold standard of PRP in the long term. The effect of PRP for PDR regression may not be as long-lasting as previously thought: Protocol S revealed that 45% of eyes that underwent complete PRP had recurrence of neovascularization requiring additional treatment at a median of 7 months. Reasons for this apparent discrepancy are unclear. The clinical acceptance of Protocol S results in our day-to-day practice will depend on how frequently a patient can be monitored in follow-ups.

The treatment paradigm for PDR as a result of the findings of Protocol S is definitely changing. The results indicate an alternate highly effective treatment modality in scenarios where complete or adequate PRP cannot be given secondary to media opacity, such as significant cataract, corneal edema, hyphema, or vitreous hemorrhage. Under these circumstances, intravitreal ranibizumab (or bevacizumab or aflibercept) may be the initial choice by default. Until long-term effects of ranibizumab (after the injections are discontinued) are better elucidated, PRP may be a better treatment option than ranibizumab in patients who have a history of poor compliance with follow-up visits or who are unable to return for monthly visits, and who have limited access to medical care. Patients with a recent cerebrovascular accident or myocardial infarction should be considered for PRP over anti-VEGF injections.

Intravitreal injection of ranibizumab may be a superior choice in terms of preserving peripheral visual function while preserving central VA similarly as when PDR eyes with or without CI-DME are treated with PRP. Despite the more favorable safety profile of ranibizumab, cost may remain a determinant in choosing to treat a patient with anti-VEGF injection or PRP. If intravitreal anti-VEGF is used, strict compliance with follow-up is necessary, which creates another factor driving treatment choice in addition to cost. The results of longer-term follow-up will demonstrate whether DR will progress after the discontinuation of anti-VEGF therapy.

DME prospective trials have shown that both aflibercept 2 mg and ranibizumab 0.3 mg can decrease the severity of DR, but it is uncertain if these doses will be equally effective as 0.5 mg of ranibizumab, which was used in Protocol S.

Future Directions

The treatment for PDR may undergo radical change as did treatment for DME as long-term information concerning ranibizumab-treated eyes in Protocol S becomes available. Many questions remain unanswered. We need to know, for example, the long-term recurrence rate of proliferative changes after initial PDR regression in the injection group to select the best option for a given patient. Also, treating pre-proliferative eyes with anti-VEGF agents may slow development of DME but additional studies are needed.

Cost also remains a concern. A recent cost analysis revealed that although the cost differential between intravitreal ranibizumab and PRP may not be significant at 2 years follow-up, over a lifetime, this differential may increase significantly [21]. Other less expensive anti-VEGF agents may one day decrease this difference [24]. Though prospective studies have only been completed on ranibizumab, longer duration-of-action anti-VEGF molecules and sustained release devices and pumps are currently under development with the hope of further decreasing treatment burden by minimizing the number of injections and office visits needed to maintain treatment benefit.

The 5-year results of Protocol S may alter our practice pattern for PDR. We remain cautious in changing the treatment pattern in all our patients with PDR on the basis of 2-year results of Protocol S due to the time-limited effects of anti-VEGF injections, as we do not yet know how DR progresses after anti-VEGF is discontinued. At this time in our practice, PRP remains the standard of care. Combination therapy with anti-VEGF initially, followed by PRP to consolidate the benefits of anti-VEGF injection, may be a reasonable alternative in PDR eyes with CI-DME or eyes with media opacities, followed by additional PRP if PDR recurs after injections are discontinued.

References

1 Diabetic Retinopathy Study Group: Photocoagulation treatment of proliferative diabetic retinopathy. Clinical application of Diabetic Retinopathy Study (DRS) findings, DRS Report Number 8. The Diabetic Retinopathy Study Research Group. Ophthalmology 1981;88: 583–600.

2 Indications for photocoagulation treatment of diabetic retinopathy: Diabetic Retinopathy Study Report no. 14. The Diabetic Retinopathy Study Research Group. Int Ophthalmol Clin 1987;27: 239–253.

3 Subash M, et al: The effect of multispot laser panretinal photocoagulation on retinal sensitivity and driving eligibility in patients with diabetic retinopathy. JAMA Ophthalmol 2016;134:666–672.

4 Fong DS, Girach A, Boney A: Visual side effects of successful scatter laser photocoagulation surgery for proliferative diabetic retinopathy: a literature review. Retina 2007;27:816–824.

5 Zhang Z, et al: Changes in choroidal thickness after panretinal photocoagulation for diabetic retinopathy: a 12-week longitudinal study. Invest Ophthalmol Vis Sci 2015;56:2631–2638.

6 Zhu Y, et al: Changes in choroidal thickness after panretinal photocoagulation in patients with type 2 diabetes. Retina 2015;35:695–703.

7 Lee SH, et al: Changes of choroidal thickness after treatment for diabetic retinopathy. Curr Eye Res 2014;39:736–744.

8 Gentile RC, et al: Risk factors for ciliochoroidal effusion after panretinal photocoagulation. Ophthalmology 1996; 103:827–832.

9 Hessemer V, Schmidt KG: Influence of panretinal photocoagulation on the ocular pulse curve. Am J Ophthalmol 1997; 123:748–752.

10 Aiello LP, et al: Vascular endothelial growth factor in ocular fluid of patients with diabetic retinopathy and other retinal disorders. N Engl J Med 1994;331: 1480–1487.

11 Bressler SB, et al: Five-year outcomes of ranibizumab with prompt or deferred laser versus laser or triamcinolone plus deferred ranibizumab for diabetic macular edema. Am J Ophthalmol 2016;164: 57–68.

12 Diabetic Retinopathy Clinical Research Network, Elman MJ, et al: Randomized trial evaluating ranibizumab plus prompt or deferred laser or triamcinolone plus prompt laser for diabetic macular edema. Ophthalmology 2010;117: 1064–1077.e35.

13 Writing Committee for the Diabetic Retinopathy Clinical Research Network, Gross JG, et al: Panretinal photocoagulation vs intravitreous ranibizumab for proliferative diabetic retinopathy: a randomized clinical trial. JAMA 2015;314: 2137–2146.
14 Ip MS, et al: Long-term effects of ranibizumab on diabetic retinopathy severity and progression. Arch Ophthalmol 2012;130:1145–1152.
15 Korobelnik JF, et al: Intravitreal aflibercept for diabetic macular edema. Ophthalmology 2014;121:2247–2254.
16 Campochiaro PA, et al: Neutralization of vascular endothelial growth factor slows progression of retinal nonperfusion in patients with diabetic macular edema. Ophthalmology 2014;121:1783–1789.
17 Gross JG, Glassman AR: A novel treatment for proliferative diabetic retinopathy: anti-vascular endothelial growth factor therapy. JAMA Ophthalmol 2016; 134:13–14.
18 Gregori NZ, Feuer W, Rosenfeld PJ: Novel method for analyzing snellen visual acuity measurements. Retina 2010; 30:1046–1050.
19 Avery RL, Gordon GM: Systemic safety of prolonged monthly anti-vascular endothelial growth factor therapy for diabetic macular edema: a systematic review and meta-analysis. JAMA Ophthalmol 2016;134:21–29.
20 Diabetic Retinopathy Clinical Research Network, Wells JA, et al: Aflibercept, bevacizumab, or ranibizumab for diabetic macular edema. N Engl J Med 2015;372:1193–1203.
21 Lin J, Chang JS, Smiddy WE: Cost evaluation of panretinal photocoagulation versus intravitreal ranibizumab for proliferative diabetic retinopathy. Ophthalmology 2016;123:1912–1918.
22 Ho AC, Zhang J, Ehrlich JS: Ranibizumab for diabetic macular edema: long-term open-label extension of the phase III RIDE and RISE trials. Invest Ophthalmol Vis Sci 2014;55:1704.
23 Brown DM, et al: Long-term outcomes of ranibizumab therapy for diabetic macular edema: the 36-month results from two phase III trials: RISE and RIDE. Ophthalmology 2013;120:2013–2022.
24 Arevalo JF, et al: Intravitreal bevacizumab for proliferative diabetic retinopathy: results from the Pan-American Collaborative Retina Study Group (PACORES) at 24 months of follow-up. Retina, 2016.

Neelakshi Bhagat
Institute of Ophthalmology and Visual Science
Rutgers New Jersey Medical School
Doctors Office Center, 90 Bergen Street, Newark, NJ 07103 (USA)
E-Mail bhagatne@njms.rutgers.edu

Bandello F, Zarbin MA, Lattanzio R, Zucchiatti I (eds): Management of Diabetic Retinopathy.
Dev Ophthalmol. Basel, Karger, 2017, vol 60, pp 143–159 (DOI: 10.1159/000459702)

Surgical Management and Techniques

Marco Codenotti · Lorenzo Iuliano · Gisella Maestranzi
Department of Ophthalmology, Vita-Salute University, San Raffaele Scientific Institute, Milan, Italy

Abstract

Technical advancements have substantially extended the indications for surgery in diabetic retinopathy (DR) during the last 40 years, from the traditional indications including non-clearing vitreous hemorrhage, traction retinal detachment (RD), and traction-rhegmatogenous RD, to epiretinal membrane (ERM), vitreomacular traction, diffuse macular edema, neovascular glaucoma, and anterior hyaloid fibrovascular proliferation. The goals of vitreoretinal surgery in DR are multiple: clearing media opacities, release of traction (anteroposterior and/or tangential), segmentation and/or removal of traction bands, peeling of ERMs, hemostasis, laser photocoagulation, and tamponade of retinal breaks with gas or silicone oil. The best management is achieved with integrated care provided by physicians with expertise in medical management of diabetes and surgical care of DR. In this chapter, the indications for surgery, preoperative considerations, surgical techniques, and complications, together with their management, will be discussed.

Introduction

Since the first human pars plana vitrectomy (PPV) was successfully performed in 1970 by Robert Machemer for a diabetic patient with a non-clearing vitreous hemorrhage (VH), surgery for diabetic retinopathy (DR) has improved tremendously. The DR Vitrectomy Study (DRVS) systematically investigated the role of early vitrectomy for severe non-clearing VH and severe fibrovascular proliferation in diabetic patients. The DRVS demonstrated that early intervention increased the likelihood of retaining the vision of 20/40 or better compared to conservative management [1–4]. Results were not uniformly positive, however, as there was a relatively high incidence of severe complications (e.g., loss of light perception was 20% in the DRVS study of severe non-clearing VH). Technological innovations (e.g., introduction of intraoperative laser photocoagulation, improved fiberoptic illumination with the evolution of bimanual dissection, development of small-gauge instrumentation) substantially reduced the rate of complications and extended the indications for surgery in DR beyond the initial indications of severe non-clearing VH, traction retinal detachment (RD), and traction-rhegmatogenous RD, to epiretinal membrane (ERM), vitreomacular traction, diffuse macular edema, neovascular glaucoma (NVG), and anterior hyaloid fibrovascular proliferation [5]. Somewhat more controversial indications include non-tractional macular edema and combined vitrectomy with cataract surgery. Despite the abundant data available in literature, due to the tremendous individual variation in case of complexity and patient needs, this information is not necessarily decisive in patient management and serves primarily as a useful adjunct to surgeons caring for such patients. Thus, surgeons must individualize treatment decisions based on individual features of the case and their own clinical experience.

The goals of vitreoretinal surgery in DR are multiple. These include clearing media opacities, releasing traction (anteroposterior and/or tangential), segmentation and removal of traction bands, peeling of ERMs, hemostasis, laser photocoagulation, and tamponade of retinal breaks with gas or silicone oil. The best management is achieved with integrated care provided by physicians with expertise in medical management of diabetes and surgical care of DR. In this chapter, the indications for surgery, preoperative considerations, surgical techniques and complications, together with their management, will be reviewed.

Pre-Operative Assessment

Systemic Conditions

Appropriate perioperative glycemic control has shown to reduce infection, neuropathy, renal failure, and improve survival in diabetic patients. Control of dyslipidemia with statins has also been associated with better vitrectomy outcomes. Therefore, collaboration with internal medicine physicians is essential to optimize the preoperative blood pressure and glycometabolic markers. Other comorbidities such as cardiovascular or renal disease must be evaluated and managed preoperatively [1–4]. Antiplatelet and/or anticoagulant agents do not increase the risk of intraoperative or postoperative VH, but they do increase the risk of retrobulbar hemorrhage. One can avoid this complication altogether by administering retrobulbar anesthesia using a blunt-tipped cannula via a limbal conjunctival incision, which can be created under topical anesthesia with the patient sedated. One might also consider administering 2 parabulbar injections instead of a retrobulbar block [6]. Alternatively, one could consider (after consultation with the referring internal medicine specialist or endocrinologist) stopping anti-platelet or anti-coagulant therapy, but this step is rarely necessary and should be avoided if possible. Since anti-platelet agents have a long-lasting effect, one generally must stop these medications for at least 1 week and preferably 2 weeks before surgery if that course of action is necessary. This aspect of management must be discussed with the patient preoperatively.

Preoperative Investigation

B-mode ultrasound (US) is useful in patients with media opacities to assess the retina for areas of traction or rhegmatogenous detachment and for anterior hyaloid fibrovascular proliferation (with prominent peripheral anteroposterior RD and dragging onto the pars plana) in severe cases in which the diagnosis cannot be made at the slit lamp (e.g., due to cataract or hyphema). We suggest performing preoperative US, even in eyes in which one may have a reasonable idea of the fundus details. Fluorescein angiography (FA) is useful in assessing the extent of retinal non-perfusion and in detecting any significant macular ischemia or occult retinal neovascularization. Spectral domain optical coherence tomography (SD-OCT) is now the best technique to study the outer retina. SD-OCT imaging of the outer retinal microarchitecture, namely integrity of the external limiting membrane and ellipsoid zone, has been shown to correlate with postoperative best-corrected visual acuity, while central foveal thickness and enlargement of the foveal avascular zone only exhibit a weak correlation. Recently developed OCT angiography is currently under investigation regarding its potential to describe and predict surgical outcomes [5–7]. En-face OCT imaging may also be of help in selected case of diabetic macular edema (DME), where the tractional component may not be as clearly evident on standard transverse SD-OCT imaging [8]. Imaging data can be very helpful for establishing realistic patient expectations prior to surgery.

Preoperative Medications

The advent of anti-vascular endothelial growth factor (VEGF) pharmacotherapy has revolutionized the treatment of many retinal diseases [9]. Preoperative injection of anti-VEGF medication 7 days prior to surgery has shown promising results [10]. However, incorporation of this approach has been limited due to fear of the so called "crunch syndrome," that is a sudden worsening of tractional RD and development of denser fibrotic connections between the retina and overlying tissue, making it harder to identify tissue planes [6]. This complication is especially critical in the more systemically ill diabetic patient, who often needs to delay or cancel surgery due to systemic complications. Although published evidence is limited, expert opinion suggests limiting the use of intravitreal anti-VEGF agents to no more than 3 days before surgery [5–7].

Preoperative insertion of a dexamethasone (DEX) implant provides some advantages in selected cases. DEX implants facilitate the regression and consolidation of neovascularization, in addition to inhibiting other inflammatory cytokines. Unlike anti-VEGF agents, there is no increased risk of systemic complications or tractional response, and tissue planes are more distinct and not converted into flat fibrovascular tissue [6]. Despite these benefits, its preoperative use is controversial, since caution needs to be taken as the implant may become mobile within the vitreous cavity during vitrectomy. It is difficult to complete a core and vitreous base vitrectomy with hyaloid delamination while sparing the implant, which is usually aspirated by the vitrectomy probe. The longer favorable effects (e.g., reduction of macular edema) are hence interrupted.

Techniques

The key surgical steps to treat DR involve performing a core vitrectomy, removing all vitreous opacities, excision of the posterior hyaloid face, and relieving all areas of traction. Areas of fibrovascular proliferation are segmented or dissected with the vitrectomy probe or with scissors. Bimanual techniques with chandelier illumination may be required in eyes with very adherent, extensive proliferation, particularly if it extends toward the equator and periphery. Proliferation in the periphery is particularly challenging because the retina is thinner and more prone to tear, and the angles required for manipulation are more cumbersome. When removal of the fibrovascular tissue is achieved without iatrogenic breaks, photocoagulation is applied to the periphery up to the ora serrata and to the attached retina outside the area centralis. An air-fluid exchange at the end of the procedure with prone positioning for a few days is indicated when foveal elevation or folds are prominent to help reduce postoperative metamorphopsia. Nasal areas of traction that do not threaten to involve the posterior pole do not need to be removed as long as there is no rhegmatogenous component or iatrogenic break [5–7].

New Vitrectors

New vitrectors in 23-, 25-, and 27-gauge with optimized fluidics and cutting rates of up to 10,000 cuts/minute allow for very efficient vitreous removal with minimized traction on the retina [11]. This technology offers several advantages over 20-gauge instrumentation: decreased surgical time, enhanced comfort in the postoperative period, and less conjunctival scarring. Furthermore, since the diabetic eye is more prone to neovascularization and vascular ingrowth at the sclerotomy entry sites and vitreous base [12, 13], smaller sclerotomies may help reduce inflammation and the associated neovascularization. Furthermore, port optimization of the vitreous cutter with a wider port closer to the tip has allowed more surgical precision (e.g., placement of the probe tip close to the retina for excision of epiretinal proliferation) and fewer intraoperative complications. Despite the advantages provided by minimally invasive vitrectomy surgery, some authors still believe in the role of 20-gauge system in conditions where affordability of the newer machine and instruments can be an issue. Furthermore, in the case of large intraocular maneuvers or the need to reach the extreme retinal periphery, smaller gauge instruments may flex too much and become damaged in contrast to 20-gauge instruments, which are relatively more rigid. Precise intraocular pressure (IOP) control afforded by modern machines such as the Constellation (Alcon) minimizes bleeding during surgery and reduces the need for endodiathermy. The introduction of curved laser probes with or without illumination allow for complete photocoagulation up to the ora even in phakic eyes. Intraoperative OCT can be very useful to assess thickened posterior hyaloid, vitreomacular traction, lamellar holes, ERMs, and macular edema in eyes with VH. These new techniques permit long-term stabilization of vitrectomized diabetic eyes with significantly reduced frequency of iatrogenic and non-iatrogenic complications.

Staining

Triamcinolone acetonide and dyes such as indocyanine green, trypan blue, brilliant blue G, membrane dual, and brilliant peel are used to enhance visualization of cortical gel, ERM, and internal limiting membrane (ILM). The routine use of chromodissection in diabetic vitrectomy is, however, left to surgeon's preference. Triamcinolone acetonide is a synthetic non-soluble steroid that is used to stain the vitreous and the hyaloid. It is particularly useful in case of vitreoschisis, when remnants of the cortical vitreous are attached to the retina despite the apparent induction of a posterior vitreous detachment (PVD). Trypan blue is an anionic hydrophilic azole dye that selectively stains ERMs. Brilliant blue selectively stains the ILM. The use of green dyes (indocyanine or infracyanine) has decreased due to their suspected toxicity [14]. The newer dual blue dye is a mixture of brilliant and trypan blue and makes it possible to stain together all the vitreoretinal interface structures.

Relief of Tangential Traction

The relief of tangential traction is a key step in diabetic vitrectomy, and this objective is achieved by segmentation, delamination, or "en bloc" dissection, or, more frequently, with a combination of all these approaches.

The use of microincisional instruments, particularly 27-gauge vitrectomy probes, is advantageous, since it allows for manipulations that were not possible with larger vitrectomy instruments. These newer manipulations involve utilizing the vitrectomy probe to blunt dissect tissue, segment membranes as scissors, and use the lift and cut technique. For the latter technique, the probe is used with suction to lift membranes, creating a space between the membrane and subjacent retina, and then the tissue is shaved. This sequence is repeated until all the tissue is removed [5, 7].

Segmentation: a large sheet of fibrous tissue (tangential traction) is cut into smaller islands, and each island of the remaining tissue connected to 1 or 2 fibro- vascular attachments to subjacent retina is subsequently removed.

Delamination: a large sheet of fibrous tissue (tangential traction) is removed by cutting those fibrovascular attachments, one-by-one. The dissection could begin either from the periphery (outside-in) or from the disc side (inside-out) or a combination of both, based on the availability of the proper cleavage plane and the height of underlying RD. The concept of a second or double layer is crucial: as mentioned earlier, in the case of vitreoschisis the false appearance of a cleavage plane is caused by the splitting of hyaloid. One part of the hyaloid induces traction, and the other part remains attached to the retina.

"En Bloc" Dissection: "en bloc" dissection (or excision) is the removal of large sheet of fibrous tissue (tangential traction) in a single sheet by interrupting the punctate attachments of the fibrovascular proliferation to the subjacent retina using a bimanual dissection approach. Bimanual dissection is done by using forceps in one hand, scissors in the other, and using chandelier illumination through a fourth port. The availability of 29-gauge fiberoptic illumination allows one to place 2 fibers in the vitreous cavity, which creates brighter, more uniform illumination than that provided by a single 25-gauge fiberoptic chandelier. The anteroposterior traction is left intact on 3 sides, and using this attachment to fibrous tissue as a third instrument, the membrane is delaminated in an outside-in or inside-out fashion, depending on the anatomy. With the availability of small gauge instrumentation, it is often unnecessary to use scissors, as most of the tangential dissection is achieved using just the vitrectomy probe. Often, the tip of the cutter can be placed in the right cleavage plane, and then by the cutting action, the tissue can be segmented followed by delamination and thereby achieve total relief from tangential traction.

Viscodissection: in selected cases with adherent fibrovascular proliferation, hyaluronic acid injection can be useful to gently separate the fibrovascular tissue from the retina, particularly if a localized area of posterior hyaloid separation from the retina can be identified. The viscodissection cannula is placed in this area of separation, and gentle injection forces separation of the retina and epiretinal tissue. Low viscosity hyaluronic acid preparations are less likely to create pressure-induced retinal breaks than high viscosity preparations. This technique can be particularly helpful in cases of traction-rhegmatogenous RD in which there is no separation of the hyaloid and detached retina and in which the detached retina is atrophic and thus likely to tear with the application of tangential force.

Fluid-Gas Exchange, Endolaser, and Tamponade

All retinal breaks must be identified and, in the case of multiple breaks, marked using diathermy before fluid-gas exchange, followed by endolaser. A curved laser probe is appropriate in phakic eyes. Tamponade devices include silicone oil (e.g., 1,300 cSt oil or higher viscosity oil, such as 5,700 cSt, that has less chance of emulsification) and gas (e.g., SF6 [sulfur hexafluoride] or longer acting gas such as C3F8 [perfluoropropane]). Any leaking sclerotomy must be closed by placing one interrupted 6–0 or 7–0 (best for sclera) or 7–0 (for conjunctiva) absorbable suture. After the first surgery, 1,300 cSt silicone oil is usually removed 4–6 months. Higher viscosity oils may be retained for a longer duration.

Intraoperative Complications

Corneal Edema: corneal edema can cause poor visibility during prolonged surgical procedures or when the IOP has been elevated for a substantial period of time. Frequent lubrication of the corneal epithelium with viscous fluid (e.g., goniosol) instead of balanced salt solution and decreasing the duration of elevated IOP can reduce the chance. Corneal epithelial debridement may be necessary to improve the visualization of posterior segment, but this maneuver should be carried out with caution in diabetic eyes since it can result in a persistent non-healing epithelial defect due to diabetic corneal neuropathy [15, 16].

Cataract Formation: intraoperative cataract formation can be an iatrogenic complication (lens touch, fluid-gas exchange) or may occur spontaneously during surgery. The rate of osmotic cataract formation intraoperatively can be reduced with the addition of 3 mL of 50% dextrose to 500 mL of BSS or, alternatively, by using BSS-Plus as infusion fluid [17].

Intraocular Bleeding: intraoperative bleeding in diabetic eyes is a frequent problem, especially in eyes with active neovascularization and in patients with uremia. In severe cases, completing the procedure can become very difficult. Bleeding commonly occurs during peeling of fibrovascular membranes or induction of PVD, or it may be due to a sudden decrease in IOP while exchanging instruments. The latter is less likely if self-sealing cannulas are used with 23-, 25-, or 27-gauge instrumentation. Preoperative treatment with an anti-angiogenic agent reduces the likelihood of uncontrolled bleeding during membrane dissection, but can be associated with progressive traction as noted above. Increasing the IOP for a brief period of time or use of intraocular diathermy is useful to stop the intraocular bleeding.

Iatrogenic Breaks: iatrogenic breaks can occur during dissection of fibrovascular membranes. The break should be encircled with laser spots, and an adequate internal tamponade should be used. It is essential to relieve all traction around retinal breaks. At the end of the case, one should perform scleral indentation and examination of the peripheral retina using a wide-angle viewing system or indirect ophthalmoscopy and scleral depression to look for tears or breaks at the end of surgery. Also, it is helpful to perform fluid-air exchange at the end of the case, even if no breaks are identified, to ensure there is no vitreous incarceration in the sclerotomies. Furthermore, creation of beveled sclerotomies for cannula insertion helps to prevent vitreous extrusion from the sclerotomy site during cannula removal.

Postoperative Complications

RD: rhegmatogenous RD is a typical complication of diabetic vitrectomy, usually caused by iatrogenic retinal tears. The rate of detachment ranges from 4.3 to 8.1%, and is lower in cases with no epiretinal dissection [18, 19]. When postoperative RD occurs, one must identify the etiologic retinal break(s), relieve all traction around the break(s) (e.g., due to vitreoretinal traction or due to residual ERM), and seal the break(s), usually with laser photocoagulation.

Reproliferation: inadequate treatment of ischemic retina during vitrectomy can lead to reproliferation of diabetic fibrovascular membranes. They are usually managed by supplemental external photocoagulation, but may require transscleral cryotherapy with or without revision of vitrectomy. In advanced cases, diabetic reproliferation may simulate proliferative vitreoretinopathy, which is occasionally seen after surgery for rhegmatogenous RD [5].

Vitreous Hemorrhage: vitreous hemorrhage following diabetic vitrectomy is a common occurrence and has been reported in 7–63% of patients, almost half of which present on the first postoperative day [20, 21]. The specific management has been discussed in the VH section.

Epiretinal Membrane: ERM can be a relatively benign complication. Surgical management should be considered in case of thickened ERMs, causing marked macular distortion with visual symptoms.

Elevated IOP: increased IOP is a frequent event after surgery, both early and late. It can be caused by the tamponade device or by obstruction of the trabecular meshwork by neovascularization or debris. It must be promptly treated since the amount and duration of IOP elevation tolerated by a diabetic subject is often lower than in healthy patients because of compromised circulation. Occasionally, diabetic patients present with no light perception after vitreous surgery and have seemingly innocuously elevated IOP (e.g., 30 mm Hg) due to impaired retina/choroidal circulation. Prompt reduction of IOP in these cases (e.g., via anterior chamber paracentesis or with medication) can restore vision even to very high levels of visual acuity.

Rubeosis Iridis: the rate of NVG following diabetic vitrectomy is now far lower than was reported in the years immediately following the introduction of vitrectomy for DR. This important change is due to the frequent use of panretinal photocoagulation (PRP) intraoperatively (a technique that was not available during the early years of vitreoretinal surgery) with or without preoperative anti-VEGF therapy and possibly due to better overall control of diabetes in the study population [22].

Phthisis Bulbi: recent data have also shown a significantly reduced rate of phthisis, ranging from 0 to 1% following diabetic vitrectomies. Eyes with multiple surgeries with detached retina are at risk [23].

Anterior Hyaloidal Fibrovascular Proliferation: this complication involves growth of retinal neovascularization in the vitreous base area and usually follows vitreoretinal surgery with a scleral buckle for proliferative DR in phakic eyes, although it can occur in severe cases with no history of surgery. Typically, the patient presents with VH and progresses to peripheral RD. The condition can be identified at slit lamp examination by the presence of neovascularization in the retrolenticular space and on fundus examination by the presence of peripheral retinal traction and anteroposterior displacement of the retina. US biomicroscopy demonstrates the anterior fibrovascular proliferation clearly, and so does B-scan US. The presence of this condition is important to recognize the progression to phthisis bulbi without treatment. Treatment typically involves lensectomy, vitrectomy, direct dissection of the fibrovascular tissue, and silicone oil infusion. Placement of cannulas/instruments through the pars plana must be done with care to avoid creating peripheral retinal breaks.

Vitreous Hemorrhage

Vitreous hemorrhage is a frequent complication of DR, and usually indicates the presence of active retinal neovascularization, although occasionally it is due to PVD from inactive neovascular tissue. Vitreous hemorrhage is debilitating for the patient due to induced decreased visual acuity, and also creates a challenge for the ophthalmologist as it prevents precise assessment of the status of retinal disease.

Management

The duration, clinical context, and functional needs of the patient are of paramount importance in guiding the management of VH. The first episode always requires special consideration, as it may indicate the progression from non-proliferative to proliferative DR. On some occasions, VH may be the first presentation of DR or even of diabetes mellitus. In either case, VH suggests the presence of aggressive disease.

Vitreous hemorrhage during PRP is defined as a hemorrhage occurring within 4 weeks of a PRP session. This type of VH occurs frequently because the laser scars shrink the neovascular tissue, which can rupture and bleed. Vitreous hemorrhage in a vitrectomized eye is a frequent event that occurs in eyes that undergo surgery for any DR indication. It may be frustrating for the patient, who may feel that the recent surgical procedure was of no benefit, even though the long-term benefits of vitrectomy with excision of the posterior hyaloid in reducing the progression of DR and the severity of macular edema are well recognized.

Timing of Surgery: criteria for the timing of surgery in cases that have VH and no other pathology, such as rubeosis iridis or RD involving the macula, are flexible and several factors need to be considered in the decision-making process. In general, type 1 patients require more attention since they usually present more aggressive disease [1–4, 24]. The first episode of VH must be given special consideration. If the view of the fundus is obscured by VH, an initial US evaluation is fundamental to assess the anatomy of the retina and the presence of extensive fibrovascular proliferation with or without retinal traction. A clinical and US follow-up should be frequent during the first month after presentation. In patients who have not received complete PRP previously and who have not improved (non-clearing VH) during the first month of observation, surgery should be scheduled promptly (Fig. 1). Hyphema, iris neovascularization or increased IOP are signs

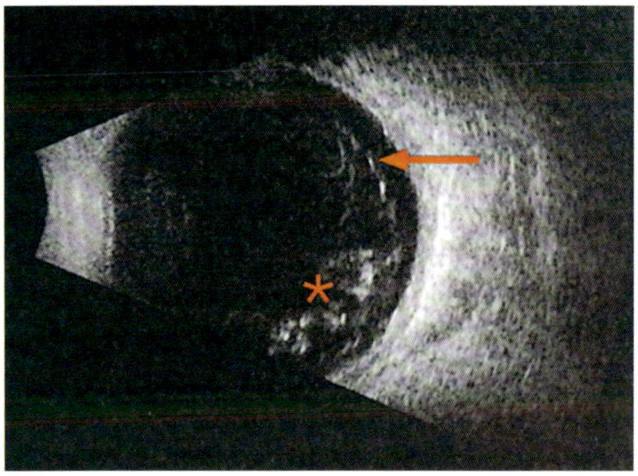

Fig. 1. Ultrasound (US) scan of vitreous hemorrhage. US scan shows a blood clot in the vitreous cavity (asterisk) and a hyaloid detachment (arrow). The hyaloid may be distinguished from the retina by means of reducing the acoustic gain, since the retina continues to be visible even at lower gain levels.

that mandate prompt surgery with little, if any, observation period for spontaneous clearing of the VH. Fellow eye status must always be performed, since bilateral aggressive disease is common.

Vitreous hemorrhage during PRP does not necessarily indicate an immediate need for additional laser treatment. The management strongly depends on the amount of PRP already performed since a dense VH occurring after only a few laser spots have been applied is considered as a case of VH in which essentially no PRP has been provided and is managed as outlined earlier. In a case of almost completed PRP, an initial weekly clinical and US follow-up should be planned, and surgery can be considered after at least 1–2 months unless the patient is monocular and has an urgent visual need in which case earlier intervention may be contemplated. Owing to the fact that blood settles in the inferior sectors with time, thus preventing the laser treatment to the inferior retina, it is usually recommended to start the PRP in the inferior quadrants.

Vitreous hemorrhage occurring after vitrectomy is usually benign, since rapid spontaneous blood reabsorption is frequent. US monitoring is fundamental to rule out any other condition after surgery (e.g., RD). Reassuring the patient is usually enough, and surgery can be considered if the VH does not clear after a suitable period of observation (e.g., more than 1 month).

Other general aspects considered for surgery are: the fellow eye status (quicker surgery for single-eye patients as noted earlier), the subject's occupational needs, the patient's age/overall health status, and compliance with follow-up.

Role of Anti-VEGF Agents

Intravitreous injection of anti-VEGF agents (e.g., aflibercept, bevacizumab, ranibizumab) results in the rapid regression of retinal neovascularization, as early as 24 h following injection. The effect, however, is transient, and neovascularization tends to reperfuse. Currently, intravitreous anti-VEGF agents do not have a significant role in the treatment of diabetic VH other than as a preoperative adjuvant to vitrectomy [25].

Data from meta-analyses suggest that pre-operative intravitreal anti-VEGF agents reduce the chance of intraoperative bleeding, iatrogenic breaks, and the operative time. Moreover, pre-operative anti-VEGF agents have been demonstrated to reduce the risk of early hemorrhage recurrence (first days/weeks after surgery; relative risk 0.35 in favor of anti-VEGF). The benefit of reducing the risk of recurrence is, however, low after some months (late recurrence) [26, 27]. Generally, if they are to be provided, one injects intravitreal anti-VEGF agents several days (1–5) before surgery.

Technique

Standard technique for VH is small-gauge (23-, 25-, or 27-gauge) 3-port PPV. Further treatments (endophotocoagulation, membrane peeling) can be performed according to the status and surgical need. Cataract surgery can also be performed concurrently. The choice of instrument gauge is made according to the retinal status prevision based on US, which should be done as part of the preoperative evaluation in cases of dense VH (vs. cases in which the VH is confined primarily over the macula with a good view of the periphery).

Aspirating blood from the surface of detached retina should be done with caution. Clot removal can be started from the attached retina: it is suggested to start from the periphery and do a "carpet rolling" maneuver towards the area of traction to remove the clot. Sometimes removal of a clot can be as difficult as the original membrane dissection, as blood tends to adhere to the same epicenters of the neovascular tissue.

Florid DR

Florid DR (FDR) is a particularly aggressive form of juvenile proliferative retinopathy, with a predilection for females, bilateral affliction, and a rapid course that may lead to blindness in a short time [28].

Management
FDR is frequently complicated by tractional detachment [29], traction DME, and VH. The initial presentation of FDR may be managed by a prompt PRP, but urgent surgical consultation is needed as soon as fibrous tissue or extensive proliferation develops. Progressive fibrovascular proliferation is a specific subtype of proliferative DR, occurring in subjects despite maximum PRP. The disease characteristics may be considered similar to FDR and can be managed similarly (Fig. 2).

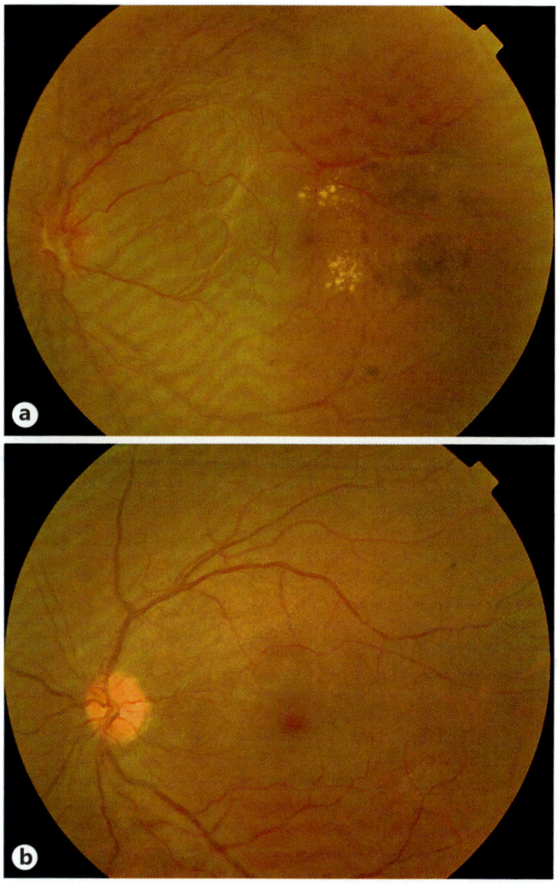

Fig. 2. Florid diabetic retinopathy. Neovascular tissue at the disc and elsewhere is evident (**a**), together with a fibrous tissue at the posterior pole causing a tractional retinal detachment. Pigmentary changes and hard exudates are also visible. Six months after surgery (**b**), all the fibrous tissues are excised, and the neovascularization regressed. The retina is attached with marked reduction of exudates and edema.

Role of Anti-VEGF Agents
Although no randomized clinical trial data are available to guide practice, most experts recommend that if intravitreal anti-VEGF agents are to be used, they should be administered no later than 3–4 days before surgery. These agents tend to be preferred in cases characterized by severe vascular proliferation and avoided in cases with traction RD or traction-induced macular edema.

Technique
Both FDR and progressive fibrovascular proliferation are indications for vitrectomy and may often coexist with tractional RD. Less commonly, vitrectomy is performed in cases with macula dragging or media opacity due to fibrovascular tissue overlying the macula. Vitrectomy always requires concurrent delamination or reduction of

the fibrovascular tissue, RD repair, and extensive PRP. Tamponade of retinal breaks with gas or silicone oil is always required.

Tractional RD

Tractional RD involving the macula is a classic primary indication for vitrectomy. With improved techniques and outcomes, tractional RD threatening the macula has also become a common indication for vitrectomy, but it is important to note that tractional RD not involving or threatening the macula can be safely observed in many cases [29]. OCT can be useful even in eyes with significant opacities and can provide valuable preoperative information [30]. It is not uncommon for eyes with VH to have localized areas of RD discovered during surgery, a reason why ultrasonography should be performed in all eyes in which the fundus is not clearly visible.

Technique

The objectives of vitrectomy are to relieve retinal traction, detach and remove the posterior hyaloid, remove fibrovascular tissue, and treat areas of retinal ischemia to prevent VEGF production and consequent neovascularization of the retina or iris.

Special Conditions

Combined Traction-Rhegmatogenous RD. These are the most complex and challenging diabetic surgeries, as they require advanced techniques for removing the fibrovascular tissue from detached and mobile retina, closing retinal breaks, and reattaching the retina. After the complete release of all tractions, fluid-air exchange is performed, followed by laser PRP around breaks and across the peripheral retina. The tamponade of choice may be then injected. Silicone oil is used in eyes with multiple large retinal breaks (pre-existing or iatrogenic) or possible unidentified breaks, eyes undergoing multiple retinotomies or retinectomy, or those with residual vitreoretinal traction [5].

Diabetic Macular Edema

DME is usually managed with a medical treatment (laser and/or intravitreal anti-VEGF or steroid injections). In some cases, however, medical treatment is unable to achieve a resolution, and a surgical treatment should be offered. Cases of DME should not be considered exclusively "medical" or "surgical," owing to the multifactorial etiology of fluid accumulation.

There are particular subtypes of DME in which surgery plays a fundamental therapeutic role. Obvious indications for surgery include tractional DME due to ERM or to a taut posterior hyaloid. These conditions, in some cases, may prevent medical treatment from being effective. An ERM may reduce the pharmacodynamics of intravitreal anti-VEGF drugs or may worsen the effects of laser photocoagulation, contracting the hyaloid and increasing the edema. In addition, there are cases in which surgery may be of help even in case of non-tractional DME, but this issue is controversial [31]. En-face OCT can distinguish particular subtypes of tractional DME that do not demonstrate significant traction on SD-OCT. Tangential fine folds of the ILM (even in non-tractional DME) may be observed, which resolve after ILM peeling, leading to edema improvement [8].

Management

Different rationales for the surgical treatment of DME have been proposed recently.

- Removal of the anteroposterior component of tangential vitreoretinal traction
- Removal of traction exerted on Müller cells, which causes cellular hypertrophy, proliferation, and vascular leakage [32, 33]
- Removal of traction on vascular tissue, which leads to intraretinal leakage [34–36]

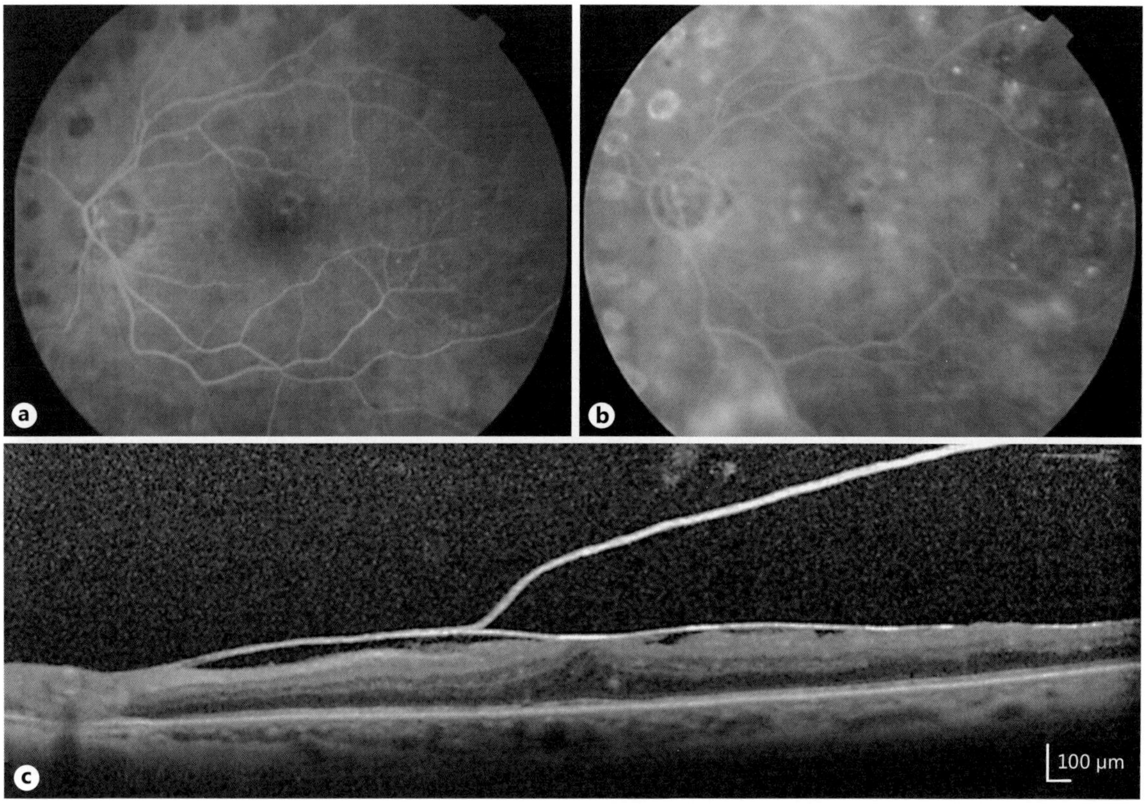

Fig. 3. Macular edema with taut and thickened posterior hyaloid. Early (**a**) and late (**b**) fluorescein angiography images showing macular edema with a taut and thickened hyaloid. Diffuse leakage with ill-defined margins is evident at the posterior pole, especially in the late phases (**b**). The thickened hyaloid associated with vitreoschisis is evident in the OCT scan (**c**).

- Removal of traction that creates retina-RPE separation, which impairs the normal RPE pump effect [34–36]
- Suppress the release of inflammatory cytokines, such as basic fibroblast growth factor, induced by mechanical stresses on the same cells [37]
- Enhancement of oxygenation in the vitreous cavity [38]
- Removal of ERMs and ILM. The glycated diabetic ILM acts as a semipermeable membrane, retaining leaked proteins within the retina. The rise in the oncotic pressure sustains fluid ingress from the vitreous into the retina [39]

Patterns of Vitreoretinal Interface: the different presentation patterns of vitreoretinal attachment may be helpful in making a decision for surgery [40]. Imaging techniques (SD-OCT and FA) are critical in aiding the surgeon to identify the interface status.

The different possibilities include:

- *Attached vitreous with taut and thickened hyaloid.* This pattern causes diffuse macular edema without clear leakage points on FA. The traction is principally tangential, and the OCT shows an edematous retina with a very thickened hyaloid, even partially detached or with vitreoschisis (Fig. 3). Surgery is considered to

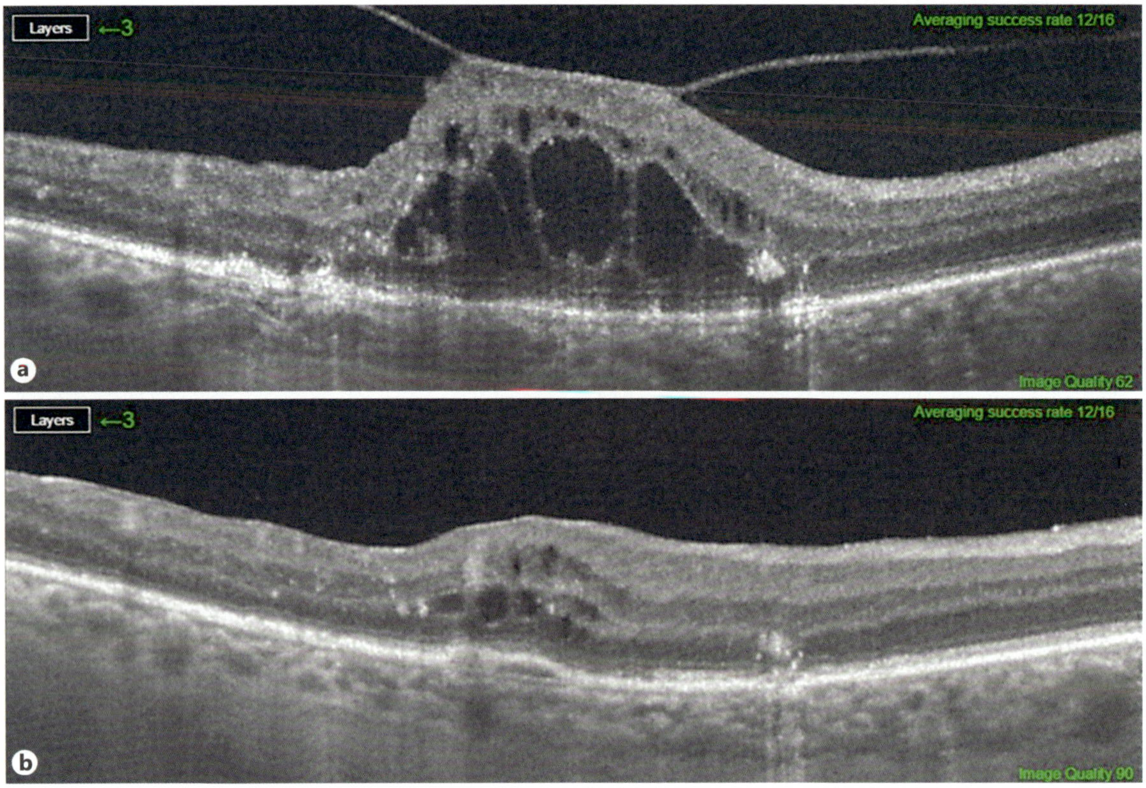

Fig. 4. Tractional diabetic macular edema. Macular edema with concomitant vitreomacular traction is present (**a**) with clear foveal distortion due to the hyaloid traction. The cystic component of edema is significantly reduced after surgical relief of traction (**b**).

be the most effective treatment, particularly in reducing the edema.

- *Attached vitreous and evidence of vitreoretinal traction.* In this pattern, the traction is anteroposterior and/or oblique. Fewer data from literature are available, but surgery with relief of traction and excision of the hyaloid usually resolves the edema (Fig. 4).
- *Attached vitreous and absence of traction.* Although the mechanism is not clear, different studies have demonstrated the efficacy of surgery in reducing the edema and improving the visual acuity in these circumstances. Possible mechanisms include removal of subtle traction not evident with OCT or with direct observation and/or improved vitreous cavity oxygenation. In this pattern, surgery may be considered but should be offered cautiously.

The vitreous is usually attached in the diabetic eyes, particularly to areas of neovascularization not associated with the optic disc; hence, the abovementioned conditions are more common. However, a PVD may be present. Several situations may present to the retina surgeon:

- *PVD and ERM.* Several studies show a successful outcome after vitrectomy and ERM removal. Probably the anatomical improvement is due to the release of ERM traction more than to other mechanisms, similar to non-diabetic ERMs (Fig. 5).
- *PVD and ERM absence.* The benefit of surgery is not clear in this situation. Surgery is

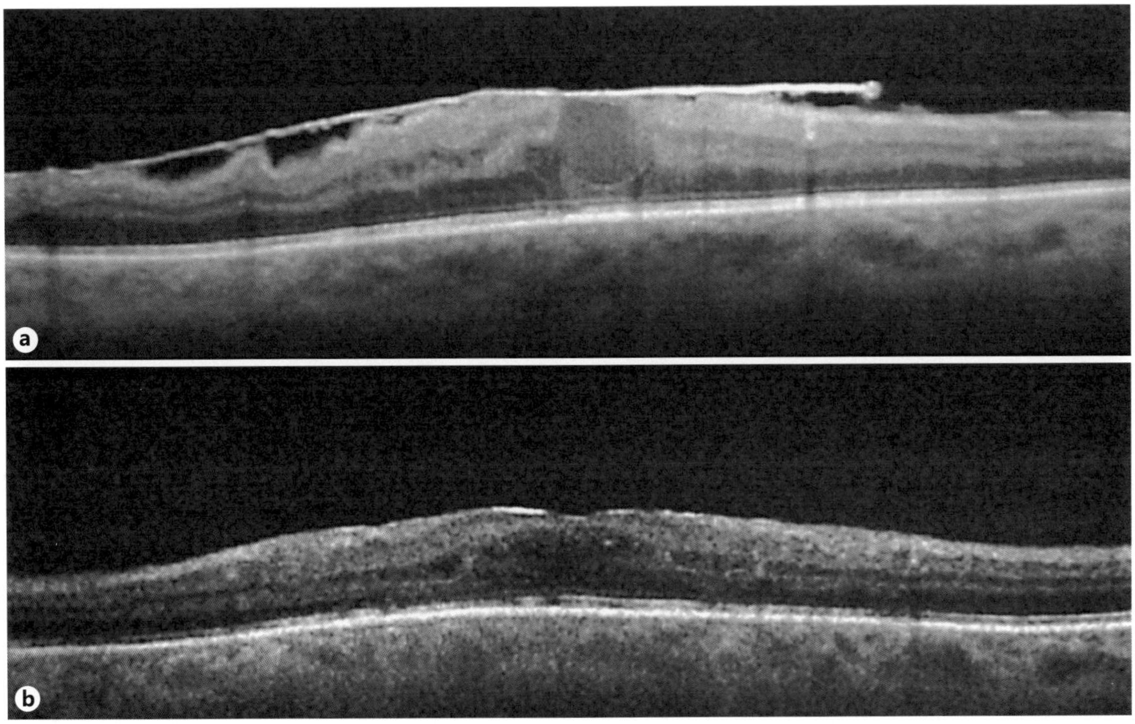

Fig. 5. Epiretinal membrane (ERM). Typical ERM associated with diabetic retinopathy (**a**). In this condition, the cystic and exudative components of diabetic maculopathy are less visible, and probably the anatomical improvement after surgery (**b**) is due to the traction removal more than to other mechanisms, similar to idiopathic ERM cases.

not routinely recommended for this type of DME. Usually, vitrectomy in such patients is reserved for cases of DME unresponsive to other treatments. Some retinal specialists consider DME medically unresponsive (refractory) in the absence of anatomical or functional improvement after at least posterior pole laser photocoagulation, 1 cycle of 3 monthly anti-VEGF injections, and 1 DEX implant injection (Fig. 6). Evidence from the RIDE and RISE studies using intravitreal ranibizumab, however, indicates that patients who do not seem to respond to 3 initial monthly intravitreal injections often show gradual response with continued monthly injections during a 2-year period of follow-up.

Intravitreal Ocriplasmin

Ocriplasmin has the ability to liquefy the vitreous, induce separation of the posterior hyaloid from the ILM, and induce a PVD in a statistically significant number of patients with idiopathic macular hole. The utility of this agent in diabetic patients has not been studied in randomized clinical trials. Current studies on patients with vitreomacular adhesion and traction suggest that the majority of patients would not achieve a PVD with a single injection. In DME, the release of traction, complete or partial, is associated with a reduction in DME, which in several cases has resulted in improved vision. Randomized clinical trials are being conducted to investigate the role of ocriplasmin in treating DME.

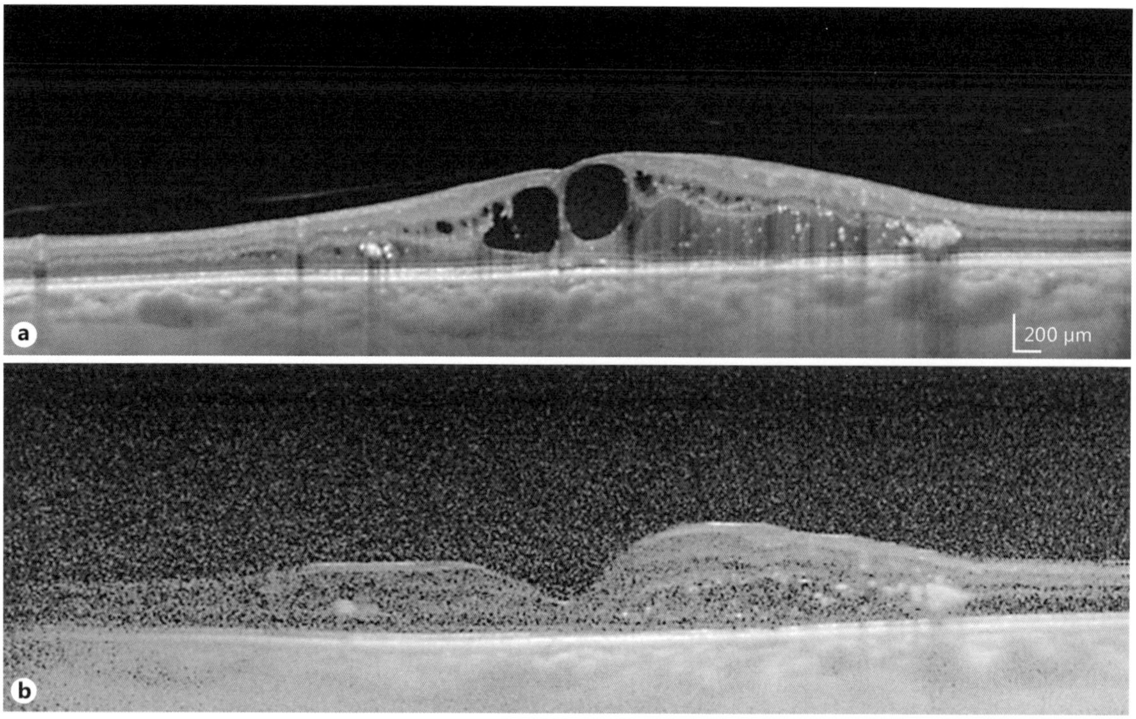

Fig. 6. Non-tractional diabetic macular edema (DME). Surgical treatment of non-tractional DME (**a**) may be beneficial for different reasons. In this case (**b**), the reduction of the cystic and exudative components is striking, and restoration of the foveal contour is evident 7 days after surgery.

Technique

DME is electively treated with a complete vitrectomy, with the release of traction in the area centralis. This usually means a PVD induction with hyaloid excision and ERM peeling. The adjunctive role of ILM peeling is controversial. The ILM of diabetic eyes can contain modified fibroblasts with contractile properties. Its removal may theoretically reduce the contractive stimulus, even if not visible with SD-OCT [41]. Furthermore, it may prevent a relapse of ERM formation, since the ILM peeling removes a scaffold for secondary membrane growth [42]. Since data from the published literature are not conclusive, ILM peeling should not be considered mandatory and probably should be limited to selected cases in which the surgeon identifies significant ILM traction on the retina (e.g., persistent inner retinal wrinkling after ERM and hyaloid excision) or a full-thickness macular hole [31]. Some studies indicate that DME with intraretinal cysts larger than 390 μm should not be treated with combined vitrectomy and ILM peeling because this may induce subfoveal atrophy, defined as the "Floor Effect," and subsequent visual deterioration [43]. A macular hole may also be present. As compared with idiopathic macular holes, these holes have a larger RD area around the hole. There may be broad or multiple focal vitreomacular adhesions at or close to the hole edge. The final visual acuity may not improve despite successful hole closure, and this fact should be discussed with the patient [44]. Gas or silicone oil tamponade is almost always done in cases with a macular hole.

Neovascular Glaucoma

NVG can be the end-stage result of severe proliferative DR that has been treated inadequately, but it may also occur despite extensive application of PRP in severely affected patients (typically young type 1 diabetic patients with fulminant progressive PDR and in older type 2 diabetic patients with coexisting systemic vascular disease and severe ischemia).

Management
If the media is clear, NVG can often be managed with intravitreal anti-VEGF agents combined with PRP and glaucoma surgery [45]. Topical cycloplegic, anti-glaucoma, and steroid medications (if not contraindicated) are also initiated. It may be appropriate to refer such patients for cardiovascular evaluation to rule out vascular causes of ischemia, such as carotid stenosis, particularly if NVG has developed despite previous extensive application of PRP.

Technique
Media opacities (e.g., cataract, corneal edema, and/or VH) may prevent laser treatment. In eyes with reasonable visual potential, such patients should consider PPV preceded by intravitreal injection of antiangiogenic agents, particularly if fibrovascular proliferation with traction RD is not present. The anti-VEGF agents reduce intraoperative bleeding, particularly in the anterior chamber from the iris or angle.

During vitrectomy, special attention should be directed to the vitreous base, which must be meticulously shaved. Aggressive photocoagulation is applied with emphasis on the peripheral retina extending treatment all the way to the ora serrata. Cryoretinopexy can be applied in cases in which peripheral laser cannot be done, for example, due to hemorrhage adherent to the surface of the peripheral retina despite vitreous shaving. The vitrectomy procedure can be combined with glaucoma surgery.

Cataract Surgery

If a significant cataract is present that hinders adequate intraoperative visualization, concomitant removal with in-the-bag intraocular lens (IOL) implantation by phacoemulsification is ideal.

Management
Combined cataract and vitreoretinal surgery (phacovitrectomy) is a debated procedure, since the risk of having more postoperative inflammation is increased with combined surgeries [46]. Despite this concern, phacovitrectomy is commonly performed to improve the intraoperative visualization during vitreoretinal surgery, to facilitate postoperative monitoring of the retina, to restore the patient's vision as rapidly as possible, and to reduce the burden of performing a separate cataract surgery in the future. Some surgeons prefer to perform phacovitrectomy in older people (even for eyes with primarily clear lenses) to avoid the inevitable second surgery that is associated with vitrectomy-induced progression of nuclear sclerosis. Other surgeons plan a combined surgery only when the cataract compromises the quality of visualization during surgery. Published reports indicate similar visual and anatomical outcomes with combined or sequential surgeries [47, 48].

Technique
Standard or microincisional phacoemulsification with IOL implantation is the standard procedure. It is performed immediately before vitrectomy, after placing the trocars. Some surgeons (especially those working with contact viewing systems) prefer to place a 10–0 nylon corneal suture, to avoid leakage from the anterior chamber during posterior segment surgery. Performing cataract surgery prior to vitrectomy in ischemic eyes can be risky due to the progressive development of iris and angle neovascularization. There are dissenting views as to when to perform phacoemulsification with vitrectomy and subsequent

secondary IOL placement versus concomitant phacoemulsification and IOL surgery with vitrectomy. In the latter case, the IOL can be placed initially, and then the PPV can be performed, or the phacoemulsification can be done and the IOL placed at the end of the procedure. The advantage of the latter technique is increased visibility of the periphery in an aphakic state during the dissection parts of vitrectomy [7].

Final Considerations

Surgery for DR remains challenging but has substantially advanced, thanks to the improved surgical instrumentation. Careful preoperative and operative planning, including the choice of instruments, gauge, and method of tamponade is critical for successful surgery, often enabling meaningful visual rehabilitation even in severe cases. The final recommendations for surgeon approaching DR are:

- Do not consider surgery as the last-step therapy, early intervention is often associated with better visual outcomes
- Avoid delay in laser treatment
- Avoid delay in vitreous hemorrhage treatment
- Strongly emphasize the systemic work-up: you are treating an ocular complication of a systemic disease, not an isolated ocular disease

References

1 Early vitrectomy for severe vitreous hemorrhage in diabetic retinopathy. Two-year results of a randomized trial. Diabetic Retinopathy Vitrectomy Study report 2. The Diabetic Retinopathy Vitrectomy Study Research Group. Arch Ophthalmol 1985;103:1644–1652.

2 Early vitrectomy for severe proliferative diabetic retinopathy in eyes with useful vision. Clinical application of results of a randomized trial – Diabetic Retinopathy Vitrectomy Study Report 4. The Diabetic Retinopathy Vitrectomy Study Research Group. Ophthalmology 1988;95: 1321–1334.

3 Early vitrectomy for severe proliferative diabetic retinopathy in eyes with useful vision. Results of a randomized trial – Diabetic Retinopathy Vitrectomy Study Report 3. The Diabetic Retinopathy Vitrectomy Study Research Group. Ophthalmology 1988;95:1307–1320.

4 Early vitrectomy for severe vitreous hemorrhage in diabetic retinopathy. Four-year results of a randomized trial: diabetic Retinopathy Vitrectomy Study Report 5. Arch Ophthalmol 1990;108: 958–964.

5 Sharma T, Fong A, Lai TY, Lee V, Das S, Lam D: Surgical treatment for diabetic vitreoretinal diseases: a review. Clin Exp Ophthalmol 2016;44:340–354.

6 Oellers P, Mahmoud TH: Surgery for proliferative diabetic retinopathy: new tips and tricks. J Ophthalmic Vis Res 2016;11:93–99.

7 Berrocal MH, Acaba LA, Acaba A: Surgery for diabetic eye complications. Curr Diab Rep 2016;16:99.

8 Abe S, Yamamoto T, Kashiwagi Y, Kirii E, Goto S, Yamashita H: Three-dimensional imaging of the inner limiting membrane folding on the vitreomacular interface in diabetic macular edema. Jpn J Ophthalmol 2013;57:553–562.

9 Figueroa MS, Contreras I, Noval S: Antiangiogenic drugs as an adjunctive therapy in the surgical treatment of diabetic retinopathy. Curr Diabetes Rev 2009;5: 52–56.

10 di Lauro R, De Ruggiero P, di Lauro R, di Lauro MT, Romano MR: Intravitreal bevacizumab for surgical treatment of severe proliferative diabetic retinopathy. Graefes Arch Clin Exp Ophthalmol 2010;248:785–791.

11 Hubschman JP, Gupta A, Bourla DH, Culjat M, Yu F, Schwartz SD: 20-, 23-, and 25-gauge vitreous cutters: performance and characteristics evaluation. Retina 2008;28:249–257.

12 Jaffe GJ, Lewis H, Han DP, Williams GA, Abrams GW: Treatment of postvitrectomy fibrin pupillary block with tissue plasminogen activator. Am J Ophthalmol 1989;108:170–175.

13 Rice TA, Michels RG, Maguire MG, Rice EF: The effect of lensectomy on the incidence of iris neovascularization and neovascular glaucoma after vitrectomy for diabetic retinopathy. Am J Ophthalmol 1983;95:1–11.

14 Shukla D, Kalliath J, Neelakantan N, Naresh KB, Ramasamy K: A comparison of brilliant blue G, trypan blue, and indocyanine green dyes to assist internal limiting membrane peeling during macular hole surgery. Retina 2011;31:2021–2025.

15 Chen WL, Lin CT, Ko PS, Yeh PT, Kuan YH, Hu FR, et al: In vivo confocal microscopic findings of corneal wound healing after corneal epithelial debridement in diabetic vitrectomy. Ophthalmology 2009;116:1038–1047.

16 Virata SR, Kylstra JA, Singh HT: Corneal epithelial defects following vitrectomy surgery using hand-held, sew-on, and noncontact viewing lenses. Retina 1999; 19:287–290.

17 Haimann MH, Abrams GW: Prevention of lens opacification during diabetic vitrectomy. Ophthalmology 1984;91: 116–121.

18 Hsu YJ, Hsieh YT, Yeh PT, Huang JY, Yang CM: Combined tractional and rhegmatogenous retinal detachment in proliferative diabetic retinopathy in the anti-VEGF era. J Ophthalmol 2014;2014: 917375.
19 Kamura Y, Sato Y, Deguchi Y, Yagi F: Iatrogenic retinal breaks during 20-gauge vitrectomy for proliferative diabetic retinopathy. Clin Ophthalmol 2013;7:29–33.
20 Khuthaila MK, Hsu J, Chiang A, DeCroos FC, Milder EA, Setlur V, et al: Postoperative vitreous hemorrhage after diabetic 23-gauge pars plana vitrectomy. Am J Ophthalmol 2013;155:757–763, 763.e1–e2.
21 Lee BJ, Yu HG: Vitreous hemorrhage after the 25-gauge transconjunctival sutureless vitrectomy for proliferative diabetic retinopathy. Retina 2010;30: 1671–1677.
22 Zhao LQ, Zhu H, Zhao PQ, Hu YQ: A systematic review and meta-analysis of clinical outcomes of vitrectomy with or without intravitreal bevacizumab pretreatment for severe diabetic retinopathy. Br J Ophthalmol 2011;95:1216–1222.
23 Tao Y, Jiang YR, Li XX, Gao L, Jonas JB: Long-term results of vitrectomy without endotamponade in proliferative diabetic retinopathy with tractional retinal detachment. Retina 2010;30:447–451.
24 El Annan J, Carvounis PE: Current management of vitreous hemorrhage due to proliferative diabetic retinopathy. Int Ophthalmol Clin 2014;54:141–153.
25 Avery RL, Pearlman J, Pieramici DJ, Rabena MD, Castellarin AA, Nasir MA, et al: Intravitreal bevacizumab (Avastin) in the treatment of proliferative diabetic retinopathy. Ophthalmology 2006;113: 1695.e1–e15.
26 Smith JM, Steel DH: Anti-vascular endothelial growth factor for prevention of postoperative vitreous cavity haemorrhage after vitrectomy for proliferative diabetic retinopathy. Cochrane Database Syst Rev 2015;8:CD008214.
27 Simunovic MP, Maberley DA: Anti-vascular endothelial growth factor therapy for proliferative diabetic retinopathy: a systematic review and meta-analysis. Retina 2015;35:1931–1942.
28 Ahmad SS, Ghani SA: Florid diabetic retinopathy in a young patient. J Ophthalmic Vis Res 2012;7:84–87.
29 Charles S, Flinn CE: The natural history of diabetic extramacular traction retinal detachment. Arch Ophthalmol 1981;99: 66–68.
30 Massin P, Duguid G, Erginay A, Haouchine B, Gaudric A: Optical coherence tomography for evaluating diabetic macular edema before and after vitrectomy. Am J Ophthalmol 2003;135:169–177.
31 Nakajima T, Roggia MF, Noda Y, Ueta T: Effect of internal limiting membrane peeling during vitrectomy for diabetic macular edema: systematic review and meta-analysis. Retina 2015;35:1719–1725.
32 Schubert HD: Cystoid macular edema: the apparent role of mechanical factors. Prog Clin Biol Res 1989;312:277–291.
33 Bringmann A, Wiedemann P: Involvement of Müller glial cells in epiretinal membrane formation. Graefes Arch Clin Exp Ophthalmol 2009;247:865–883.
34 Wolfensberger TJ, Gregor ZJ: Macular edema – rationale for therapy. Dev Ophthalmol 2010;47:49–58.
35 Smiddy WE, Green WR, Michels RG, de la Cruz Z: Ultrastructural studies of vitreomacular traction syndrome. Am J Ophthalmol 1989;107:177–185.
36 Augustin A, Loewenstein A, Kuppermann BD: Macular edema. General pathophysiology. Dev Ophthalmol 2010; 47:10–26.
37 Lindqvist N, Liu Q, Zajadacz J, Franze K, Reichenbach A: Retinal glial (Müller) cells: sensing and responding to tissue stretch. Invest Ophthalmol Vis Sci 2010; 51:1683–1690.
38 Holekamp NM: The vitreous gel: more than meets the eye. Am J Ophthalmol 2010;149:32–36.
39 Saravia M: Persistent diffuse diabetic macular edema. The role of the internal limiting membrane as a selective membrane: the oncotic theory. Med Hypotheses 2011;76:858–860.
40 Talcott KE, Modjtahedi BS, Eliott D: Surgical management of diabetic macular edema. Int Ophthalmol Clin 2015;55: 123–136.
41 Gentile RC, Milman T, Eliott D, Romero JM, McCormick SA: Taut internal limiting membrane causing diffuse diabetic macular edema after vitrectomy: clinicopathological correlation. Ophthalmologica 2011;226:64–70.
42 Gandorfer A, Messmer EM, Ulbig MW, Kampik A: Resolution of diabetic macular edema after surgical removal of the posterior hyaloid and the inner limiting membrane. Retina 2000;20:126–133.
43 Romano MR, Romano V, Vallejo-Garcia JL, Vinciguerra R, Romano M, Cereda M, et al: Macular hypotrophy after internal limiting membrane removal for diabetic macular edema. Retina 2014;34: 1182–1189.
44 Yeh PT, Cheng CK, Chen MS, Yang CH, Yang CM: Macular hole in proliferative diabetic retinopathy with fibrovascular proliferation. Retina 2009;29:355–361.
45 Olmos LC, Sayed MS, Moraczewski AL, Gedde SJ, Rosenfeld PJ, Shi W, et al: Long-term outcomes of neovascular glaucoma treated with and without intravitreal bevacizumab. Eye (Lond) 2016;30:463–472.
46 Shinoda K, O'hira A, Ishida S, Hoshide M, Ogawa LS, Ozawa Y, et al: Posterior synechia of the iris after combined pars plana vitrectomy, phacoemulsification, and intraocular lens implantation. Jpn J Ophthalmol 2001;45:276–280.
47 Lahey JM, Francis RR, Kearney JJ: Combining phacoemulsification with pars plana vitrectomy in patients with proliferative diabetic retinopathy: a series of 223 cases. Ophthalmology 2003;110: 1335–1339.
48 Lahey JM, Francis RR, Kearney JJ, Cheung M: Combining phacoemulsification and vitrectomy in patients with proliferative diabetic retinopathy. Curr Opin Ophthalmol 2004;15:192–196.

Lorenzo Iuliano
Department of Ophthalmology
Vita-Salute University, San Raffaele Scientific Institute
Via Olgettina, 60, IT–20132 Milan (Italy)
E-Mail iuliano.lorenzo@hsr.it

Bandello F, Zarbin MA, Lattanzio R, Zucchiatti I (eds): Management of Diabetic Retinopathy.
Dev Ophthalmol. Basel, Karger, 2017, vol 60, pp 160–164 (DOI: 10.1159/000460275)

Enzymatic Vitreolysis for Vitreomacular Traction in Diabetic Retinopathy

Stanislao Rizzo · Daniela Bacherini

Department of Surgery and Translational Medicine, Careggi University Hospital, Eye Clinic, University of Florence, Florence, Italy

Abstract

Vitreomacular traction (VMT) is one of many possible factors involved in the etiology of diabetic macular edema (DME). Pharmacologic vitreoretinal separation is a potential alternative to vitrectomy for VMT in diabetic retinopathy. Small case series have been published on the use of enzymatic vitreolysis in tractional DME, and demonstrate that the enzymatic release of the posterior vitreous cortex is more likely following the injection of plasmin enzyme. Further prospective and randomized clinical trials are necessary to evaluate the clinical relevance of ocriplasmin for vitreomacular traction in diabetic retinopathy, and additional studies are needed to determine more accurately which patients might benefit most from this treatment and how often and at what concentration ocriplasmin should be administered.

Vitreomacular interface abnormalities have long been considered a key element involved in a wide spectrum of retinal diseases including macular hole, vitreomacular traction syndromes, epiretinal membrane (ERM) pathogenesis, retinal detachment, and most recently, neovascular age-related macular degeneration and diabetic retinopathy [1]. Vitreomacular traction (VMT) is one of many possible factors involved in the etiology of diabetic macular edema (DME). VMT can coexist with DME, and it is likely that VMT can worsen DME (Fig. 1).

Undoubtedly the vitreous play a role in the pathogenesis of some cases of DME. In fact DME may improve with spontaneous posterior vitreous detachment (PVD) [2], and the incidence of DME is lower in eyes with PVD compared to those without PVD [3]. Many studies indicate that vitreomacular separation may promote the spontaneous resolution of DME with subsequent improvement in visual acuity [4]. In addition, the vitreoretinal interface may play a role in the pathogenesis of proliferative diabetic retinopathy (PDR). The posterior hyaloid seems to act as a scaffold for neovascular proliferation, and vitrectomy eliminates the support structure for further proliferation. In diabetic eyes, posterior vitreous separation has long been believed to reduce the progression of PDR [5]. Furthermore, a high prevalence of vitreomacular interface abnormalities has been reported in eyes

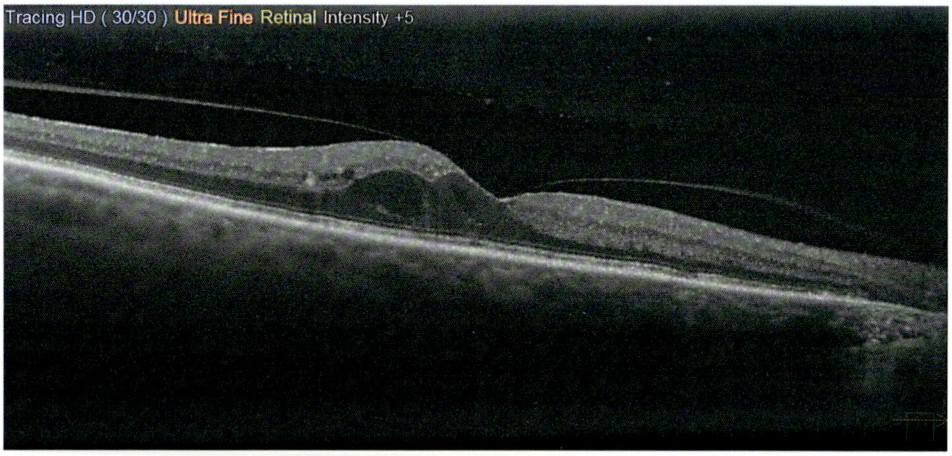

Fig. 1. An optical coherence tomography linear scan showing vitreomacular traction, which may contribute to the development of diabetic macular edema.

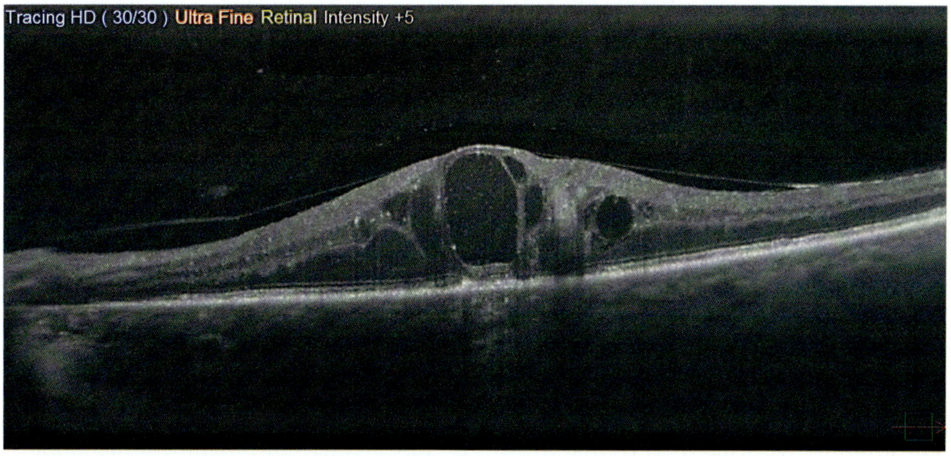

Fig. 2. An optical coherence tomography linear scan showing cystoid macular edema with a thickened posterior hyaloid diffusely attached to the retinal surface.

with DME that persists after focal laser treatment [6] (Fig. 2).

There are limited data on the prevalence of VMT in patients with DME, and published studies have used different diagnostic criteria and retinal imaging methodologies. A recent meta-analysis evaluated 7 studies on the prevalence of VMT in eyes with DME and revealed that vitreomacular traction was present in 28.7% of 188 eyes undergoing PPV and in 12.0% of 326 nonsurgical cases. There was insufficient evidence to calculate the prevalence of vitreous attachment in DME [7]. A recent study determined the prevalence and associated findings using spectral domain optical coherence tomography (SD-OCT) in 198 patients undergoing macular laser for center-involving DME: ERM or partial vitreomacular separation was found on SD-OCT scanning in 25%

of patients undergoing laser for center-involving DME. In 20% of all patients, these tractional elements were either present in the central subfield scan, or the traction was contiguous with the central macular thickening [8].

Surgical intervention to remove the posterior hyaloid has been effective in decreasing the risk for DME. Lewis first described a beneficial effect of vitrectomy with the release of a thickened and taut posterior hyaloid traction on the macula [9]. Subsequently, many studies have shown the benefit of vitrectomy and the removal of the posterior hyaloid on morphologic and functional results [10, 11].

Pharmacologic vitreoretinal separation is a potential alternative to vitrectomy for VMT in diabetic retinopathy. The term pharmacologic vitreolysis refers to the use of exogenous agents (enzymes) to liquefy the vitreous gel and to induce PVD by altering the biochemical state of the macromolecules responsible for maintaining vitreous structure and vitreoretinal adhesion. Small case series have been published on the use of enzymatic vitreolysis in tractional DME. A few studies using plasmin indicate that it is likely to have a beneficial effect in DME. The efficacy of intrasurgical autologous plasmin enzyme (APE) in causing PVD was evaluated in a prospective study in 12 eyes of 11 patients with DME secondary to posterior vitreous cortex contraction. APE was useful for inducing a PVD and facilitating surgery. It did not interfere with the final retinal thickness, and the final visual acuity statistically improved at the end of the 1-year follow-up period. A prospective interventional study was conducted to assess the preoperative factors associated with PVD following intravitreal autologous plasmin injection in 25 eyes of 25 patients affected by DME associated with VMT. PVD was achieved in 10 eyes (41.7%). In diabetic eyes with VMT, the induction of PVD after plasmin injection is influenced by the thickness and reflectivity of the posterior hyaloid face: eyes with a thinner, less reflective posterior hyaloid face are more likely to develop PVD [12]. Another study evaluated the outcome of vitreolysis using intravitreal autologous plasmin in 50 patients with diffuse DME in comparison to triamcinolone acetonide (TA). Vitreolysis using plasmin injection resulted in an effective diminution of central macular thickness with improvement of best-corrected visual acuity, and this effect was long lasting and safer than intravitreal injection of TA, as there was no concomitant increase of intraocular pressure [13]. A prospective study was performed to evaluate the effectiveness of intravitreal injection of autologous plasmin (0.2 mL) without vitrectomy as a treatment for refractory diffuse DME: the macular edema improved in all injected eyes (100%), with complete resolution in 7 patients (44%). The authors observed that intravitreal injection of autologous plasmin reduced DME in cases that did not respond to conventional laser photocoagulation, improved visual acuity in a short time, and the results were maintained with medium-term follow-up [14]. In conclusion, several small case series show that enzymatic release of the posterior vitreous cortex is more likely following intravitreal injection of plasmin enzyme.

Ocriplasmin has an identical enzymatic profile to plasmin enzyme with better diffusion characteristics, and for this reason, it should allow similar rates of PVD induction and VMT release. It is important to take into account other contributing factors in DME such as macular ischemia, other vasogenic abnormalities, and systemic factors. Furthermore, timing could play an important role, and it would be important to know the clinical value of injecting ocriplasmin early after the onset of DME. In addition, we can hypothesize that ocriplasmin treatment in patients with VMT and DME could result in more than just greater VMT resolution; it might also result in a reduced need for anti-VEGF drug injections.

Ocriplasmin (molecular weight 27.2 kDa) is a recombinant human protein that is a truncated form of the human plasmin with protease activity against substrates in the vitreous structure and vitreoretinal interface, including collagen, fibronectin, and laminin. It is indicated in adults for the treatment of VMT, including when associated with idiopathic macular hole of diameter ≤400 microns. Ocriplasmin has been evaluated clinically in a number of trials. Its efficacy was demonstrated in 2 multicenter, randomized, double-masked, placebo-controlled, 6-month studies in patients with VMT (TG-MV-006 and TG-MV-007). The integrated data show that 26.5% of patients in the ocriplasmin group compared with 10.1% in the placebo group achieved VMT resolution at day-28 ($p < 0.001$). The difference was maintained from day-7 through month-6. Haller et al. [15] studied the effect of ocriplasmin in a subgroup of patients in the MIVI study. The best outcome was found in patients younger than 65 years of age and with absence of ERM, occurrence of phakic eyes, VMT <1,500 μm in diameter, and presence of full thickness macular hole <250 μm diameter.

Based on the information provided before, a potential application of enzymatic vitreolysis with ocriplasmin could be in treating DME with VMT. MIVI-II-DME, a multicenter, double-masked, randomized, and sham-controlled trial, evaluated the efficacy of ocriplasmin to induce complete PVD and vitreous liquefaction to prevent DME. The phase II multicenter study compared multiple doses of intravitreal ocriplasmin for nonsurgical PVD induction for the treatment of patients with DME. The primary outcome was the proportion of patients with total PVD 14 days after the 25, 75, or 125 μg of ocriplasmin and sham injection. According to study results posted at clinicaltrials.gov, there were no statistically significant differences of PVD induction between 25, 75, or 125 μg versus the sham group [16].

Several studies have demonstrated increased nonenzymatic glycation in vitreous from patients with diabetic retinopathy. Using near-infrared laser-excited Fourier-transform (FT) Raman spectroscopy (RS) on vitreous specimens obtained at surgery from 7 patients with PDR, Sebag et al. [17] revealed that human vitreous obtained from subjects with diabetes may be distinguished from control vitreous by FT-RS and that the peaks characterizing the diabetic samples are possibly due to nonenzymatic glycation. For this reason, it is reasonable to hypothesize that diabetic vitreous has altered susceptibility to enzymatic degradation. Additional prospective randomized clinical trials are needed to evaluate the clinical relevance of ocriplasmin for VMT in diabetic retinopathy, and further studies are needed to determine more accurately which patients could benefit most from this treatment, and how often and at what concentration it should be administered.

References

1 Agarwal D, Gelman R, Prospero Ponce C, Stevenson W, Christoforidis JB: The vitreomacular interface in diabetic retinopathy. J Ophthalmol 2015;2015:392983.

2 Yamamoto T, Akabane N, Takeuchi S: Vitrectomy for diabetic macular edema: the role of posterior vitreous detachment and epimacular membrane. Am J Ophthalmol 2001;132:369–377.

3 Nasrallah FP, Jalkh AE, Van Coppenolle F, et al: The role of the vitreous in diabetic macular edema. Ophthalmology 1988;95:1335–1339.

4 Hikichi T, Fujio N, Akiba J, Azuma Y, Takahashi M, Yoshida A: Association between the short-term natural history of diabetic macular edema and the vitreomacular relationship in type II diabetes mellitus. Ophthalmology 1997;104:473–478.

5 Akiba J, Arzabe CW, Trempe CL: Posterior vitreous detachment and neovascularization in diabetic retinopathy. Ophthalmol 1990;97:889–891.

6 Ghazi NG, Ciralsky JB, Shah SM, Campochiaro PA, Haller JA: Optical coherence tomography findings in persistent diabetic macular edema: the vitreomacular interface. Am J Ophthalmol 2007;144:747–754.

7 Jackson TL, Nicod E, Angelis A, Grimaccia F, Prevost AT, Simpson AR, Kanavos P: Vitreous attachment in age-related macular degeneration, diabetic macular edema, and retinal vein occlusion: a systematic review and metaanalysis. Retina 2013;33:1099–1108.

8 Akbar Khan I, Mohamed MD, Mann SS, Hysi PG, Laidlaw DA: Prevalence of vitreomacular interface abnormalities on spectral domain optical coherence tomography of patients undergoing macular photocoagulation for centre involving diabetic macular oedema. Br J Ophthalmol 2015;99:1078–1081.

9 Lewis H, Abrams GW, Blumenkranz MS, Campo RV: Vitrectomy for diabetic macular traction and edema associated with posterior hyaloidal traction. Ophthalmology 1992;99:753–759.

10 Gandorfer A, Messmer EM, Ulbig MW, Kampik A: Resolution of diabetic macular edema after surgical removal of the posterior hyaloid and the inner limiting membrane. Retina 2000;20:126–133.

11 Diabetic Retinopathy Clinical Research Network Writing Committee, Haller JA, Qin H, Apte RS, et al: Vitrectomy outcomes in eyes with diabetic macular edema and vitreomacular traction. Ophthalmology 2010;117:1087–1093.e3.

12 Elbendary AM, Elwan MM, Azzam HA, Eldeeb DR: Predictability of vitreous detachment following intravitreal plasmin injection in diabetic macular edema associated with vitreomacular traction. Curr Eye Res 2011;36:534–539.

13 Elsawy MF: Intravitreal autologous plasmin as a therapeutic modality for diffuse diabetic macular edema. Clin Ophthalmol 2012;6:2063–2068.

14 Diaz-Llopis M, Udaondo P, Arevalo F, Salom D, Garcia-Delpech S, Quijada A, Romero FJ: Intravitreal plasmin without associated vitrectomy as a treatment for refractory diabetic macular edema. J Ocul Pharmacol Ther 2009;25:379–384.

15 Haller JA, Stalmans P, Benz MS, Gandorfer A, Pakola SJ, Girach A, Kampik A, Jaffe GJ, Toth CA; MIVI-TRUST Study Group: Efficacy of intravitreal ocriplasmin for treatment of vitreomacular adhesion: subgroup analyses from two randomized trials. Ophthalmology 2015;122:117–122.

16 ThromboGenics: A Multicenter Study to Compare Multiple Doses of Intravitreal Microplasmin versus Sham Injection for Treatment of Patients with Diabetic Macular Edema (DME) (MIVI-II). http:// clinicaltrials.gov/show/NCT00412451. NLM identifier: NCT00412451.

17 Sebag J, Nie S, Reiser K, Charles MA, Yu NT: Raman spectroscopy of human vitreous in proliferative diabetic retinopathy. Invest Ophthalmol Vis Sci 1994;35:2976–2980.

Daniela Bacherini
Department of Surgery and Translational Medicine
Careggi University Hospital, Eye Clinic, University of Florence
Largo Piero Palagi, 1, IT–50139 Florence (Italy)
E-Mail daniela.bacherini@gmail.com

Bandello F, Zarbin MA, Lattanzio R, Zucchiatti I (eds): Management of Diabetic Retinopathy.
Dev Ophthalmol. Basel, Karger, 2017, vol 60, pp 165–174 (DOI: 10.1159/000459706)

Diabetic Macular Edema: Emerging Strategies and Treatment Algorithms

Elad Moisseiev · Anat Loewenstein

Department of Ophthalmology, Tel Aviv Medical Center, Sackler Faculty of Medicine, Tel Aviv University, Tel Aviv, Israel

Abstract

Diabetic macular edema (DME) is the most common cause of vision loss in diabetic patients, and its management is often a long process requiring frequent monitoring and therapeutic interventions. During the past several decades, numerous treatments have been developed for the treatment of DME. Although many of them have been found to be effective and safe, there is relatively little comparative data, and no established guidelines for the optimal treatment approach exist. In this chapter, the evolution of DME therapies is reviewed, and the current common practice patterns are discussed. Available data from clinical trials on the commonly used agents, as well as comparative studies and combination therapies are reviewed. Additionally, recent advances and novel treatment options that are currently being investigated are also discussed.

Introduction

Diabetic retinopathy (DR) is recognized as the leading cause of vision loss in adults (between the ages of 20 and 74 years) and the most common cause of blindness in the working-age population in the developed world [1, 2]. The prevalence of diabetes mellitus is continuously increasing worldwide, in both developing and developed countries, and the prevalence of DR and associated vision loss is also therefore continuously growing [3, 4]. The prevalence of DR is relatively high, and it has been estimated that at any time 10.2% of diabetic patients have some form of vision threatening retinopathy [5]. Diabetic macular edema (DME) is the most common manifestation of DR leading to vision loss and can complicate any stage of DR [6]. It has been estimated that at any time, 6.8% of diabetic patients have some degree of DME [5]. Therefore, DME accounts for a significant proportion of global visual impairment and has been the focus of considerable research efforts so that treatment options can be developed. Advances made in recent years have led to a variety of treatment options for DME, which allow for visual recovery and reduction of vision loss for many of these patients. The purpose of this chapter is to review the existing treatment algorithms for DME and the emerging treatment strategies that hold promise for improving the management of this common condition.

Evolution of DME Treatments

The first proven effective treatment for DME was macular laser photocoagulation, which was demonstrated by the ETDRS to achieve a 50% reduction of visual loss and increased rates of edema resolution and visual improvement [7]. Laser therapy was the mainstay of DME treatment since the 1980s for approximately 25 years. About a decade ago, vascular endothelial growth factor (VEGF) was recognized as an important therapeutic target in DME, and several prospective randomized controlled trials demonstrated the superiority of the intravitreal injection of ranibizumab (Lucentis, Genentech, San Francisco, CA, USA), an anti-VEGF agent over macular laser for the treatment of DME [8–10]. The RISE and RIDE studies established the safety and efficacy of anti-VEGF therapy for DME, with approximately 40% of patients achieving visual improvement of more than 15 letters, and a high rate of DME resolution and improvement of DR [11], and paved the way for its approval as a first-line treatment for DME. Moreover, the DRCRnet Protocol I results showed that deferring macular laser treatment is preferable to its prompt application, as patients assigned to receive prompt laser + ranibizumab had a slightly worse visual outcome compared to those assigned to prompt ranibizumab and deferred laser treatment [12–14]. Additionally, the VIVID and VISTA studies demonstrated the superiority of aflibercept (Eylea, Regeneron Pharmaceuticals, Inc., Tarrytown, NY, USA) over macular laser for the treatment of DME [15]. These results have led to a marked reduction in the use of macular laser therapy for DME, and at present, it is reserved for a minority of patients who have non-central DME as a first line therapy.

It should be noted that bevacizumab (Avastin, Genentech, San Francisco, CA, USA) is another anti-VEGF agent that is frequently used for the treatment of DME. Although it has not been approved by the FDA for this purpose, it is used off-label for economic reasons.

Additionally, intravitreal injection of steroids is also an effective treatment for DME. Initial studies used triamcinolone acetonide, which although less potent than dexamethasone, has a longer half-life that makes it suitable for intravitreal administration. The first studies on this treatment modality were conducted before the advent of anti-VEGF agents and have established the safety and efficacy of intravitreal steroids for the treatment of DME [16, 17]. Furthermore, it should be noted that in the DRCRnet Protocol I, treatment with triamcinolone acetonide was equivalent to treatment with ranibizumab in the subset of pseudophakic eyes [12]. Although intravitreal injection of steroids has been proven to be an effective treatment for DME, this approach is limited by ocular complications of cataract progression and intraocular pressure (IOP) elevation, and the need for repeated injections. Therefore, research has been directed at creating a long-lasting slow-release injectable corticosteroid implant that will be as efficacious and allow a longer duration of action with a better safety profile. Two types of slow-release steroid implants had been developed and approved by the FDA for the treatment of DME: a degradable dexamethasone implant (Ozurdex, Allergan Inc., Irvine, CA, USA) and a non-degradable fluocinolone acetonide implant (Iluvien, Alimera Sciences Inc., Alpharetta, GA, USA) [18, 19].

Ozurdex is a biodegradable intravitreal implant, made of a copolymer (polylactic-co-glycolic acid) loaded with 700 µg of dexamethasone. As the polylactic-co-glycolic acid slowly hydrolyzes to lactic and glycolic acids, the dexamethasone is released in a slow and stable manner, allowing for up to 6 months duration of action. The efficacy of Ozurdex in DME was first demonstrated in a phase 2 study that included 171 eyes with persistent DME that were treated with a single injection of Ozurdex 700 µg, Ozurdex 350 µg or sham. After 6 months, 30% of patients treated with Ozurdex 700 µg had improved by 2 or more lines of vision, compared to 19% of patients treated with

Ozurdex 350 μg, and 23% of patients in the sham group. The patients treated with Ozurdex 700 μg also had significantly reduced central macular thickness (CMT) [20]. A subsequent study compared Ozurdex with macular laser and macular laser alone in a large cohort of patients with DME and showed that a significant proportion of patients treated with Ozurdex had gained 2 or more lines of vision up to 9 months [21].

The MEAD study was a multi-center randomized controlled trial in which 1,048 patients with DME were randomized into treatment with 700 μg Ozurdex, 350 μg Ozurdex, or sham injection and followed for 3 years with re-treatments possible at 6 months intervals. An improvement of 3 or more lines in visual acuity (VA) was achieved in 22.2% of patients treated with 700 μg Ozurdex, 18.5% of patients treated with 350 μg Ozurdex and only 12.0% of patients in the sham group. The reduction in CMT was also significantly greater in the Ozurdex-treated groups than the sham group. About a third of the Ozurdex treated patients had an IOP elevation, but these were transient and only 2 patients in the entire study required trabeculectomy. Cataract progression was documented in 67.9% of patients treated with 700 μg Ozurdex, 64.1% of patients treated with 350 μg Ozurdex and only 20.4% of patients in the sham group [18]. This study provided high-quality evidence for the efficacy of this therapeutic modality as a first line treatment for DME.

It is important to emphasize that the MEAD study design allowed re-injection with Ozurdex only at 6-month intervals, which is the maximal period of action the implant was originally designed to have. Subsequent data from smaller studies and real-world use of Ozurdex has shown that the response to this therapeutic modality is individual, and that in many patients, signs of decreasing efficacy, such as a decrease in VA, an increase in CMT, or recurrence of DME, that warrant re-treatment occur earlier than 6 months. In a recent retrospective study reporting the real-life results achieved with repeated Ozurdex injections for the treatment of DME in a multi-center series of 128 eyes, the mean interval between injections was found to vary over time, and was under 6 months during the first year [22]. Also, a large survey that assessed the real-life practice patterns of more than 100 retina specialists in France reported that when used for the treatment of DME, Ozurdex is administered on an average 2.4 times per year with a mean interval of 4.9 months between injections [23]. Additional smaller series focused on Ozurdex treatment for DME also reported that it is usually repeated before 6 months [24, 25]. Therefore, using a patient-specific tailored approach, the results achieved with treating DME with Ozurdex can be optimized.

Since intravitreal steroids are associated with increased rates of cataract progression and glaucoma, anti-VEGF agents are currently more commonly used as the first line of treatment for DME. However, it should be emphasized that steroid therapy may be an excellent alternative, especially in pseudophakic patients or in patients in whom anti-VEGF therapy is contraindicated (such as those who had a recent stroke or myocardial infarction, patients with severe cardiovascular risk factors, and pregnant patients). They are also a good option for non-compliant patients who may not keep the close monitoring required with anti-VEGF therapy. Although Ozurdex is less frequently used for the first-line treatment of DME than anti-VEGF injections [26], it should be emphasized that it is not an inferior treatment. In the BEVORDEX study, patients with DME were treated with either 700 μg Ozurdex or bevacizumab injections and compared. After 12 months, 40% of the bevacizumab-treated eyes and 41% of the Ozurdex-treated eyes had an improvement of 2 or more lines of vision. None of the bevacizumab-treated eyes lost more than 2 lines of vision, while 11% of those treated with Ozurdex did lose vision due to cataract progression. However, patients in the bevacizumab group received a mean of 8.6 injections over 12 months, compared to only 2.7 injections in the Ozurdex group [27].

The results were later reported to have been maintained over 2 years of follow up [28]. These results indicate that intravitreal injections of Ozurdex may be as effective as anti-VEGF agents for the treatment of DME, offering similar results with fewer injections but a higher rate of cataract progression.

The change in DME therapy from the time when macular laser was the only option to the era of intravitreal injections is notable not only for the change of treatment modality, but also more importantly, for the availability of multiple treatment options. Intravitreal injections can be used to administer a variety of drugs, which include the 3 anti-VEGF agents discussed above, as well as triamcinolone acetonide and the slow-release steroid implants. The treatment regimen and timing of repeated injections are also variable, and may change over time as a patient's response to treatment can also change. In addition, new treatment modalities are also constantly being developed and include new drugs with different mechanisms of action, subthreshold micropulse laser and even vitrectomy techniques. This multitude of options also allows for numerous treatment switches and combinations.

In the 2016 Global Trends in Retina Survey, over 90% of retina specialists reported that they use an anti-VEGF agent as the first treatment for patients with DME [26]. However, it should be noted that other treatments are also approved and in use as the first line of DME therapy. Except for the above mentioned data that showed superiority of intravitreal ranibizumab and aflibercept injections over macular laser, there are very few comparative studies on DME treatments, and no high quality evidence that one option is better than another in a clinically meaningful sense. The plethora of treatment possibilities make their comparison virtually impossible, as a clinical trial designed to compare them (and their potential combinations) would need to include more than 10 different arms, an extremely large number of patients, and be very difficult to mask and monitor. For this reason, although effective treatments for DME exist and are frequently used clinically, there is no established consensus on DME management, and the choice of treatment varies between patients and is influenced by their responses, their treating ophthalmologists' preferences, as well as regional regulatory and economic reasons.

Existing DME Treatment Algorithms

There is an abundance of level-one evidence for the efficacy of anti-VEGF agents for the treatment of DME. However, it should be acknowledged that the randomized controlled studies that established their efficacy included monthly treatment regimens for 2 years [10, 11, 15]. There are a few studies that followed patients for longer periods of time, the most notable being the DRCRnet Protocol I trial, which included 5 years of follow-up and showed that with a pro re nata (PRN) treatment regimen the number of intravitreal injections needed gets smaller with time and that long-term visual improvement can be maintained in this way [13, 14].

Although monthly anti-VEGF is an excellent treatment strategy for DME patients, it is generally not continued indefinitely. Patients are often switched to PRN regimens after the resolution of DME, but there is always the need for monitoring and risk of recurrence. One appealing strategy is to use a treat-and-extend regimen (TER), which is customized to the patient based on the response to treatment, starting with monthly injections and increasing the intervals once maximal clinical response has been achieved. This approach offers several important advantages, such as the need for fewer visits, fewer recurrences, and better long-term disease stability [29]. In the RETAIN study, patients with DME were randomized to be treated by a TER regimen with or without laser or by a PRN regimen. The results showed similar VA gain in all 3 arms, but it was achieved with a 40% reduction in the number of visits for patients in the TER groups [30].

The European Vitreo-Retinal Society collected data on the initial management of over 2,500 patients from multiple centers. The results of this study showed that the best results were achieved with anti-VEGF therapy or with vitrectomy, better than those reported with intravitreal steroids, macular laser, or subthreshold laser [31]. In a more organized attempt to create a treatment algorithm for DME, a Canadian expert panel suggested categorizing DME as "center involving" or "non-center involving." If the macular center is not involved, management should include observation or laser therapy according to the historic ETDRS guidelines. If the center is involved and there is a decrease in VA, intravitreal anti-VEGF therapy should be initiated [32]. In addition to this simplified algorithm, the panel also considered common clinical scenarios that are frequently encountered:

- Mild DME with preserved vision (better than 20/30) and minimal intraretinal cysts on optical coherence tomography (OCT) – such patients should be followed closely, and treatment with anti-VEGF injections initiated if VA decreases, OCT demonstrates worsening, or the patient is very symptomatic.
- DME with central thickening, but no macular traction – such patients should be managed with intravitreal anti-VEGF injections. It is recommended to continue with monthly injections as long as DME persists, and then switch to PRN or TER algorithms. Any recurrence of fluid should warrant repeated injection. It was noted that in pseudophakic patients, intravitreal steroids are also an option for these cases.
- DME with macular traction – such patients should be treated with anti-VEGF injections, but if the DME and traction persist, vitrectomy should be considered.

Another important aspect of DME therapy that should be emphasized is the systemic glucose control. It has been shown that the most important risk factors for DME are duration of diabetes and glycemic control [6, 33]. For example, the DCCT trial demonstrated that, among patients with type I diabetes mellitus, strict glycemic control achieved a 58% reduction in DME compared to conventional control [34].

An even more complicated problem than the choice of initial DME therapy is the management of patients with inadequate response. There are several reports of improved anatomical and functional outcomes in DME patients who did not respond to one anti-VEGF agent and were then switched to another anti-VEGF agent or received intravitreal steroid therapy [35–40]. However, the definition of treatment failure, the timing of treatment change, and the choice of an alternative treatment are variable, and there are no clear guidelines for them, and no high-quality evidence from randomized controlled trials. Although the timing of treatment change is controversial, analysis of the DRCRnet Protocol I data suggests that the long-term response may be predicted based on that achieved early with the first 3 injections. Based on these results, it has been recommended that if no improvement is seen after 3 injections, a change of treatment should be considered [41]. Further studies on this issue may lead to a more established treatment change pattern.

The multitude of treatment options available for DME attests to the considerable research efforts directed towards this goal, but also indirectly indicates that there is no single optimal treatment that has been consistently shown to be the most effective. Furthermore, the pathogenesis of DME is complex and includes multiple mechanisms, the most notable of which are angiogenesis and inflammation. The oxidative stress induced by metabolic changes of diabetes mellitus causes tissue hypoxia and results in the upregulation of hypoxia inducible factor 1α. This in turn upregulates the production of VEGF, which is responsible for numerous aspects of DR pathogenesis such as increased retinal vascular permeability, vasodilation, attraction of mononuclear leukocytes to the retina, and pathologic retinal neovascularization [42]. In addition, numerous inflammatory cytokines have been shown to be upregulated in response to the oxidative stress and metabolic changes induced by diabetes mellitus. These include interleukin (IL)-6, IL-8, tumor necrosis factor α (TNFα), nuclear factor kappa-light-chain-enhancer of activated B cells, protein kinase C, monocyte chemotactic protein, and nitric oxide synthase. These induce inflammation and other para-inflammatory processes such as activation of the complement pathway, attraction of leukocytes and macrophages to the retina, leukostasis, and breakdown of the blood-retina barrier [43]. It should be noted that each individual treatment option, regardless of its efficacy, is not able to fully resolve DME and keep it that way long-term. Therefore, it is plausible to speculate that a combination of therapies may achieve better results than any monotherapy option [44]. However, although there are relatively few studies that evaluated combination therapies, such as anti-VEGF and steroid agents together, none have demonstrated any superiority of the combination therapy over monotherapy [45–49].

Emerging DME Treatment Strategies

As the optimal treatment regimens using available therapies are still being explored, novel therapeutic options are constantly being developed. These include new drugs that target different pathways, new laser technologies such as subthreshold micropulse laser, and surgical techniques, which may be incorporated into the treatment strategies in future.

There are a large number of new pharmaceutical agents that are being explored for DME treatment that target VEGF and other key factors in pathways involved in its pathogenesis [50]. One such example is Ziv-aflibercept, a recombinant fusion protein that inhibits VEGF and was shown to be safe and effective for the treatment of DME [51]. There is also considerable research into designed ankyrin repeat proteins, which are genetically engineered antibody mimetic proteins that inhibit VEGF and have a long duration of action [52]. Squalamine is a new anti-angiogenic aminosterol that inhibits VEGF and platelet-derived growth factor, and basic fibroblast growth factor. It is currently being evaluated for DME treatment [53]. Inhibitors of TNFα and angiopoietin-2 are also being explored as therapy for DME.

In addition to new drugs, new methods of drug delivery are also being developed. For example, a recent study has investigated the use of topical 1.5% dexamethasone γ-cyclodextrin nanoparticle eye drops in patients with DME and reported improvement in VA and reduction in CMT comparable to those achieved with a subtenon injection of triamcinolone, although with a higher rate of IOP elevation [53]. There is also growing interest in devices to allow for sustained release of intravitreal medicines. The Triamcinolone Acetonide I-vation Sustained Drug Delivery System (SurModics) is an implant with a helical design that allows for a larger surface area for drug delivery. This non-biodegradable device is self-anchoring within the sclera and has adjustable drug elution rates. The I-vation device has been evaluated for DME treatment, but was discontinued due to a high rate of IOP elevation. Other devices that allow long-term therapeutic coverage include the Micropump™ (Replenish Inc.), a refillable reservoir that is surgically implanted in the subconjunctival space and has a flexible cannula that can be placed in the anterior or posterior segment and adjusted to control the release of the drug from the reservoir into the eye through the cannula, and the Port Drug Delivery System (Genentech/ForSight Vision 4 Inc.), a surgically-implanted reservoir that is accessible by a special needle that allows flushing out its contents and refilling it with a fresh dose of drug [54].

Subthreshold laser is different from the conventional laser, as it may have a longer wavelength (e.g., 810 nm, although 577 nm devices are also used), and it is delivered in a micropulse fashion (duty cycle: 5–15%). When used correctly, micropulse laser does not cause a visible burn in the retina, and it causes no detectable retinal damage on fundus photography, autofluorescence, OCT, microperimetry, fluorescein angiography, or histology. Several studies have demonstrated that subthreshold micropulse laser is an effective treatment for patients with DME and suggested its superiority over standard macular laser [55–60]. The role of subthreshold laser in DME treatment is still unclear, and future large-scale randomized controlled trials are required to elucidate it. However, as it has proven efficacy and an excellent safety profile, it is likely to become a part of the standard management of DME.

Vitrectomy is usually reserved for patients with chronic, persistent and diffuse DME, after medical therapies have failed to achieve adequate improvement, and there are no established guidelines for the use of surgery for DME treatment. However, as surgical techniques and instrumentation are constantly being refined and improved, there is a growing body of evidence that vitrectomy may be a safe and effective treatment for DME, even in earlier stages of the condition. Recent series on vitrectomy for DME treatment using small gauge instrumentation report favorable results with anatomical and functional improvements lasting over 1 year postoperatively and with most patients enjoying a gain of 2–3 lines of vision [61–64]. Marked visual recovery has also been reported in cases where vitrectomy was the primary treatment [31].

Conclusion

Currently, the strongest evidence favors anti-VEGF therapy as the first line treatment for most patients with DME. Although there are no formal guidelines, the vast majority of ophthalmologists use this as the first approach for DME treatment, typically starting with monthly anti-VEGF injections until the maximal response has been achieved and then continuing with PRN or TER protocols. It should be noted that, in some studies, ranibizumab and aflibercept have been shown to achieve better results than bevacizumab and that in pseudophakic patients similar improvement may be achieved with steroidal therapy. Systemic control of glucose levels and other cardiovascular risk factors should always be included. Macular laser photocoagulation is currently seldom used and is typically reserved for cases with non-central DME or for patients who have not had adequate response to medical therapy. When the response is inadequate, switching treatment modalities such as changing from an anti-VEGF to Ozurdex, can be considered, possibly quite early in the course of the disease, or one may attempt to use a combination of treatments. In patients with significant cardiovascular disease and in patients who cannot commit to monthly follow-up or monthly monitoring, Ozurdex can be considered as the first line treatment. At present, the best approach is to tailor the treatment to the individual patient, using their clinical response to understand their optimal treatment modality and frequency of repeated interventions. In the near future, numerous new options may become available for the treatment of DME.

References

1 Cheung N, Mitchell P, Wong TY: Diabetic retinopathy. Lancet 2010;376:124–136.

2 Prokofyeva E, Zrenner E: Epidemiology of major eye diseases leading to blindness in Europe: a literature review. Ophthalmic Res 2012;47:171–188.

3 Shaw JE, Sicree RA, Zimmet PZ: Global estimates of the prevalence of diabetes for 2010 and 2030. Diabetes Res Clin Pract 2010;87:4–14.

4 World Health Organization: Diabetes Action Now: An initiative of the World Health Organization and the International Diabetes Federation. Switzerland, World Health Organization, 2004.
5 Yau JW, Rogers SL, Kawasaki R, Lamoureux EL, Kowalski JW, Bek T, Chen SJ, Dekker JM, Fletcher A, Grauslund J, Haffner S, Hamman RF, Ikram MK, Kayama T, Klein BE, Klein R, Krishnaiah S, Mayurasakorn K, O'Hare JP, Orchard TJ, Porta M, Rema M, Roy MS, Sharma T, Shaw J, Taylor H, Tielsch JM, Varma R, Wang JJ, Wang N, West S, Xu L, Yasuda M, Zhang X, Mitchell P, Wong TY; Meta-Analysis for Eye Disease (META-EYE) Study Group: Global prevalence and major risk factors of diabetic retinopathy. Diabetes Care 2012;35:556–564.
6 Lee R, Wong TY, Sabanayagam C: Epidemiology of diabetic retinopathy, diabetic macular edema and related vision loss. Eye Vis (Lond) 2015;2:17.
7 Photocoagulation for diabetic macular edema. Early treatment diabetic retinopathy study report number 1. Early treatment diabetic retinopathy study research group. Arch Ophthalmol 1985; 103:1796–1806.
8 Massin P, Bandello F, Garweg JG, Hansen LL, Harding SP, Larsen M, Mitchell P, Sharp D, Wolf-Schnurrbusch UE, Gekkieva M, Weichselberger A, Wolf S: Safety and efficacy of ranibizumab in diabetic macular edema (RESOLVE study): a 12-month, randomized, controlled, double-masked, multicenter phase II study. Diabetes Care 2010;33: 2399–2405.
9 Mitchell P, Bandello F, Schmidt-Erfurth U, Lang GE, Massin P, Schlingemann RO, Sutter F, Simader C, Burian G, Gerstner O, Weichselberger A; RESTORE Study Group: The RESTORE study: ranibizumab monotherapy or combined with laser versus laser monotherapy for diabetic macular edema. Ophthalmology 2011;118:615–625.
10 Nguyen QD, Shah SM, Khwaja AA, Channa R, Hatef E, Do DV, Boyer D, Heier JS, Abraham P, Thach AB, Lit ES, Foster BS, Kruger E, Dugel P, Chang T, Das A, Ciulla TA, Pollack JS, Lim JI, Eliott D, Campochiaro PA; READ-2 Study Group: Two-year outcomes of the ranibizumab for edema of the mAcula in diabetes (READ-2) study. Ophthalmology 2010;117:2146–2151.
11 Nguyen QD, Brown DM, Marcus DM, Boyer DS, Patel S, Feiner L, Gibson A, Sy J, Rundle AC, Hopkins JJ, Rubio RG, Ehrlich JS; RISE and RIDE Research Group: Ranibizumab for diabetic macular edema: results from 2 phase III randomized trials: RISE and RIDE. Ophthalmology 2012;119:789–801.
12 Diabetic Retinopathy Clinical Research Network, Elman MJ, Aiello LP, Beck RW, Bressler NM, Bressler SB, Edwards AR, Ferris FL 3rd, Friedman SM, Glassman AR, Miller KM, Scott IU, Stockdale CR, Sun JK: Randomized trial evaluating ranibizumab plus prompt or deferred laser or triamcinolone plus prompt laser for diabetic macular edema. Ophthalmology 2010;117:1064–1077.e35.
13 Diabetic Retinopathy Clinical Research Network, Elman MJ, Qin H, Aiello LP, Beck RW, Bressler NM, Ferris FL 3rd, Glassman AR, Maturi RK, Melia M: Intravitreal ranibizumab for diabetic macular edema with prompt versus deferred laser treatment: three-year randomized trial results. Ophthalmology 2012;119: 2312–2318.
14 Elman MJ, Ayala A, Bressler NM, Browning D, Flaxel CJ, Glassman AR, Jampol LM, Stone TW; Diabetic Retinopathy Clinical Research Network: Intravitreal Ranibizumab for diabetic macular edema with prompt versus deferred laser treatment: 5-year randomized trial results. Ophthalmology 2015; 122:375–381.
15 Brown DM, Schmidt-Erfurth U, Do DV, Holz FG, Boyer DS, Midena E, Heier JS, Terasaki H, Kaiser PK, Marcus DM, Nguyen QD, Jaffe GJ, Slakter JS, Simader C, Soo Y, Schmelter T, Yancopoulos GD, Stahl N, Vitti R, Berliner AJ, Zeitz O, Metzig C, Korobelnik JF: Intravitreal aflibercept for diabetic macular edema: 100-week results from the VISTA and VIVID studies. Ophthalmology 2015; 122:2044–2052.
16 Martidis A, Duker JS, Greenberg PB, Rogers AH, Puliafito CA, Reichel E, Baumal C: Intravitreal triamcinolone for refractory diabetic macular edema. Ophthalmology 2002;109:920–927.
17 Gillies MC, Sutter FK, Simpson JM, Larsson J, Ali H, Zhu M: Intravitreal triamcinolone for refractory diabetic macular edema: two-year results of a double-masked, placebo-controlled, randomized clinical trial. Ophthalmology 2006;113:1533–1538.
18 Boyer DS, Yoon YH, Belfort R Jr, Bandello F, Maturi RK, Augustin AJ, Li XY, Cui H, Hashad Y, Whitcup SM; Ozurdex MEAD Study Group: Three-year, randomized, sham-controlled trial of dexamethasone intravitreal implant in patients with diabetic macular edema. Ophthalmology 2014;121:1904–1914.
19 Campochiaro PA, Hafiz G, Shah SM, Bloom S, Brown DM, Busquets M, Ciulla T, Feiner L, Sabates N, Billman K, Kapik B, Green K, Kane F; Famous Study Group: Sustained ocular delivery of fluocinolone acetonide by an intravitreal insert. Ophthalmology 2010;117:1393–1399.e3.
20 Haller JA, Kuppermann BD, Blumenkranz MS, Williams GA, Weinberg DV, Chou C, Whitcup SM; Dexamethasone DDS Phase II Study Group: Randomized controlled trial of an intravitreous dexamethasone drug delivery system in patients with diabetic macular edema. Arch Ophthalmol 2010;128:289–296.
21 Callanan DG, Gupta S, Boyer DS, Ciulla TA, Singer MA, Kuppermann BD, Liu CC, Li XY, Hollander DA, Schiffman RM, Whitcup SM; Ozurdex PLACID Study Group: Dexamethasone intravitreal implant in combination with laser photocoagulation for the treatment of diffuse diabetic macular edema. Ophthalmology 2013;120:1843–1851.
22 Malclès A, Dot C, Voirin N, Agard É, Vié AL, Bellocq D, Denis P, Kodjikian L: Real-life study in diabetic macular edema treated with dexamethasone implant: the reldex study. Retina 2016, Epub ahead of print.
23 Querques G, Darvizeh F, Querques L, Capuano V, Bandello F, Souied EH: Assessment of the real-life usage of intravitreal dexamethasone implant in the treatment of chronic diabetic macular edema in France. J Ocul Pharmacol Ther 2016;32:383–389.
24 Matonti F, Pommier S, Meyer F, Hajjar C, Merite PY, Parrat E, Rouhette H, Rebollo O, Guigou S: Long-term efficacy and safety of intravitreal dexamethasone implant for the treatment of diabetic macular edema. Eur J Ophthalmol 2016; 26:454–459.
25 Aknin I, Melki L: Longitudinal study of sustained-release dexamethasone intravitreal implant in patients with diabetic macular edema. Ophthalmologica 2016; 235:187–188.

26 Rezaei KA, Stone TW (eds): 2015 Global Trends in Retina Survey. San Francisco, American Society of Retina Specialists, 2016.
27 Gillies MC, Lim LL, Campain A, Quin GJ, Salem W, Li J, Goodwin S, Aroney C, McAllister IL, Fraser-Bell S: A randomized clinical trial of intravitreal bevacizumab versus intravitreal dexamethasone for diabetic macular edema: the BEVORDEX study. Ophthalmology 2014;121:2473–2481.
28 Fraser-Bell S, Lim LL, Campain A, Mehta H, Aroney C, Bryant J, Li J, Quin GJ, McAllister IL, Gillies MC: Bevacizumab or dexamethasone implants for DME: 2-year results (the BEVORDEX study). Ophthalmology 2016;123:1399–1401.
29 Freund KB, Korobelnik JF, Devenyi R, Framme C, Galic J, Herbert E, Hoerauf H, Lanzetta P, Michels S, Mitchell P, Monés J, Regillo C, Tadayoni R, Talks J, Wolf S: Treat-and-extend regimens with anti-VEGF agents in retinal diseases: a literature review and consensus recommendations. Retina 2015;35:1489–1506.
30 Prünte C, Fajnkuchen F, Mahmood S, Ricci F, Hatz K, Studnička J, Bezlyak V, Parikh S, Stubbings WJ, Wenzel A, Figueira J; RETAIN Study Group: Ranibizumab 0.5 mg treat-and-extend regimen for diabetic macular oedema: the RETAIN study. Br J Ophthalmol 2016; 100:787–795.
31 Adelman R, Parnes A, Michalewska Z, Parolini B, Boscher C, Ducournau D: Strategy for the management of diabetic macular edema: the European vitreoretinal society macular edema study. Biomed Res Int 2015;2015:352487.
32 Hooper P, Boucher MC, Colleaux K, Cruess A, Greve M, Lam WC, Shortt S, Tourville E: Contemporary management of diabetic retinopathy in Canada: from guidelines to algorithm guidance. Ophthalmologica 2014;231:2–15.
33 Ding J, Wong TY: Current epidemiology of diabetic retinopathy and diabetic macular edema. Curr Diab Rep 2012;12: 346–354.
34 Retinopathy and nephropathy in patients with type 1 diabetes four years after a trial of intensive therapy. The diabetes control and complications trial/epidemiology of diabetes interventions and complications research group. N Engl J Med 2000;342:381–389.
35 Hanhart J, Chowers I: Evaluation of the response to ranibizumab therapy following bevacizumab treatment failure in eyes with diabetic macular edema. Case Rep Ophthalmol 2015;6:44–50.
36 Dhoot DS, Pieramici DJ, Nasir M, Castellarin AA, Couvillion S, See RF, Steinle N, Bennett M, Rabena M, Avery RL: Residual edema evaluation with ranibizumab 0.5 mg and 2.0 mg formulations for diabetic macular edema (REEF study). Eye (Lond) 2015;29:534–541.
37 Do DV, Nguyen QD, Vitti R, Berliner AJ, Gibson A, Saroj N, Soo Y, Boyer DS: Intravitreal aflibercept injection in diabetic macular edema patients with and without prior anti-vascular endothelial growth factor treatment: outcomes from the phase 3 program. Ophthalmology 2016;123:850–857.
38 Katz G, Moisseiev E, Goldenberg D, Moisseiev J, Lomnicky Y, Abend Y, Trester G, Levkovitch-Verbin H: Ranibizumab for persistent diabetic macular edema after bevacizumab treatment. Eur J Ophthalmol 2016, Epub ahead of print.
39 Shah AR, Xi M, Abbey AM, Yonekawa Y, Faia LJ, Hassan TS, Ruby AJ, Wolfe JD: Short-term efficacy of intravitreal dexamethasone implant in vitrectomized eyes with recalcitrant diabetic macular edema and prior anti-VEGF therapy. J Ophthalmic Vis Res 2016;11: 183–187.
40 Maturi RK, Bleau L, Saunders J, Mubasher M, Stewart MW: A 12-Month, single-masked, randomized controlled study of eyes with persistent diabetic macular edema after multiple anti-VEGF injections to assess the efficacy of the dexamethasone-delayed delivery system as an adjunct to bevacizumab compared with continued bevacizumab monotherapy. Retina 2015;35:1604–1614.
41 Gonzalez VH, Campbell J, Holekamp NM, Kiss S, Loewenstein A, Augustin AJ, Ma J, Ho AC, Patel V, Whitcup SM, Dugel PU: Early and long-term responses to anti-vascular endothelial growth factor therapy in diabetic macular edema: analysis of protocol I data. Am J Ophthalmol 2016;172:72–79.
42 Ozaki H, Hayashi H, Vinores SA, Moromizato Y, Campochiaro PA, Oshima K: Intravitreal sustained release of VEGF causes retinal neovascularization in rabbits and breakdown of the blood-retinal barrier in rabbits and primates. Exp Eye Res 1997;64:505–517.
43 Stewart MW: Corticosteroid use for diabetic macular edema: old fad or new trend? Curr Diab Rep 2012;12:364–375.
44 Amoaku WM, Saker S, Stewart EA: A review of therapies for diabetic macular oedema and rationale for combination therapy. Eye (Lond) 2015;29:1115–1130.
45 Ahmadieh H, Ramezani A, Shoeibi N, Bijanzadeh B, Tabatabaei A, Azarmina M, Soheilian M, Keshavarzi G, Mohebbi MR: Intravitreal bevacizumab with or without triamcinolone for refractory diabetic macular edema; a placebo-controlled, randomized clinical trial. Graefes Arch Clin Exp Ophthalmol 2008;246: 483–489.
46 Soheilian M, Garfami KH, Ramezani A, Yaseri M, Peyman GA: Two-year results of a randomized trial of intravitreal bevacizumab alone or combined with triamcinolone versus laser in diabetic macular edema. Retina 2012;32:314–321.
47 Faghihi H, Roohipoor R, Mohammadi SF, Hojat-Jalali K, Mirshahi A, Lashay A, Piri N, Faghihi Sh: Intravitreal bevacizumab versus combined bevacizumab-triamcinolone versus macular laser photocoagulation in diabetic macular edema. Eur J Ophthalmol 2008;18:941–948.
48 Soheilian M, Ramezani A, Obudi A, Bijanzadeh B, Salehipour M, Yaseri M, Ahmadieh H, Dehghan MH, Azarmina M, Moradian S, Peyman GA: Randomized trial of intravitreal bevacizumab alone or combined with triamcinolone versus macular photocoagulation in diabetic macular edema. Ophthalmology 2009;116:1142–1150.
49 Sheth S, Rush R, Natarajan S, Gillies M: Intravitreal triamcinolone acetonide versus combined intravitreal bevacizumab and dexamethasone in diffuse diabetic macular oedema. Clin Exp Ophthalmol 2011;39:673–681.
50 Das A, McGuire PG, Rangasamy S: Diabetic macular edema: pathophysiology and novel therapeutic targets. Ophthalmology 2015;122:1375–1394.

51 Andrade GC, Dias JR, Maia A, Farah ME, Meyer CH, Rodrigues EB: Intravitreal INJECTIONS of ziv-aflibercept for diabetic macular edema: a Pilot Study. Retina 2016;36:1640–1645.
52 Campochiaro PA, Channa R, Berger BB, Heier JS, Brown DM, Fiedler U, Hepp J, Stumpp MT: Treatment of diabetic macular edema with a designed ankyrin repeat protein that binds vascular endothelial growth factor: a phase I/II study. Am J Ophthalmol 2013;155:697–704, 704.e1–e2.
53 Ohira A, Hara K, Jóhannesson G, Tanito M, Ásgrímsdóttir GM, Lund SH, Loftsson T, Stefánsson E: Topical dexamethasone γ-cyclodextrin nanoparticle eye drops increase visual acuity and decrease macular thickness in diabetic macular oedema. Acta Ophthalmol 2015;93:610–615.
54 Humayun M, Santos A, Altamirano JC, Ribeiro R, Gonzalez R, de la Rosa A, Shih J, Pang C, Jiang F, Calvillo P, Huculak J, Zimmerman J, Caffey S: Implantable microPump for drug delivery in patients with diabetic macular edema. Transl Vis Sci Technol 2014;3:5.
55 Luttrull JK, Sinclair SH: Safety of transfoveal subthreshold diode micropulse laser for fovea-involving diabetic macular edema in eyes with good visual acuity. Retina 2014;34:2010–2020.
56 Mansouri A, Sampat KM, Malik KJ, Steiner JN, Glaser BM; Medscape: Efficacy of subthreshold micropulse laser in the treatment of diabetic macular edema is influenced by pre-treatment central foveal thickness. Eye (Lond) 2014;28: 1418–1424.
57 Lavinsky D, Cardillo JA, Melo LA Jr, Dare A, Farah ME, Belfort R Jr: Randomized clinical trial evaluating mETDRS versus normal or high-density micropulse photocoagulation for diabetic macular edema. Invest Ophthalmol Vis Sci 2011;52:4314–4323.
58 Nakamura Y, Mitamura Y, Ogata K, Arai M, Takatsuna Y, Yamamoto S: Functional and morphological changes of macula after subthreshold micropulse diode laser photocoagulation for diabetic macular oedema. Eye (Lond) 2010;24: 784–788.
59 Sivaprasad S, Sandhu R, Tandon A, Sayed-Ahmed K, McHugh DA: Subthreshold micropulse diode laser photocoagulation for clinically significant diabetic macular oedema: a three-year follow up. Clin Exp Ophthalmol 2007; 35:640–644.
60 Chen G, Tzekov R, Li W, Jiang F, Mao S, Tong Y: Subthreshold micropulse diode laser versus conventional laser photocoagulation for diabetic macular edema: a Meta-Analysis of Randomized Controlled Trials. Retina 2016;36:2059–2065.
61 Kumagai K, Hangai M, Ogino N, Larson E: Effect of internal limiting membrane peeling on long-term visual outcomes for diabetic macular edema. Retina 2015;35:1422–1428.
62 Lee DH, Kim YJ, Yoon YH: Minimally invasive microincision vitrectomy surgery with an intraoperative dexamethasone implant for refractory diabetic macular edema. Ophthalmologica 2016; 235:150–156.
63 Bonnin S, Sandali O, Bonnel S, Monin C, El Sanharawi M: Vitrectomy with internal LIMITING membrane peeling for tractional and nontractional diabetic macular edema: long-term Results of a Comparative Study. Retina 2015;35: 921–928.
64 Navarrete-Sanchis J, Zarco-Bosquets J, Tomas-Torrent JM, Diago T, Ortega-Evangelio L: Long-term effectiveness of vitrectomy in diabetic cystoid macular edema. Graefes Arch Clin Exp Ophthalmol 2015;253:713–719.

Elad Moisseiev, MD
Department of Ophthalmology
Tel Aviv Medical Center
Weitzman 6 St., IL–64239 Tel Aviv (Israel)
E-Mail elad_moi@netvision.net.il

Bandello F, Zarbin MA, Lattanzio R, Zucchiatti I (eds): Management of Diabetic Retinopathy.
Dev Ophthalmol. Basel, Karger, 2017, vol 60, pp 175–189 (DOI: 10.1159/000459707)

Application of Clinical Trial Results to Clinical Practice

Marco A. Zarbin · Neelakshi Bhagat · Lekha K. Mukkamala

Institute of Ophthalmology and Visual Science, Rutgers-New Jersey Medical School, Rutgers University, Newark, NJ, USA

Abstract

Two critical questions one must answer as one applies the results of a clinical trial to clinical practice are: (1) Regardless of whether the trial result is likely to be replicated or reproduced in a second large-scale trial, are the results likely to be reproduced in one's practice? (2) Regardless of whether the experimental treatment was better than the alternative on average for a population of patients, are the results clinically important for a given patient in one's practice? To determine if a study result is likely to be reproduced in one's clinical practice, it may be helpful to answer 5 questions: (1) Have steps been taken to minimize bias? (2) Is the result likely due to the treatment? (3) Is the result unlikely due to chance? (4) Is the study population representative of one's patients? (5) Is the totality of evidence consistent? If the answer to all 5 questions is "yes," then we posit that the trial result is likely to be reproduced in one's practice. If not, the likelihood of reproducibility is low. If the answer is yes to all questions except the last, then reproducibility in one's practice is not clear and depends on the strength of the prior versus the current evidence. If the prior evidence is strong, such as multiple pivotal randomized clinical trials, and if the current trial result is not consistent with the previous studies, then the current result may not be reproduced in one's practice. To determine if a study result is clinically important, a 3-step approach is suggested. Step 1. Decide, a priori, what a clinically meaningful difference between 2 treatments would be. This choice defines regions of beneficial, harmful, and trivial outcomes. Step 2. Identify the confidence intervals (CIs). Determine whether the 95% CI mostly includes the range of clinically beneficial outcomes and lies outside the range of clinically harmful outcomes. If these conditions are met, the result is probably clinically important, but the result may or may not be statistically significant. Put the CIs and the regions of benefit/harm together to make a decision about clinically important effects. Step 3. Assess the proportion of eyes with clinically meaningful changes in vision. The proportion of "responders" among patients receiving a given treatment reflects the likelihood of one's patient having a clinically meaningful response to the treatment. In summary, not all statistically significant results are reproduced, even those of carefully designed clinical trials. Determining if a study result is likely to be reproduced in one's practice is even more problematic. The 5-question test may help in this regard. The 5-question test attempts to

Supported in part by the New Jersey Lions Eye Research Foundation.

assess whether steps have been taken to: minimize bias; avoid confounding; ensure adequate statistical power to support precision in the estimates of population parameters; insure external validity of the trial result; and determine whether there is a convergence of evidence consistent with the trial's major findings. To determine if a statistically significant result is likely to be clinically important, a 3-step approach may be useful, focusing on CIs and the proportion of eyes with clinically meaningful changes in vision. Application of clinical trial results to clinical practice requires critical analysis of the extant literature and good clinical judgment.

Introduction

The number of published ophthalmic clinical trials has increased substantially during the past 30 years (Fig. 1). Between 1980 and 1985, the mean number of ophthalmic clinical trials published annually was 94, and since 2010 an average of 797 trial results have been published annually [1]. An average of 9 retina trial results was published annually from 1980 to 1985, and since 2010 the mean number of retina trials published annually is 161. As we have become inundated with clinical trial data, we are now confronted with the challenging task of applying these data to our clinical practice in a rational manner [2]. Similar challenges have arisen in other medical specialties [3, 4]. Two critical questions one must answer as one applies the results of a clinical trial to clinical practice are: (1) Regardless of whether the trial result is likely to be replicated or reproduced in a second large-scale trial, are the results likely to be reproduced in one's practice? (2) Regardless of whether the experimental treatment was better than the alternative on an average for a population of patients, are the results clinically important for a given patient in one's practice?

Although we may use the terms reproduce and replicate interchangeably colloquially, they are not synonymous [5]. Replicability refers to the ability to obtain an identical result when an experiment is repeated under conditions identical to those of the initial experiment. Replicability is likely to be inversely proportional to the number of experimental variables and the stochastic nature of biological processes [5]. Frequentist statistical analysis (the type of statistics typically used to analyze clinical trial data, including stipulation of a null hypothesis and type 1 and 2 error rates, and calculation of means and CIs, etc.) of clinical trial data generally assumes replicability of a trial result. Replicability in clinical trials, however, is virtually impossible even for parallel trials. (The parallel studies, for example, may have identical enrollment criteria and treatment alternatives, but they do not have identical patients.) Reproducibility refers to the property that a result will recur even if experimental conditions vary to some degree from experiment to experiment [5]. If a trial's findings are so dependent on precise experimental conditions that replication of the study is needed to reproduce the trial result, then the result may be idiosyncratic and less important compared to a result that can be reproduced by a variety of independent, non-identical approaches [5]. Reproducibility of a trial result demonstrates external validity of the finding (i.e., the result can be generalized to "real-world" patients, who may not fit all the enrollment criteria of the trial). Casadevall and Fang [5] have noted that, "controlling variables to achieve greater reproducibility in the trial result often will cause the trial to diverge from the heterogeneity of true clinical practice." As enrollment criteria are made increasingly restrictive to ensure replicability of the trial result, for example, the external validity of the trial result is likely to decrease. Investigators can increase the chance of generating trial results that are reproducible by increasing the number of individual measurements, which increases the power of the trial and the likelihood of a reproducible result. Clinicians are generally interested in the reproducibility of a trial result rather than its replicability [5].

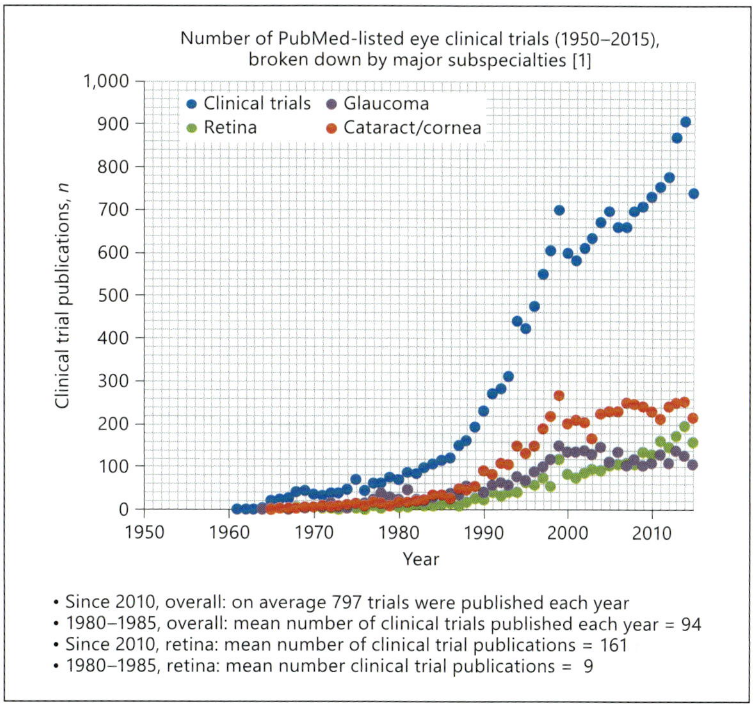

Fig. 1. The number of clinical trials in ophthalmology has increased exponentially since 1980.

Two Problems Relevant to the Application of Clinical Trial Results to Clinical Practice

The application of clinical trial results to clinical practice is confounded by restrictive enrollment criteria [6], conflicts of interest (declared and undeclared) [6], publication bias [7], biological variability, and experimental design limitations [8]. Two problems relevant to the interpretation of clinical trial results are, first, that not all statistically significant results are reproduced, and, second, that not all statistically significant results are clinically important [2]. Before exploring these issues further, it may be helpful to review some concepts underlying statistical significance.

Frequentist Statistics: *p* versus Alpha [9, 10]

What is the *p* value? The *p* value is the probability of observing a given outcome (or a more extreme outcome) under the condition posited by the null hypothesis (H_0) and given the statistical model used to predict the distribution of outcomes under H_0. If the *p* value is very small, it implies that, given the statistical model used, the likelihood of achieving the observed outcome (or a more extreme outcome) is very low assuming H_0 is true. The *p* value does not indicate whether H_0 is valid though. To illustrate this point, consider the case of a coin toss in which one side of the coin is marked "heads," and the other side is marked "tails." If a coin is "fair," one expects to obtain "heads" in 10 of 20 tosses ($p_{\text{heads}} = 0.5$). If H_0 represents the coin being "fair" and if one simulates 10,000 such trials, then one observes "heads" in 10 of 20 tosses in 1,753/10,000 trials ($p_{\text{heads}} = 0.175$). The distribution of outcomes obtained by these trials is termed the null distribution, and "heads" in 10 of 20 tosses is the most common result obtained but not the only result (Fig. 2). If one is presented with an unknown coin and observes "heads" in 16 of 20 coin tosses, can one conclude the coin is "fair" or should one

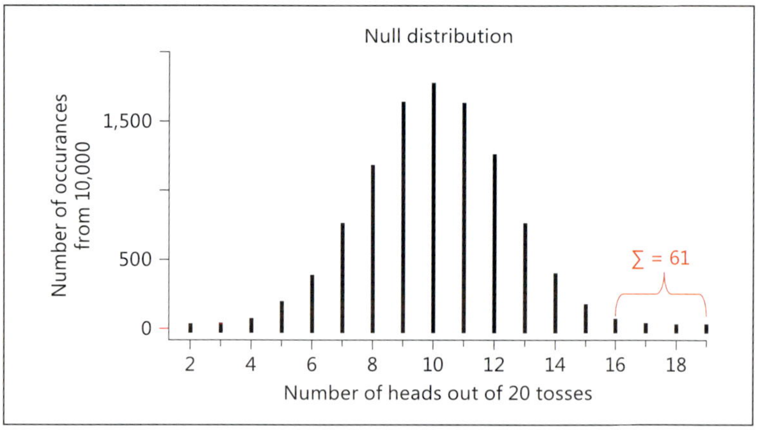

Fig. 2. The null distribution. Adapted from: http://labstats.net/articles/pvalue.html. Please see text for details.

conclude that it is a "trick" coin? Examination of the null distribution demonstrates that even a "fair" coin gives heads 16 or more times in 20 tosses in 61/10,000 trials or 0.61% of the time ($p_{\text{heads } \geq 16/20 \text{ tosses}} = 0.0061$). Given this information, one cannot know whether the coin is "fair" and an unlikely event occurred (in which case, one would accept H_0) or whether the coin is a "trick" coin (in which case, one would reject H_0 and conclude the coin is not "fair"). The p value does not indicate which of these opposite conclusions is correct. Thus, a low p value does not clarify whether an unlikely event has been observed and H_0 is valid or that one should reject H_0. The decision strategy for whether one should accept or reject H_0, given the p value, is based on α, the type 1 error rate also known as the "significance level."

What is the "significance level"? In practice, one is particularly concerned about rejecting H_0 when it is valid, termed a type 1 error. A classic example involves the trial of a man accused of murder. If H_0 represents the man being innocent, then a type 1 error occurs if one condemns the innocent man to death by having concluded incorrectly that he is guilty. Alpha is the type 1 error rate. Specification of α is subjective, and its magnitude is determined primarily by how willing one is to reject H_0 if it is valid. That decision is a matter of clinical judgment, not statistics. When α (the significance level) is greater than the p value (the probability of observing a given outcome or more extreme outcome under H_0 and a given statistical model of the distribution of possible outcomes), then one is willing to reject H_0 recognizing that one may be adopting an incorrect conclusion in doing so. Where one sets the level of α should depend on the consequences of a type 1 error. Would we be concerned, for example, that 1 of every 20 (α = 0.05) convicted murderers was put to death despite their innocence? Thus, α is the error rate of rejecting H_0 even though it is valid, and p is the probability of observing an outcome (or more extreme outcome) assuming H_0 is valid. They are different quantities and are calculated in very different ways (Fig. 3).

A trial result is "statistically significant" if the p value is less than α. If one rejects H_0, one has concluded that if the trial were to be repeated many times, one would see a difference between the compared cohorts (e.g., "treated" vs. "observed") of this magnitude or greater less than 5% of the time assuming: (1) H_0 (there is no difference between the cohorts) is valid; (2) the statistical model of the expected distribution of outcomes is valid; (3) the p value is <0.05, and (4) $\alpha = 0.05$.

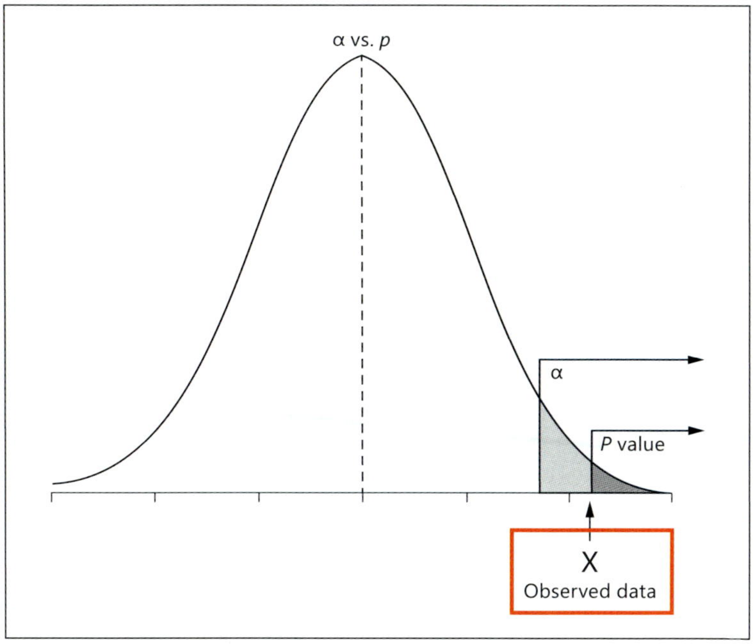

Fig. 3. Distinction between alpha. the type I error rate, and p, the probability of a given outcome or more extreme outcome than X, assuming the null hypothesis is correct and given the statistical model used to predict the distribution of outcomes under the null hypothesis [9]. Reproduced with kind permission. Please see text for details.

Reproducibility of Study Results

In the VIEW 1 trial involving patients with age-related macular degeneration and choroidal new vessels, intravitreal injection of 2 mg aflibercept every 4 weeks (n = 304) gave a statistically significant 2.8-letter better visual outcome compared to 0.5 mg ranibizumab (n = 301; Fig. 4). In VIEW 2, although not statistically significant, the direction of benefit was reversed (2.1-letter better outcome for 0.5 mg ranibizumab [n = 291] vs. 2 mg aflibercept [n = 309]) [11]. In the RIDE trial, among the subgroup with diabetic macular edema and entry-level best-corrected visual acuity (BCVA) <20/200, intravitreal injection of 0.3 mg ranibizumab yielded a mean 8.8-letter gain in BCVA (n = 10), whereas in the parallel RISE trial, the same dose yielded a mean 17.3-letter gain (n = 18) [12]. Even if all conditions are identical for the 2 studies (and they never are since, at a minimum, the 2 studies will differ because they do not enroll exactly the same patients), there is a certain probability that by random or biological variation, the results will differ. Thus, variation in the outcome of parallel studies is not uncommon.

Poor reproducibility of results is a significant problem in the peer-reviewed clinical science and the basic science literature. Aarts et al. [13] reported that only 39% of 100 studies published in the psychological science literature were reproduced successfully. It might seem reasonable to posit that basic science research would not be subject to this degree of irreproducibility, given the greater control over experimental conditions and less ambiguous outcomes than are possible with psychological studies or large-scale clinical trials. Begley and Ellis [14], however, reported that only 11% of 53 published landmark preclinical studies in cancer were reproducible, and Prinz et al. [15] noted that only approximately 25% of 67 published seminal basic research pharmacology studies were reproducible. Ioannidis [16] reported that more than 1 in 6 highly cited original research studies reporting an effective intervention were contradicted by subsequent studies. Some sources of this variability might include bi-

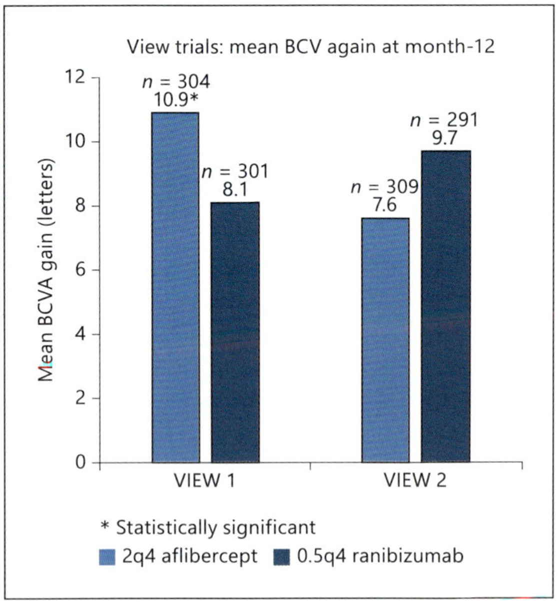

Fig. 4. Visual outcomes with intravitreal aflibercept (2 mg, every 4 weeks) vs. ranibizumab (0.5 mg, every 4 weeks) in the VIEW 1 and VIEW 2 trials [11]. Reproduced with kind permission. Please see text for details.

ological variability, changing standards of care or methods of measurement, or scientific misconduct, but in most cases the most likely explanation for failure to reproduce a study result involves differences in experimental design. Macleod et al. [8] reported that among 2,671 published basic science papers, randomized assignment to different treatment groups (to avoid selection bias, that is, assignment of healthiest animals to treatment vs. control) was reported in approximately 25%. Researchers assessed the outcome of the intervention in a masked fashion (to reduce bias of ascertainment) in approximately 30% of the studies. Sample size was calculated in advance (to avoid repeated testing of accumulated data and inadequate power to detect true differences between groups) in approximately 1% of studies. Investigators declared potential conflicts of interest (allowing independent assessment of investigator bias) in approximately 12% of studies. These limitations in experimental design occurred no less frequently in high-impact journals or in papers from highly regarded institutions. Thus, clinical and basic science research require similar safeguards to avoid the pitfalls of bias, confounding, and multiple testing, all of which may contribute to the publication of results that are not reproduced. The importance of reproducibility increases in proportion to the importance of the experimental result, particularly if the result challenges established paradigms [5].

Five Questions to Assess Likelihood of Reproducing a Trial Result in Clinical Practice

To reduce the risks associated with generalizing the results of a single study to one's clinical practice, it is desirable to reproduce the results. The United States Food and Drug Administration, for example, generally expects 2 well designed studies for drug registration. Unfortunately, most clinicians do not have the opportunity to reproduce large-scale studies. To determine whether a study's results are likely to be reproduced in one's practice, it may be useful to ask 5 questions [2]. The premise underlying this approach is that the likelihood that a single research finding is true depends on the prior evidence, the design of the study, and the level of statistical significance, that is, pre-specified type 1 error versus *p* value [9, 10]. Note that in the previous discussion of statistical inference, there was no mention of prior evidence as part of the decision strategy for rejecting H_0, which is characteristic of frequentist statistics, an inferential method in which an event's probability is the limit of its relative frequency in a large number of independent trials. In practice, many physicians adopt a different perspective when analyzing clinical data, a perspective in which any given result, from the laboratory or from clinical examination, is interpreted in the context of all other available results regarding a given patient. In other words, the valence accorded to any given result is influenced by the totality of data available. Thus, if a patient's laboratory data include a markedly elevated prothrombin/partial thromboplastin time (PT/PTT), yet the patient does not exhibit signs of a bleeding diathesis, consume an anticoagulant, or have some known predisposing risk factor such as a rheumatological disease, a clinician is more likely to repeat the PT/PTT (expecting the repeat value to be normal) rather than to order fresh frozen plasma to manage the abnormal laboratory result. This perspective might be termed a Bayesian perspective. In Bayesian analysis, the probability that a hypothesis is true depends not only on new relevant data, but also on the prior probability of the hypothesis being true based on previously available information distinct from the new data generated by the current experiment. Bayes's rule allows one to change the probability estimate that a hypothesis is correct as additional evidence is obtained. Bayes's theorem can be expressed as:

$$P(H|E) = [P(E|H) \times P(H)]/P(E),$$

where:

H is the given hypothesis that may be affected by evidence,

$P(H)$ is the prior probability that H is true before E is observed,

E is evidence not used in calculating the prior probability,

$P(H|E)$ is the posterior probability, that is, the probability that H is true after E is observed,

$P(E|H)$ is the likelihood of observing E given H,

and $P(E)$ is the marginal likelihood of E.

In the case of the patient in whom an elevated PT/PTT is suspected, $P(H_{\text{bleeding problem}})$ is low, so the probability that he has a bleeding diathesis given the elevated PT/PTT, $P(H_{\text{bleeding problem}}|E_{\text{abnormal PT/PTT}})$, is low.

It is hypothesized that the 5-question test will help one to determine if a study result is likely to be reproduced in one's clinical practice. The questions are as follows.

1. Have steps been taken to minimize bias? These steps include concealed treatment allocation (i.e., neither the physician nor the patient knows which treatment will be assigned to the patient at the time the assignment is proposed), double masking, and randomized assignment to a given treatment cohort. Failure to mask the patient, the examiner, and the treating physician generally leads to overestimation of the treatment effect [17, 18]. Trials that are not double masked (i.e., single-masked studies) overestimate treatment effects with odds ratios exaggerated by 17% on average [17].

2. Is the result likely due to the treatment? A confounding variable (e.g., history of stroke) correlates with both the dependent variable (e.g., treatment assignment to an anti-vascular endothelial growth factor agent) and the independent variable (e.g., incidence of stroke while using the agent) and, if unrecognized, can corrupt estimation of the magnitude of a relationship between the dependent and independent variables. Confounding is best, but not always [19], controlled by randomized assignment to treatment.

3. Is the result unlikely due to chance? Have enough patients been enrolled to provide a reliable estimate of the treatment effect? As variability in the treatment outcome (e.g., standard deviation) increases and the difference between the outcomes of the compared cohorts decreases (e.g., mean values of the outcome statistic), an increasingly large number of patients have to be enrolled to avoid accepting H_0 when it is false (termed as type 2 error or β) and rejecting H_0 when it is true (type 1 error, α). Small sample size generally results in low statistical power (1-β), that is, the ability to reject H_0 when it is false. Button et al. [20] pointed out that low power reduces the likelihood that a statistically significant result is a true effect (i.e., reproducible). Also, when an underpowered study identifies a true effect, the effect's magnitude is likely to be exaggerated (such studies are less capable of identifying statistically significant differences between cohorts

when they are small), and thus, the magnitude of the effect is less likely to be replicated [20]. Low event rates generally signify inadequate sample size, and low event rate results are less likely to be replicated. The use of composite outcomes to reduce the sample size needed to achieve a given statistical power may provide increased precision around the numerical estimate of the treatment effect, but there is greater uncertainty in the interpretation of the trial result [21]. A composite outcome comprises combinations of outcomes, each of which either occurs or does not occur (dichotomous outcomes) and each of which is equally important to the patient and contributes similarly to treatment differences (i.e., a favorable treatment is more beneficial for all the components than a less favorable treatment). In defining a composite outcome as "need for laser photocoagulation or vitrectomy," for example, the dichotomous outcomes are laser and vitrectomy. In contrast to the composite outcome, the relative risks of the dichotomous components may have large CIs due to the relatively small number of patients in each subgroup. Furthermore, composite endpoints may mask a difference in 2 treatments that is clinically important. If, for example, treatment A is associated with 6 cases of stroke in 100 patients, and treatment B is associated with 6 cases of transient ischemic attack in 100 patients, then there is no treatment difference for the composite endpoint of "stroke or TIA" between treatments A and B (6% in each case). Despite this fact, the incidence of stroke with A is 6% and with B is 0%, a difference that many clinicians would regard as clinically important. In this case, the composite outcome does not increase the statistical power and may even be considered to have reduced the power by masking a clinically important difference in outcome between treatments A and B. Is the analysis pre-specified or post hoc? Post-hoc analyses tend to be less reliable and more subject to bias than pre-specified analyses. If the p value is much less than the pre-specified type 1 error (alpha), then one may have greater confidence in rejecting H_0 for reasons outlined earlier. Similarly, if the CI clearly excludes the null result, the range of outcomes is unlikely to be due to chance. Regardless of whether or not the CI excludes the null result, a large CI indicates that the estimate of the treatment effect is not precise.

4. Is the study population representative of one's patients? If the study population is not representative, then the study results are less likely to be generalizable to one's practice.

5. Is the totality of evidence consistent? One way to counterbalance the influence of biological variability on the reproducibility of trial results is to assess the totality of evidence across studies, which might include basic science, animal experiments, and human trials. Convergence of evidence strengthens one's conviction regarding the validity of a trial's results. This evidence includes not only findings from relevant previously published research but also one's clinical experience, if extensive.

If the answer to all 5 questions is "yes," then we posit that the trial result is likely to be reproduced in one's practice (Table 1). If not, the likelihood of reproducibility is low. If the answer is yes to all questions except the last, then reproducibility in one's practice is not clear and depends on the strength of the prior versus the current evidence. If the prior evidence is strong, such as multiple pivotal randomized clinical trials, and if the current trial result is not consistent with the previous studies, then the current result may not be reproduced in one's practice.

The application of the 5-question test to the Diabetic Retinopathy Vitrectomy Study (DRVS) results might be as follows. The DRVS enrolled patients with severe vitreous hemorrhage reducing BCVA to ≤5/200 for at least one month. Patients were randomly assigned to early vitrectomy versus deferral. Early vitrectomy gave better visual results than deferral ($p = 0.0001$) only for patients with type 1 diabetes mellitus by year-2 of the study (Fig. 5). The DRVS was un-

Table 1. Is a study result likely to be reproduced in your practice? Five-question test

Question	0/5 "yes"	1/5 "yes"	2/5 "yes"	3/5 "yes"	4/5 "yes"	5/5 "yes"
1 Influence of bias on study result minimized?[1]	No	✓	✓	✓	✓	✓
2 Result likely due to the treatment (no confounding)?[2]	No	No	✓	✓	✓	✓
3 Result unlikely due to chance?[3]	No	No	No	✓	✓	✓
4 Study population representative (generalizable)?[4]	No	No	No	No	✓	✓
5 Result consistent with prior objective evidence (totality of the evidence)?[5]	No	No	No	No	No	✓
Likelihood of reproducing results in your practice	Very Low	Very Low	Low	Low	Unclear	High

[1] Bias is minimized via masking (both investigators and subjects) [17, 18], detailed declaration of conflicts of interest, and submission of trial data to a publicly accessible database. [2] Best controlled by random assignment to different treatment cohorts. However, imbalances can still occur even if randomization is done [19]. Statistical significance testing only accounts for random error and not residual systematic error [22]. Visual acuity is probably heteroscedastic since the variance associated with repeated measurements of good visual acuity is probably less than that associated with low levels of visual acuity. [3] Chance outcomes can be minimized via adequate patient enrollment and testing pre-specified hypotheses with a pre-specified plan of analysis. Under these circumstances, outcomes are less likely due to chance if $p << \alpha$ and if the confidence interval lower bound is >> null result. [4] Careful attention to exclusion criteria is warranted. The rate of all-cause mortality associated with intravitreal anti-VEGF therapy, for example, is probably influenced by the patient's cardiovascular history [23] and by the degree of exposure to the anti-VEGF agent [24]. [5] Judgments about the relevance and quality of evidence are largely subjective, but these judgments are critical in placing the current trial result in an appropriate context. Adapted from the works of Zarbin [2]. Reprinted with permission.

biased (randomized trial) with a result unlikely due to chance (a large number of patients (~500) typically found in clinical practice was enrolled with $p << \alpha$). Thus, the answer to four of the 5 questions is "yes." The result, however, was not consistent with prior objective evidence (totality of the evidence). Specifically, the evidence from clinical practice strongly suggested that the no light perception rate (20%) was much higher in the trial than in practice, possibly due to surgical innovations introduced into practice during the time the trial was being conducted (e.g., intraoperative panretinal photocoagulation). As a result, many surgeons did not distinguish type 1 versus type 2 diabetes mellitus patients when recommending early vitrectomy for severe non-clearing vitreous hemorrhage because they recognized that some of the major findings of the study were unlikely to be reproduced in their practice. It is important to note that this crucial additional evidence did not come from additional randomized studies but simply from extensive observations in clinical practice. It is also important to note that few, if any, surgeons feel that an additional trial must be done to justify their "deviation" from the DRVS recommendation.

Clinical Importance of Trial Results

The issue of clinical importance is illustrated by the comparison of intravitreal aflibercept and bevacizumab treatment of diabetic macular edema at year-2 in the Protocol T trial. For patients with entry-level vision of 20/50 or worse, at year-2, there was a mean 4.7 letter better visual outcome in the aflibercept injection cohort versus the bevacizumab cohort with $p = 0.02$ and a 95% CI of (+0.5, 8.8) ETDRS letters (Table 2) [25].

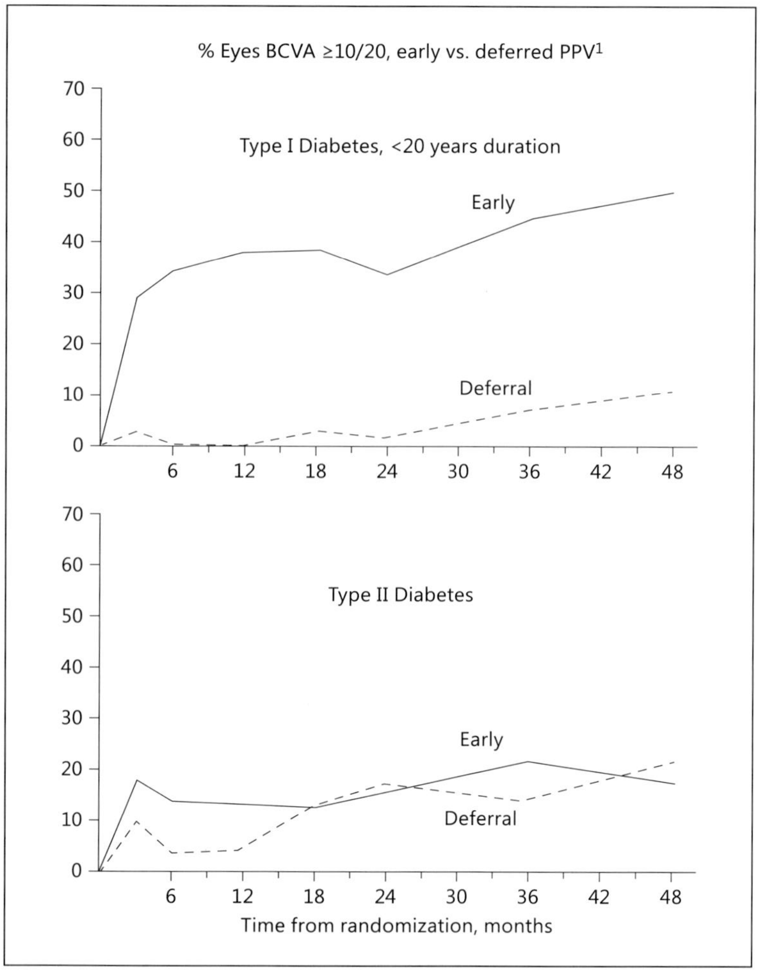

Fig. 5. Year-4 results from the DRVS trial [30]. Reproduced with kind permission. Please see text for details.

This difference was statistically significant, but was it clinically important? One may use a 3-step approach to address this question [2]. This approach is based, in large part, on the work of Batterham and Hopkins [26].

Step 1. Decide, a Priori, What a Clinically Meaningful Difference between 2 Treatments Would Be

This decision requires knowledge of the disease under study and knowledge of the patients one plans to treat. The choice is not always clear. Suppose, for example, that a 4 ETDRS letter change in vision is the smallest change in visual outcome that one considers clinically important. This choice defines regions of beneficial, harmful, and trivial outcomes (Fig. 6).

Step 2. Identify the CIs

A CI is an interval estimate of a population parameter (vs. a point estimate such as the mean). Calculation of a 95% CI produces a range of parameter values that is expected to include the parameter's true value in 95 of every 100 experiments. The CI gives a sense of precision of a point estimate (e.g., the mean gain in vision from baseline in a treatment cohort) by providing the range of average outcomes one might expect for a given

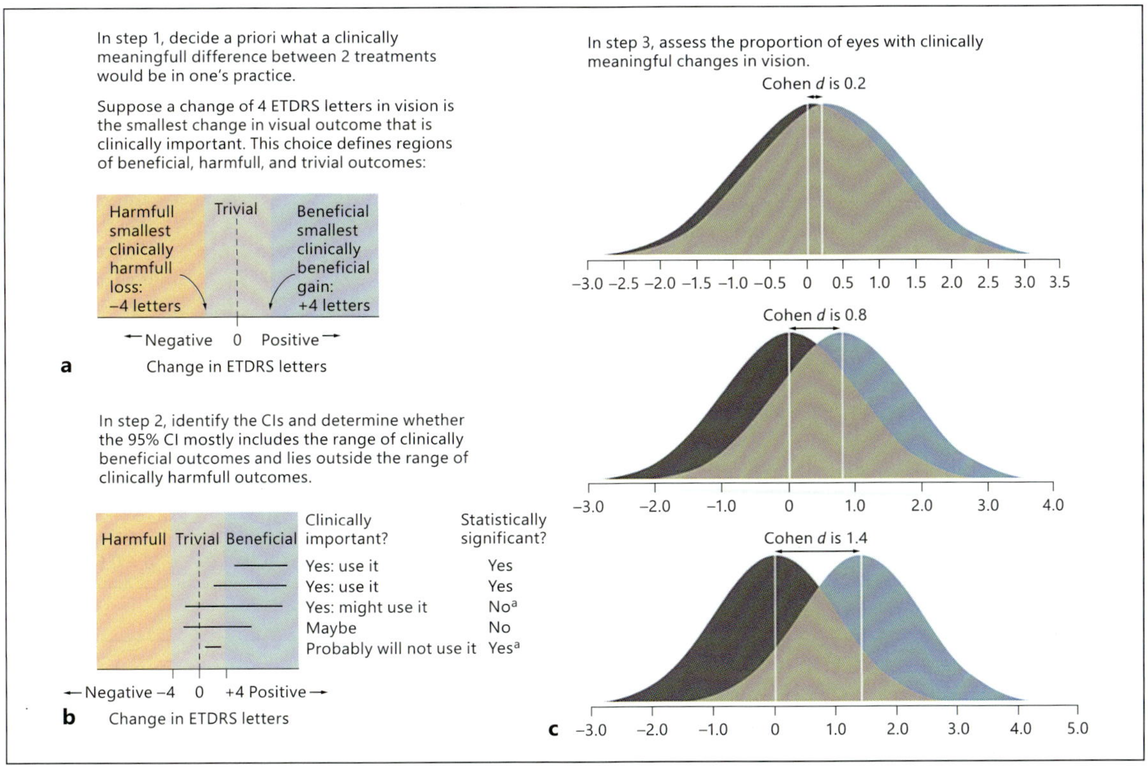

Fig. 6. A 3-Step Approach to Assessing Clinical Importance. **a** In this example, 4 Early Treatment Diabetic Retinopathy Study (ETDRS) letters would be a clinically meaningful difference. **b** If the CI lies entirely within the beneficial range of outcomes or even extends into the trivial range, the result may be both clinically important and statistically significant. If the CI lies mostly within the beneficial range but extends into the trivial range, even crossing the value of 0 (no difference between the 2 treatments), then the result may be clinically important, but it is not statistically significant if it crosses 0. If the CI lies mostly in the trivial range, crosses the value 0, and extends into the beneficial range only slightly, the treatment is not likely to be clinically important. It is not statistically significant. If the CI lies entirely within the trivial range but does not include the value 0, then the result is statistically significant but may not be clinically important. Therefore, some clinically meaningful results might not be statistically significant, and some statistically significant results might not be clinically meaningful. **c** Shown is the distribution overlap of 2 populations associated with different Cohen d coefficients. Cohen d is a quantity that indicates how large the treatment difference between 2 groups is relative to the standard deviation of the samples. Cohen d of 0.2 indicates a small treatment effect, 0.5 a moderate treatment effect, and 0.8 a large treatment effect. When Cohen d is 0.2 and the data are normally distributed, the outcome of 58% of the treatment group is greater than the mean outcome of the control group, and the outcomes of 92% of the treatment and control groups overlap. To have 1 more favorable outcome in the treatment group vs the control group (the number needed to treat [NNT]), one needs to treat approximately 17 patients. When Cohen d is 0.8, the outcome of 79% of the treatment group is greater than the mean outcome of the control group, but the outcomes of 69% of the 2 groups overlap, and the NNT is approximately 4. A Cohen effect size of 0.8 is generally accepted as a clinically meaningful outcome. To have less than 50% of the treatment and control group outcomes overlapping, Cohen d must be at least 1.4, in which case 92% of the treatment group has an outcome greater than the mean outcome of the control group, and the NNT is approximately 2. A web-based calculator for these estimations and graphs is available at http://rpsychologist.com/d3/cohend (created by Kristoffer Magnusson). Parts **a** and **b** are adapted from the study by Batterham and Hopkins. **c** is generated from http://rpsychologist.com/d3/cohend under the terms of a Creative Commons license (http://creativecommons.org/licenses/by/4.0). **a** Statistical significance is misleading. Reproduced with kind permission from [2].

Table 2. Visual outcomes at year-2 in the Protocol T trials[1]

Visual acuity	Aflibercept	Bevacizumab	Ranibizumab	A vs. B	A vs. R	R vs. A
Change from baseline (letters)	+18.1±13.8	+13.3±13.4	+16.1±12.1	+4.7 (+0.5 to +8.8) $p = 0.02$	+2.3 (−1.1 to +5.6) $p = 0.18$	+2.4 (−1.0 to +5.8) $p = 0.18$
≥10 letter improvement	74 (76)	61 (66)	67 (71)	+10 (−6 to +26) $p = 0.35$	+3 (−9 to +15) $p = 0.57$	+7 (−6 to +20) $p = 0.57$
≥10 letter decline	5 (5)	8 (9)	2 (2)	−3 (−10 to +3) $p = 0.49$	+2 (−3 to +7) $p = 0.49$	−5 (−13 to +3) $p = 0.33$
≥15 letter improvement	57 (58)	48 (52)	52 (55)	+8 (−9 to +25) $p = 0.74$	+2 (−11 to +15) $p = 0.75$	+6 (−8 to +20) $p = 0.75$
≥15 letter decline	2 (2)	4 (4)	2 (2)	−2 (−7 to +3) $p = 0.86$	0 (−4 to +4) $p = 0.86$	−2 (−6 to +3) $p = 0.86$

Values are mean ± SD or *n* (%). [1] Adapted from the works of Wells et al. [25].

intervention in a given patient population. Even for point estimates whose difference from a null result is statistically significant, the CI around the point estimate may range from almost no difference to a large difference from the null result. Furthermore, if one study has a CI indicating that 2 treatments have significantly different outcomes, and a second study indicates these treatments are not significantly different, this discrepancy does not necessarily mean the studies conflict as the CIs might have a broad overlap.

Determine whether the 95% CI mostly includes the range of clinically beneficial outcomes and lies outside the range of clinically harmful outcomes. If these conditions are met, the result is probably clinically important, but the result may or may not be statistically significant. Consider the CIs and the regions of benefit/harm together to make a decision about clinically important effects (Fig. 6). If the CI lies entirely within the beneficial range of outcomes or even extends into the trivial range, the result may be both clinically important and statistically significant. If the CI lies mostly within the beneficial range, but extends into the trivial and crosses the value of 0 or no difference, then the result may be clinically important but it is not statistically significant. If the CI lies mostly in the trivial range, crossing the value of 0, and extends minimally into the beneficial range, the result is unlikely to be clinically important and is not statistically significant. If the CI lies entirely within the trivial range but does not include the value of 0, then the result is statistically significant, but it may not be clinically important. So clinically important results can fail to reach statistical significance, and statistically significant results may not be clinically important.

Step 3. Assess the Proportion of Eyes with Clinically Meaningful Changes in Vision

The *p* value indicates the likelihood of observing a given outcome (or more extreme outcome), given H_0 and the statistical model used to describe the distribution of potential outcomes. The *p* value does not provide information on the validity of H_0. In addition, the degree of statistical significance does not imply anything about the magnitude of the difference between different treatments/cohorts of patients. If a clinically important difference in outcome is a gain of ≥4 ETDRS-letters and if the mean gain in the treatment versus the control group is +6 letters with 95% CI of (+2, +10) letters, the difference between the treatment and control groups is statistically significant and clinically meaningful. One needs to know, however, the proportion of patients achieving ≥4 letter gain, not simply the range of mean outcomes expected based on the CI. The former information is critical in counseling patients since one cannot expect all patients to experience the average outcome of the study. (If the data are normally distributed, only a minority of patients will experience the mean outcome.) Consider, for example, the following three hypothetical interactions between a doctor and his/her patient and assume the outcomes of the trials to which the doctor refers are distributed normally.

1. Doctor: "Mrs. Jones, I recommend treatment A for your diabetic macular edema because patients receiving A had a mean 4 EDTRS letter gain in vision."

Patient: "Doctor, that means half the patients had less than a 4 letter gain!"

2. Doctor: "Mrs. Jones, I do not recommend treatment B for your diabetic macular edema because patients receiving B had a mean 0 EDTRS letter gain in vision."

Patient: "But Doctor, does that not mean that half the patients had more than a 0 letter gain?"

3. Doctor: "Mrs. Jones, I recommend treatment A for your diabetic macular edema because patients receiving A had a mean 4 EDTRS letter gain in vision."

Patient: "Doctor, you may believe that a 4 letter gain is a definite improvement, but will I really notice a 4 letter gain? What is the chance I will achieve an improvement that I will think is important?"

Thus, physicians in practice are called upon to make recommendations for individual patients and not for populations of patients. The proportion of "responders" among patients receiving a given treatment reflects the likelihood of one's patient having a clinically meaningful response to the treatment. One can assess the distribution of clinically important outcomes in a trial in a number of different ways [27]. One can, for example, assess the proportion of eyes with clinically meaningful changes in vision (i.e., proportion gaining ≥15 ETDRS letters) [28], or one can compare the degree to which the distribution of outcomes for the treatment and control populations overlap [29]. Cohen's d, for example, indicates how large the treatment difference between 2 groups is relative to the standard deviation of the samples. Cohen's $d = 0.2$ indicates a small treatment effect; $d = 0.5$ is a moderate treatment effect; and $d = 0.8$ is a large treatment effect (Fig. 6) [27, 29]. Distribution-based approaches such as these provide a measure of the treatment effect, but, unlike CIs, they do not measure whether the treatment effect is statistically significant or not. Also, distribution-based approaches to assess clinically meaningful changes in outcome do not take into account risks or costs associated with the treatment.

Returning to the comparison of aflibercept and bevacizumab for patients with diabetic macular edema and entry-level vision of 20/50 or worse, at year-2 there was no significantly greater chance of a ≥10 letter gain or a ≥15 letter gain among the aflibercept versus bevacizumab cohorts (≥10 letter gain: mean difference +10 with 95% CI [–6, +26], $p = 0.35$; ≥15 letter gain: mean difference +8 with 95% CI [-9, +25], $p = 0.74$), nor was there a greater chance for a ≥10 letter loss or a ≥15 letter loss (≥10 letter loss: mean difference –3 with 95% CI [–10, +3], $p = 0.49$; ≥15 letter loss: mean difference –2 with 95% CI [–7, +3], $p = 0.86$). Assuming that the data from Protocol T are distributed normally, one can calculate Cohen's $d = 0.35$ for the aflibercept-bevacizumab comparison, which means there is ~86% overlap in the distribution of results of the aflibercept- and bevacizumab-treated patients at year-2, and the number needed to treat is approximately ~8 (assuming ~52% of patients in the bevacizumab group have a favorable outcome of ≥15 ETDRS letters of improvement from baseline). In other words, to achieve 1 more favorable outcome in the aflibercept group compared to the bevacizumab group, one needs to treat 8 patients. Thus, at year-2, there is a convergence of evidence that there was no clinically important difference in visual outcome between the 2 agents despite the difference in mean gain in vision from baseline with aflibercept versus bevacizumab.

Conclusions

Not all statistically significant results are reproduced, even those of carefully designed clinical trials. Determining if a study result is likely to be reproduced in one's practice is even more problematic. The 5-question test may help in this regard. The 5-question test attempts to assess whether steps have been taken to: minimize bias; avoid confounding; ensure adequate statistical power to support precision in the estimates of population parameters; insure external validity of the trial result; and determine whether there is a convergence of evidence consistent with the trial's major findings. To determine if a statistically significant result is likely to be clinically important, a 3-step approach may be useful, focusing on CIs and the proportion of eyes with clinically meaningful changes in vision. The application of clinical trial results to clinical practice requires critical analysis of the extant literature and good clinical judgment.

References

1 Zarbin M, McGuigan R: Analysis paralysis. Ophthalmol 2016;34:44–49.
2 Zarbin MA: Challenges in applying the results of clinical trials to clinical practice. JAMA Ophthalmol 2016;134:928–933.
3 Pocock SJ, Stone GW: The primary outcome is positive – is that good enough? N Engl J Med 2016;375:971–979.
4 Pocock SJ, Stone GW: The primary outcome fails – what next? N Engl J Med 2016;375:861–870.
5 Casadevall A, Fang FC: Reproducible science. Infect Immun 2010;78:4972–4975.
6 Smith GA: Review of patient inclusion exclusion criteria. 2013. http://www.fda.gov/downloads/Drugs/NewsEvents/UCM341154.pdf.
7 Kyzas PA, Denaxa-Kyza D, Ioannidis JP: Almost all articles on cancer prognostic markers report statistically significant results. Eur J Cancer 2007;43:2559–2579.
8 Macleod MR, Lawson McLean A, Kyriakopoulou A, Serghiou S, de Wilde A, Sherratt N, Hirst T, Hemblade R, Bahor Z, Nunes-Fonseca C, Potluru A, Thomson A, Baginskaite J, Egan K, Vesterinen H, Currie GL, Churilov L, Howells DW, Sena ES: Risk of bias in reports of in vivo research: a focus for improvement. PLoS Biol 2015;13:e1002273.
9 Goodman SN: Toward evidence-based medical statistics. 1: the p value fallacy. Ann Intern Med 1999;130:995–1004.
10 Goodman SN: Toward evidence-based medical statistics. 2: the Bayes factor. Ann Intern Med 1999;130:1005–1013.
11 Heier JS, Brown DM, Chong V, et al: Intravitreal aflibercept (VEGF trap-eye) in wet age-related macular degeneration. Ophthalmology 2012;119:2537–2548.
12 Nguyen QD, Brown DM, Marcus DM, et al: Ranibizumab for diabetic macular edema: results from 2 phase III randomized trials: RISE and RIDE. Ophthalmology 2012;119:789–801.
13 Open Science Collaboration: Psychology. Estimating the reproducibility of psychological science. Science 2015;349:aac4716.
14 Begley CG, Ellis LM: Drug development: raise standards for preclinical cancer research. Nature 2012;483:531–533.
15 Prinz F, Schlange T, Asadullah K: Believe it or not: how much can we rely on published data on potential drug targets? Nat Rev Drug Discov 2011;10:712.
16 Ioannidis JP: Contradicted and initially stronger effects in highly cited clinical research. JAMA 2005;294:218–228.
17 Schulz KF, Chalmers I, Hayes RJ, Altman DG: Empirical evidence of bias. Dimensions of methodological quality associated with estimates of treatment effects in controlled trials. JAMA 1995;273:408–412.
18 Schulz KF, Chalmers I, Altman DG: The landscape and lexicon of blinding in randomized trials. Ann Intern Med 2002;136:254–259.
19 Berg K, Pedersen TR, Sandvik L, Bragadottir R: Comparison of ranibizumab and bevacizumab for neovascular age-related macular degeneration according to LUCAS treat-and-extend protocol. Ophthalmology 2015;122:146–152.

20 Button KS, Ioannidis JP, Mokrysz C, et al: Power failure: why small sample size undermines the reliability of neuroscience. Nat Rev Neurosci 2013;14:365–376.

21 Tomlinson G, Detsky AS: Composite end points in randomized trials: there is no free lunch. JAMA 2010;303:267–268.

22 Schuemie MJ, Ryan PB, DuMouchel W, Suchard MA, Madigan D: Interpreting observational studies: why empirical calibration is needed to correct p-values. Stat Med 2014;33:209–218.

23 Bressler NM, Boyer DS, Williams DF, et al: Cerebrovascular accidents in patients treated for choroidal neovascularization with ranibizumab in randomized controlled trials. Retina 2012;32:1821–1828.

24 Avery RL, Gordon GM: Systemic safety of prolonged monthly anti-vascular endothelial growth factor therapy for diabetic macular edema: a systematic review and meta-analysis. JAMA Ophthalmol 2016;134:21–29.

25 Wells JA, Glassman AR, Ayala AR, et al: Aflibercept, bevacizumab, or ranibizumab for diabetic macular edema: two-year results from a comparative effectiveness randomized clinical trial. Ophthalmology 2016;123:1351–1359.

26 Batterham AM, Hopkins WG: Making meaningful inferences about magnitudes. Sportscience 2005;9:6–13.

27 Copay AG, Subach BR, Glassman SD, Polly DW Jr, Schuler TC: Understanding the minimum clinically important difference: a review of concepts and methods. Spine J 2007;7:541–546.

28 Beck RW, Maguire MG, Bressler NM, Glassman AR, Lindblad AS, Ferris FL: Visual acuity as an outcome measure in clinical trials of retinal diseases. Ophthalmology 2007;114:1804–1809.

29 Cohen J: A power primer. Psychol Bull 1992;112:155–159.

30 Early vitrectomy for severe vitreous hemorrhage in diabetic retinopathy. Four-year results of a randomized trial: Diabetic Retinopathy Vitrectomy Study Report 5. Arch Ophthalmol 1990;108:958–964.

Marco A. Zarbin
Institute of Ophthalmology and Visual Science, Rutgers-New Jersey Medical School
Rutgers University, Doctors Office Center, Room 6155
90 Bergen Street, Newark, NJ 07103 (USA)
E-Mail Zarbin@rutgers.edu

Subject Index